GALEN'S METHOD OF HEALING
PROCEEDINGS OF THE 1982 GALEN SYMPOSIUM

STUDIES IN
ANCIENT MEDICINE

EDITED BY

JOHN SCARBOROUGH

VOLUME 1

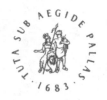

GALEN'S METHOD
OF HEALING

PROCEEDINGS OF THE 1982 GALEN SYMPOSIUM

Edited by

Fridolf Kudlien and Richard J. Durling

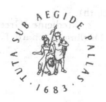

E.J. BRILL

LEIDEN · NEW YORK · KØBENHAVN · KÖLN

1991

The paper in this book meets the guidelines for permancence and durability of the Committee on Production Guidelines for Book Longevity of the Council on Library Resources.

Library of Congress Cataloging-in-Publication Data

Galen Symposium (1982: Christian-Albrechts Universität)
    Galen's method of healing: proceedings of the 1982 Galen
Symposium / herausgegeben von Fridolf Kudlien und Richard J.
Durling.
        p.   cm.—(Studies in ancient medicine, ISSN 0925-1421; v.
1)
English and German.
    Includes index.
    ISBN 90-04-09272-2 (cloth)
    1. Galen—Congresses.   2. Medicine, Greek and Roman—Congresses.
I. Kudlien, Fridolf.   II. Durling, Richard J.   III. Title.
IV. Series.
R126.G8G33   1982
610—dc20   90-27138
                                                          CIP

ISSN 0925-1421
ISBN 90 04 09272 2

PRINTED IN THE NETHERLANDS

CONTENTS

CONTENTS

INTRODUCTION

Our original plan for the Galen Symposium represented by this book was as follows: a) a contribution on the unique character of this most important clinical writing within the context of Galen's oeuvre; b) a contribution to the study of Galen's attitude to surgical treatment, where one had to remember that Galen—no surgeon himself—appears to have had an ambivalent relationship to this clinical subject, if one is to believe M. Michler; c) as philosophical considerations seemed to play an important role in MM, we anticipated a contribution on this; d) "endeixis", known in contemporary medicine as "indication", deserved special treatment as a central clinical concept; e) finally the afterlife of MM in various aspects—e.g. translations; place in later medical education—had to be examined.

Habent sua fata libelli: the basic concept could be preserved, as one can see from the present book. It underwent, however, some modifications, for various reasons. First, a fate that attends all such projects, some speakers could not come. So Michael Burnyeat, who was to have spoken on the relationship of medicine and philosophy, had to deny us. Jonathan Barnes, a specialist in ancient logic, who had already researched into the interrelationship of medicine and logic (see his contribution to the book "Science and speculation. Studies in Hellenistic theory and practice", which he edited in 1982) could speak in his stead. Pearl Kibre had to decline to participate on health grounds, but sent us the typescript of her contribution. This needed revision on grounds of content and arrangement, and this was undertaken by R. J. Durling. Gundolf Keil had agreed to lecture on medieval German translations of MM, but was forced to desist on grounds of time and difficulties with the material. As it happened, a contribution by Faye Getz could be welcomed; she was not invited to the Symposium and did not take part: Vivian Nutton informed us afterwards that Faye Getz had prepared something on a Middle English version of MM. So this aspect of the *fortuna* of MM could be taken into account.

Something else resulted from the extraordinarily intensive and fruitful discussion at the Symposium: it became clear to us, that a paper on how the Arabs dealt with the concept "endeixis" could be illuminating. Ian Cassels, with Ursula Weisser's energetic support, devoted himself to this study after the Symposium. Peter Dilg drew our attention to a Renaissance commentary to MM and promised to send a contribution to the book planned. This added a welcome complement to the remarks of Jerome Bylebyl on the role of MM in Renaissance medical teaching.

The Symposium was international in scope and so planned in two tongues, and so it was in the discussion also. The papers are printed in the languages in which they were delivered or circulated. Thanks are due to W. F. Kümmel, who referred us to our publisher Brill.

Preparation of the papers for publication has been delayed partly for unpredictable reasons. One could expect—or fear—that in the interim new research would necessitate extensive changes in the papers submitted, or even render their publication otiose. This is not so: since 1982 nobody has devoted any close scrutiny to MM. So the present volume preserves its raison d'être: a central clinical writing of Galen's, one which has had great influence is here for the first time the subject of careful investigation.

FRIDOLF KUDLIEN   RICHARD J. DURLING

VIVIAN NUTTON

STYLE AND CONTEXT IN THE *METHOD OF HEALING*

The *Method of healing*, which occupies the whole of one stubby volume in
Kühn's edition of 1825, is remarkable for two features in addition to its
length, 1021 pages. First, it offers the most sustained account of Galen's
attitude towards medical theory and practice, embracing not only a
whole range of varied diseases but also the philosophical arguments and
presuppositions that in Galen's view should govern the doctor's
therapeutic activities. Secondly, it was composed in two distinct stages,
Books 1-6, and Books 7-14, separated by at least twenty years. In this
paper I shall not be discussing Galenic medical theory, but instead I shall
first examine the evidence for the dating of the two parts of the treatise,
and then attempt to set them in the context of Galen's life and interests.
I shall point out some of the contrasts and inconsistencies between the
two halves, and consider what conclusions might be drawn from them.
Although a detailed stylistic analysis of the treatise would be premature,
given that Kühn's text is far from satisfactory and that the many manuscripts and the exceedingly complex secondary tradition have so far
deterred every scholar who has examined the work from producing an
edition of it that would satisfy the requirements of modern philology;[1]
nevertheless, one can say something about certain broader aspects of
Galen's literary art, in particular his polemics and case-histories, both of
which feature prominently in the *Method of healing*. Finally I shall use
some of the assumptions Galen makes in Books 7-14 to throw light on his
position in Rome in the later years of the second century.

It is unfortunate that for neither half of the work do we have any external evidence that would fix its date of composition exactly to within a
month or even a year. The two outside events to which Galen refers in
Books 1-6, the continued existence of the great plague in Rome (360) and

---

[1] A preliminary listing of Mss. is given in H. Diels, 'Die Handschriften der antiken
Ärzte', AAW Berlin 1905, pp. 93, 135; Syriac versions are given by R. Degen, 'Galen
im Syrischen', in V. Nutton (ed.), Galen: problems and prospects, London, Wellcome
Institute, 1981, p. 145f.; Arabic Mss. by M. Ullmann, Die Medizin im Islam, Leiden,
Cologne, Brill, 1970, p. 45, and by F. Sezgin, Geschichte des arabischen Schrifttums III,
Leiden, Brill, 1970, p. 96; addenda to Diels' Latin Mss. are given by R. J. Durling,
'Corrigenda and addenda to Diels' Galenica', *Traditio* 23 (1967) 474f.; 37 (1981) 380.
One obvious stylistic point. Hiatus is rare outside the general rules given by P. De
Lacy, CMG V 4,1,2, 52-55: I note examples at 331,17; 337,7; 499,3; 571,6; 673,3, all
of which can be avoided by transposition or simple emendation, should it be thought
necessary.

his visit to Alexandria twenty years before (53), are both imprecise. How
long an epidemic had to last before Galen exclaimed 'Would God it
would end' is an exercise in psychology, not chronology, and, despite the
confident assertions of Sarton and Singer that Galen arrived in Alexandria in A.D. 152,[2] that date can only be obtained by extrapolating back
from the *Method of healing*. Although we know that Galen did not leave
Pergamum before the death of his father in A.D. 148/9 (VI.756) and that
he returned from Alexandria in A.D. 157, we cannot tell how long Galen
spent with Pelops at Smyrna or delayed at Corinth before he followed
Numisianus to Alexandria (II.217).[3] Nor, despite his vignettes of student
life at Alexandria and of his travels in Egypt, does Galen ever give us a
date from which to calculate when he arrived there. So in order to set this
treatise in its proper context we must have recourse to the cross-
references provided by Galen within his own books, which fortunately
give a good relative chronology.

The *Method of healing* was already projected in the early 170s. Galen
told his friend Glaucon that he intended to write a substantial book on
therapeutic method, which he would give him on his return to Italy, or,
should his stay abroad be prolonged for any reason, send to him there
(XI.145). The big book was still in the future when Galen wrote *On the
differences and causes of symptoms* (VII.263), a work which was also being
planned at the time Galen wrote to Glaucon (XI.11) and which Galen
came to regard as an essential preliminary for the proper understanding
of the *Method of healing* (85). Similarly, his discussion of drugs in Books
1 to 6 demanded a detailed knowledge of what he had written in his book
on simples. All this points to a date for the *Method of healing*, 1-6, in the
170s, but how late? Certainly before the great series of Hippocratic commentaries, to which Galen intended soon to turn his mind (444), and
before the last two books of *On hygiene*, for in them Galen justified the
brevity of his description of drugs in the *Method of healing* on the grounds
that he was there writing specifically for doctors, not for laymen or even
amateurs of medicine already well versed in its fundamentals (VI.269).
Since we know that all these tracts, covering some 2,500 pages or more,
preceded *On prognosis* (written in 178, cf. CMG V 8,1,49-51), a date for
the *Method of healing*, 1-6, later than the first months of 176 is unlikely.
It can be pushed back still earlier if a cross-reference in *On dyspnoea*

---

[2] G. Sarton, Galen of Pergamon, Lawrence, University of Kansas Press, 1954, p. 18;
C. Singer, Galen, On anatomical procedures, London, Oxford University Press, 1956,
pp. xiv, 2.
[3] Galen's remarks at II.217, that he had visited Corinth to hear Numisianus, and went
from there to Alexandria, where he had heard that Numisianus was living, do not suggest
a long stay, or that he attended lectures on anatomy at Corinth.

(VII.903) is genuine, and any date later than the first months of 175 risks squeezing Galen's stay at Alexandria impossibly tightly.[4]

A possible dating criterion for tracts of the middle 170s has been found in the three treatises *On crises*, *On critical days*, and *On the differences between fevers*, which were all written before May, 175.[5] However, D. W. Peterson's attempt to use them to date the *Method of healing* is, on his own admission, inconclusive, since any argument from silence is considerably weakened by the fact that in Books 1-6, Galen did not deal at all with crises and critical days, and only in passing with fevers. He concentrated instead on defining his terms (Books 1-2) and then discussing ulcers and other lesions of continuity (3-6). There was little reason in these books for Galen to refer to his specialised works on aspects of fever and crises, even if they had already been in circulation, and although one might have expected him in any later discussion of fevers to refer to the theoretical arguments that open the *Method of healing*, this is far from being essential. We cannot then tell whether Galen fulfilled his promise to Glaucon and wrote his larger work almost immediately, or whether it was delayed for two or three years. Nevertheless, a date for Books 1-6 in the mid-170s is probable, hardly before 173, given the enormous number of pages Galen was writing between 169 and this tract, and possibly as late as 175.

The later books, 7-14, are equally hard to pin down. Galen refers to the existence of a plague (733) and his past experiences with an epidemic of anthrax (not its modern namesake) in Asia (980), but neither outbreak can be dated from historical sources. Nevertheless, it is clear from Galen's own cross-references that these books were among the last of his writings, following the second part of his tract on simples, and preceding the revision and formal 'publication' of his major tract, in two parts, on compound drugs, described according to type or to the site of the ailment.[6] The whole tract, *The Method of healing*, was thus completed in the late 190s, and possibly even later, if we accept Arabic evidence, deriving

---

[4] K. Bardong, 'Beiträge zur Hippokrates- und Galenforschung', NAW Göttingen 1942, p. 635f. The cross-reference at VII.903 bears the suspicious marks of an interpolation, particularly in the way it breaks up the flow of the argument, but, until more is known of the textual tradition of this tract, this inconcinnity could be Galen's own. If the reference to a visit to Alexandria twenty years before is intended to be chronologically precise and to refer to his arrival there (both of which suppositions may be wrong), it is hard to date this tract later than 174, given Galen's emphasis on his varied education at Alexandria.

[5] D. W. Peterson, 'Observations on the chronology of the Galenic corpus', *Bull. Hist. Med.* 51 (1977) 488, 492-495.

[6] Bardong, art. cit., above n. 4, p. 640. For the ambiguity of Galenic cross-references in the present tense, see ibid., p. 605.

ultimately from Galen's contemporary Alexander of Aphrodisias, that
Galen lived on into his eighties.[7]

Did Galen in any way attempt to revise the earlier books when he
came, twenty years later, to write Books 7-14? Only at 300-301 is there
a hint of any rewriting, but 'it is revealed in the diagnoses of affected
parts' is not a citation of the later book *On affected parts* but a general
reference to a topic that, as we know from the nearly contemporaneous
On the various stages of diseases (VII.460), was beginning to engage Galen's
interest, even though it too was not written up in full for another twenty
years. We should not, then, see Galen as a modern author polishing up
earlier books in preparation for a complete edition of his medical *Method*,
but rather as taking up again, under an older framework and title, topics
that had once interested him but which for various reasons he had not
been able to set down in writing.

A long gap between the two parts of a single treatise is not unusual for
the busy Galen. Almost twenty years elapsed between the composition of
the first eight books on simples and the last three, a gap he explained on
the grounds of pressure of work and, much more respectably for the
scholar he claimed to be, the lack of an opportunity to see some of the
mineral drugs that he wanted to include in his treatise (XII.227). It may
even have been the taking up again and completion of this long tract that
suggested to Galen that he should finish the *Method of healing*, for the latter
depended on the former for its organisation and prescription of drugs. A
closer parallel to Galen's own reason for leaving his great project half-
finished, the death of the dedicatee, Hiero, can be found in his comments
on two other tracts, *Anatomical procedures* and *On the opinions of Hippocrates
and Plato*. Both were begun c. 165 at the request of Flavius Boethus, a
wealthy consular with a keen interest in medicine, and were abandoned
a few years later when Galen heard of Boethus' unexpected death. A few
years elapsed before, in response to requests from 'those eager to learn'
(CMG V 4,1,2, 438), Galen added the last three books of *On the opinions
of Hippocrates and Plato*, during that prolific period of his life, 170-176
(CMG V 4,1,2,46-48). *Anatomical procedures* offers an even more complicated story. At first Galen wrote only two books for Boethus, in which
he summarised what he had done in his dissections. His own copy was
then destroyed in a fire, and Boethus' books perished with him, so Galen
began to rewrite and expand the whole treatise, beginning in the early
170s (II.216f.). He had already handed over for transcription the first
eleven books of his treatise (and they were already, presumably, cir-
culating among his friends) and the last four existed in his library at least

---

[7] The quotation is reported by me at CMG V 8,1, 189.

in note form when the great fire at the Temple of Peace in 192 consumed them in its flames. The last four he had then to rewrite before they could be circulated among those interested (108 Duckworth). This example shows the great length of time over which Galen could occupy himself with one topic, as well as the somewhat haphazard way in which even a major treatise could reach a wider audience.

But such was not the readership Galen had in mind for the *Method of healing*, which demanded, as an essential preliminary, a knowledge of medical terminology and ideas, and possibly clinical experience. It was not a book for the layman, or even the ordinary physician (XI.359). Hiero, to whom the first six books were dedicated, must then be assumed to have been an extremely competent practitioner, and we are told by Galen that he had a detailed knowledge of anatomy (409) and a long-standing and intimate acquaintance with Galen and other doctors (75, 114). His death put an end for the moment to the writing of the tract, although Galen may have contemplated a swift resumption within a few months.[8]

It might, however, be objected that Galen was merely using Hiero's death to cloak his own inability to finish the book, and that a personal friendship and interest in the subject should not be inferred from a dedication. Literary artifice and, above all, a desire for patronage could serve as sufficient reason to mention the exploits of a man of wealth. Cicero's 'Prior Academics', for example, begins with a fulsome eulogy of the celebrated soldier and politician, L. Licinius Lucullus, in which Cicero carefully explains that although Lucullus' career and public reputation (as a bon viveur) might not, on the face of it, suggest any interest in philosophy, to those who knew him the inner reality was far different. However, in a private letter to his friend Atticus, Cicero confesses that in truth Lucullus, and two other interlocutors, Catulus and Hortensius, were notorious for their lack of expertise in matters philosophical.[9] But although it would be wrong to rule out entirely a

---

[8] In *On the various stages of diseases*, a little tract that came after *On crises* and *On the differences between fevers* (VII.432), and which, pace Bardong, art. cit., above n. 4, p. 614, might be as early as 175, Galen referred, in the present tense, to a discussion in the *Method of healing* about the intermediate stages of diseases. Dr. I. Wille, in her edition of *On the various stages of diseases*, Kiel, 1960, Teil III, p. III, wished to connect this with a passage from Book 11 (X.748), but this would involve a massive redating of both treatises for the sake of a fleeting comment. There are two other possibilities: that the reference is to a few lines at X.289, or, given the ambiguities of Galen's use of the present (above, n. 6), that Galen was talking of something he was planning to include shortly when he took up work again on the *Method of healing*. Given the various topics he had already indicated for the subsequent books (below, p. 7 f.), the latter hypothesis seems preferable.

[9] Cicero, *Academica priora*, II.1-4; *Ad Atticum*, XIII.16, with the commentary by D. R. Shackleton Bailey.

desire for patronage on Galen's part in his choice of dedicatee, various considerations suggest that his claims to be writing with particular friends in mind (456) or to satisfy their importunities were not wildly exaggerated. Very few of them come from the Roman governing elite—Victorinus (CMG Suppl. Or. II.77) and Boethus are exceptions—, even though Galen reports many contacts there. Several of them, Epigenes, Teuthras, Apellas, and possibly Glaucon, seem to have known him in his younger days at Pergamum, while others are possibly fellow doctors in Rome. Even with Boethus Galen is on terms of friendly intimacy, acting as one of his medical advisers, instructing him in medicine, and frequently dropping his name in contexts where, were his claims untrue, his many opponents would eagerly seize upon his blatant falsehoods.[10] Furthermore, his references to his friends did not cease with the preface: Galen often adds personal touches in his exposition, or appeals to the dedicatee to confirm by his own past experience the truth of Galen's statements. All this suggests that, although he might undoubtedly have played down his desire for a patron and exaggerated the demands of his friends as a spur to writing particular tracts—a man with so fluent a pen and so definite a standpoint is unlikely to have lacked for a stimulus—, Galen did often write with friends in mind; and that Hiero's death could easily have caused him to interrupt, for the moment, the writing of a major treatise.

Other interests, other activities then intervened, and it was not for another twenty years or more that Galen fulfilled the requests of his friends, including Eugenianus, to whom he dedicated the last eight books, and produced the desired sequel. According to Galen, 458, all that he could then find were brief summaries of chapter headings, without any formal ascription or continuous exposition. This description hardly fits the first six books, which were certainly accessible to others and cited by Galen several times in the intervening years. Besides, as we have seen, there is nothing to suggest that, as we have them, they were in any way revised or touched up after they were written in the mid-170s. Similarly, although Galen may not himself have appended his name to them, it is unlikely that they circulated among his friends totally anonymously. But it is entirely possible that all that Galen had of the projected treatises were stray notes and jottings, relics of a scheme that he could no longer recall in detail. Book 6, in which he ended his discussion of the treatment of lesions of continuity, ulcers, sprains and fractures, formed a natural break before Galen passed on to consider the various types of fevers. The division at the end of Book 6 was deliberate, for,

---

[10] CMG V 8,1, 164, 200, 203.

unlike the end of Book 5 (383) and, still more obviously, Book 3 (231), there is no suggestion that it was only the length of the bookroll that forced Galen to curtail his exposition, or that it was to be continued directly in the next book.

Nevertheless, we can detect traces of what Galen was planning to say in the later books of the *Method of healing*, had they been written for Hiero, and we can see how far, twenty years later, he stuck by his original scheme. First, some topics on whose importance Galen seems to have changed his mind. At the end of Book 4, he apologises for talking only about the different types of ulcer by promising a later discussion of the indications for treatment drawn from the strength of the disease, the patient's age, the site and conformation of the affected part, and the severity or absence of pain (295). Some of these topics are mentioned in passing in Books 5 and 6 (which may be also seen as an exposition of the treatment of lesions of continuity according to particular organs), but in Books 7-14 they receive no concerted or detailed discussion, although they are often mentioned and the problem of pain and its causes is touched on in Book 12 (812ff., 850ff.). In Book 5, Galen announced that he would answer at an appropriate place the question as to who most needed treatment with milk (375), but when milk is mentioned later (474ff., 727), no answer is given, except perhaps by implication. Neither do I find a reference in the later books to his planned discussion of the proper therapy for seepage of blood (diapedesis) (332).

There may have been more major changes of plan. There is no hint of the projected section on eye diseases, and it is possible that Galen intended to pass directly from this treatment of ulcers and lesions of continuity to an account of inflammation, his λόγος φλεγμονῶν (408). It was perhaps here that Galen was to deal with tumours, sepsis and scirrhoses left after the application of strongly heating drugs (296, 335, 302, 408, 439), and the reader is led to expect something more substantial than the hurried and somewhat confused account given in Book 13 and 14 (cf. also 874). In this projected book, or books, Galen might have included a detailed description of the treatment of aneurysms (335, 381), and of various fluxes (317), of which only cursory hints are to be found in Book 13.[11]

---

[11] The artist who illustrated the famous Dresden codex of Galen, Db 92-93, of c. 1460, depicted, in the miniature that opens the whole treatise, fol. 467 r. (= E. C. v. Leersum, W. Martin, Miniaturen der Lateinischen Handschrift der Kgl. Oeffenl. Bibliothek in Dresden Db. 92-93, Leiden, Sijthoff, 1910, n. 87), two patients, one with his hand to his chest, the other, very pale and sad, resting his head on his hand, with, behind them, a servant with a flute. The flute, with its links with music, suggests that the second patient was melancholic, to be cured by sweet music, and that the illustration was intended to show Galen as a great healer of both body and mind. But, in the *Method of healing*, Galen sticks firmly to bodily ailments.

His descriptions in Book 13, and still more in Book 14, of conditions that might require surgery are curiously hurried by comparison with Galen's earlier promises and with the leisured treatment of fevers that occupies Books 7-12, and they prompt a further question about the development of the whole treatise. Was it ever intended to include detailed sections on surgery, or did Galen change his mind and decide to follow it with a separate tract entirely devoted to surgery? Book 14 certainly refers to a range of conditions, some of which demand surgery, but this book above all resembles a very hasty combination of stray thoughts and lacks any strong central core, either thematic or paradigmatic. If Galen's decision to relegate a discussion of surgery to 'the end of this treatise' (990, cf. 986) refers solely to its last five chapters, his exposition there is oddly cursory and haphazard. It is easier to believe that Galen was going to follow the wishes of his students (943) and consider surgery 'at the conclusion of the whole treatise' (in a temporal, rather than bibliographical sense) in a book that he never managed to write. It was to this unwritten treatise that he postponed his discussion of the surgical treatment for varicose veins (943) and his comments in those who wanted to treat ocular suffusion by emptying the eye of liquid (987). It was also to contain a discussion of the aims and intentions of surgery, both in general and in particular, for they should be considered together. At Book 14, chapter 13 (986), Galen took pains to state why his consideration of unnatural tumours would, for the moment, be brief: a more extensive analysis would follow later in his Χειρουργούμενα. The work, alas, was never written.

But it would be wrong to conclude from all this that Galen was constantly changing his mind or breaking his promises. Leaving aside the possibility that he had neither the time nor the opportunity to reread his first six books making careful note of what, in passing, he had once promised to say, we may suppose, with good reason, that Galen was concerned more to avoid duplicating any general themes and to expound his medical method for different diseases and conditions. In this he was successful, for there is scarcely any overlap, and the bulk of the later books (8-12) treat at length a topic deliberately postponed from Books 1-6, that of fevers. The subject of humoral imbalance, foreshadowed at 295, takes up much of Book 7, and underlies the discussion of fevers, and one of its therapies, bloodletting, is examined in Books 9 and 13, thereby fulfilling the promises made at 288 and 439. In Book 9 can also be found the exposition of the various types of evacuation from the stomach that Galen had postponed from Book 6 (439). It was also in the later books that Galen wrote in passing about the various stages of disease, a topic which, if my conjecture is right (see note 8), was in his mind about the time that Hiero died.

There is also one major change in Galen's organisation of his material between the two halves of the work: the prominence given in the later books to the paradigmatic case-history (cf. 628). In the first four books, where cases are less needed to exemplify theory, Galen was at pains to remind his readers that his was a universal method, and that individual examples only added to the length of a book and obscured the clarity of the argument (322). He later modified this precept (398, 425), and Book 6 contains a variety of stories from his clinical career. With Book 7 comes a marked change to one major exposition of a case-history per book (504-507, 535-540, 608-616 [two antithetical cases discussed together], 671-678, 792-797, 856-861) leading in Book 13 to one of Galen's great set-pieces, the humiliation of Attalus (909-916). By contrast, Book 14 has several references to Galen's cases, none of them described at any length, which may be a further indication that this last book was put together rather hurriedly. Galen's procedure in these later books of the *Method of healing* can be paralleled in the almost contemporary *On affected parts*, whose major stories, like those of Antipater (VIII.293-296) and Glaucon (VIII.361-363), are similarly rationed among its books. The result of this change is that the somewhat tedious argument of the earlier books is given relief by the exposition, in a different and more literary style, of a tale designed to interest the reader. The general point is given a specific and memorable example, and Galen's assertions of his courage, wisdom and medical pre-eminence are provided with factual backing.

To illustrate Galen's skill as a narrator of case-histories, I shall analyse first the doublet that serves as his example of synochic (continuous) fever in Book 9 (608-616; for the problem of nomenclature, cf. 602ff.), and then go on to discuss a case from *On the properties of simples* which is also given by Aretaeus of Cappadocia. It should be borne in mind in all this that Galen had enjoyed a long and deep education, that he took a more than amateur interest in the Greek literary classics, and that he was a friend of leading sophists and rhetoricians. Besides, medicine had been since the days of the Hippocratics a partly public art, and the doctor had to convince his patients and the lookers-on of his abilities by words as much as by deeds. So we should not be surprised to find Galen deploying a range of literary and rhetorical skills, and being able to vary the tone, style and tempo of his narratives to suit the occasion and to avoid monotony.[12]

He introduces his joint case-history in Book 9 with the claim that such an example is necessary on good educational grounds (608); a general method by itself is not enough to supply precise knowledge, and, besides,

---

[12] See, e.g., my comments at CMG V 8,1, pp. 59-63.

what we have seen with our own eyes provides the best example of all. Eugenianus' role in this story is complex. Not only is he the dedicatee of the book and the ostensible recipient of its teachings, but as a friend of Galen and a medical man himself, he had observed the cases that Galen now describes, and his recollections, it is implied, serve in turn to reinforce the truth of Galen's account of what happened.

The two young men who suffered from continuous fever were roughly of the same age. One was a citizen and a fitness fanatic, the other a slave and keen on physical training only in so far as was appropriate for a slave in the exercise of his duties. Galen heightens the contrasts between the two by using a series of oppositive particles, which also link the two men together in the same sentence. They offer, in Galen's eyes, a specially memorable example of continuous fever in its two forms, with or without putrefaction. Mention of examples leads Galen into a brief tirade against the ignorance of his contemporaries (609) and their preference for time-serving subservience over his own passion for learning. Emphatic particles, traditional contrasts (as between δοξοσοφία and truth) and the repetition of 'There is nothing surprising' help to set Galen apart as a man of wisdom and even modesty, for he claims merely to have assessed the discoveries of past ages and put some of them into practice. This athletics metaphor, ἀσκεῖν, provides a bridge back to the actual cases.

Galen introduces the young gymnast briefly: he was seen at the beginning of his fever at 7 p.m. and then at about 9 a.m. (The hesitant που helps to suggest that Galen is not just regurgitating his notes but is human after all). Then follows an immense sentence, seventeen lines long (610, 1-17), in which Galen describes all the symptoms, the man's pulse, temperature, urine, habits, past activity, food, colouring, and feelings, to explain why he thought it best to delay intervention. The line of thought is not lost in this periodic sentence, for Galen's clever use of particles acts as a signpost and holds everything tightly together. Shorter sentences follow, until Galen comes to describe the reappearance of various symptoms on the third night, which are all contained in a single sentence nine lines long (611,8-17). The narrative is then speeded up by a change of tenses, from the aorist to the historic present and imperfect. A certain light relief is then imparted to the narrative by the interjections of bystanders and servants, with the colloquial 'You've strangled the fever' setting off the more learned 'quenched' (612,14-15). The case concludes with Galen making repeated visits to the man as he lay in a heavy sleep, and then deliberately waking him up for food by loud shouting (613,12). Galen's elaborate and occasionally heavy medical expertise thus terminates in light humour.

The case of the second youth, whose fever is accompanied by putrefaction, is described with less dramatic variation. There is no scene setting, no change of tone or vocabulary. We are given a flat description of his symptoms and Galen's treatment, and what movement there is comes from the interjection of short, pithy sentences (614, 5; 11; 615, 4). Only once does Galen launch out into a long period (617, 9-16), significantly not in his description of the actual case, but in a general summary of the exemplary value of these cases for the treatment of continuous fevers in general. The final page (616) is taken up with a vigorous attack on those who, for whatever reason, fail to let blood, even when nature herself demands it most clearly.

In this section of Book 9, we can see how Galen works up two related cases, setting them off against each other in literary as well as medical and social ways. In the first the emphasis is less on the detailed development of symptoms as on the story, on the patient, and on Galen's relationship with him and his attendants: in the second, the medical data are more prominent, and Galen points more to the conclusions to be drawn from them for the general treatment of continuous fevers. Galen organises his material differently, and narrates the cases in different ways: the tone and style is varied in the first, the second is a straightforward technical description in flat technical language.

My second example of Galen's ability as a raconteur comes not from the *Method of healing*, but from a nearly contemporary book, *On the properties of simples*, XI.1, (XII.312-3). It is interesting not only from its content, the saga of a sufferer from a skin disease called *elephas* who was cured by drinking wine in which a viper had drowned, but from being the unique example of a case described by two ancient authors, neither of whom can be shown to have depended on the other.

It is Aretaeus of Cappadocia who, at the end of his final book on the causes of chronic diseases, IV.13, 20 = CMG II 90, 7-22, first tells the story. The sufferer, cast out into the mountains or the desert, sees the snake creep into the winejar, inject its poison, and drown. From a desire to end it all, he drinks from the jar until he collapses in a drunken stupor. On waking up, he finds his hair falling out, his fingers and nails beginning to slough off. Within a short time, his whole body has, as it were, grown a new skin; he has discarded his old skin and become another man. In this brief story, Aretaeus emphasises the man's physical condition and his regeneration above the more pitiful aspects of the story.

Galen's account, by contrast, is a much more elegant, although not necessarily a more studied, performance.[13] It is a vignette of country life,

---

[13] K. Deichgräber, 'Aretaeus von Kappadozien als medizinischer Schriftsteller', AAW Leipzig 63, 1971. The comments of P. Petit, apud 'Aretaei Cappadocis Opera omnia', ed. C. G. Kühn, Leipzig, Cnobloch, 1828, pp. 547-566, are not entirely superseded.

that occupies some twenty-four lines (XII.312, 9-313, 15). All that we are
told about the patient is that he looked and smelled horrible, and that at
the end he was cured when his tuberous skin fell off him like the shell of
a crustacean. Galen plays up the human interest of the story with a
multitude of imaginative detail. The man lived in isolation, in a hut on
a little hill, although he had previously lived with his family until he
began to pass on the disease to others. Villagers had built him his hut,
by a stream, and they came daily with enough food to keep him alive.
The wine reached him almost by accident. It had been left unattended
in the fields in high summer for the benefit of some reapers. Its bouquet
was strong, and it was not until the lad who mixed their drinks lifted up
the jar to pour its contents into the mixing bowl that the dead snake was
noticed as it dropped out of the jar.[14] There was consternation, and the
harvesters drank only water that day. But, on their way home, out of
charity and compassion, they presented the wine to the poor outcast,
thinking it better for him to die than drag out a miserable existence. But,
once having drunk, he was miraculously cured.

It can be seen from this description of the two accounts that Galen is
by far the more accomplished storyteller. He has an eye for pleasant
detail, a fund of sympathy, and a vivid imagination. The medical importance of the case is almost subsumed in the abundance of intimate (and
unnecessary) details. It is not simply that Galen's purpose, to extol the
merits of viper flesh, differs from that of Aretaeus, to describe the
disease: Galen feels free to exploit all his literary and rhetorical skills to
adorn a tale for the entertainment, as well as the instruction, of his
readers.

But there is another point of conflict between the two authors. For
Aretaeus, the story is simply a tale, a myth, something not entirely certain, but very plausible. For Galen, in *On simples*, this is an incident that
he experienced when he was a young man back home in Asia Minor
(XII.312). Is Galen stealing a good story from folk tale, or from a book,
or even from Aretaeus, and claiming it as his own?[15] And, if so, does not
this cast doubt on the credibility of any Galenic recollection of events in
which he took part? The truth is less damning. This case-history, and the
two which follow on it directly, were first recorded by Galen some thirty

---

[14] The following emendations by K. S. Kontos to Kühn's text should be noted,
Athenaion 6 (1877) 417: 313,1 ⟨οὖν⟩ (but perhaps superfluous); 313,3 ⟨εἰς⟩ κρατῆρα but
most of the Greek Mss. read κρατῆρι, rightly; 313,4 ἐξερῶντος, rightly.

[15] The problem was already seen by Petit, above, n. 13, but was first fully set out by
F. Kudlien, Der Beginn des medizinischen Denkens bei den Griechen, Zürich and Stuttgart, Artemis Verlag, 1967, p. 103f.

years before, in his *Sketch of Empiricism*, ch. 10.[16] There, if Niccolo's Latin translation is accurate—and there is nothing to suggest that it is not—Galen reported the first two cases, the second of which occurred in Mysia, not far from Galen's home at Pergamum, without any reference to his own personal experience, and claimed that it was precisely from knowing these cases (presumably either from books or hearsay) that he was enabled to devise the appropriate treatment for the third case. In his old age, Galen took his examples from his earlier book, copied them almost word for word, and, perhaps misled by the case from Mysia, introduced them all as tales from his own personal experience. Galen's error is venial, the result of a hasty re-reading, but still disconcerting.

As well as the prominent part given to case-histories in Books 7-14 of the *Method of healing*, there are other features which may be explained by the many years which passed between the writing of the two parts, and by the different circumstances of their composition. As Galen tells us (XIV.650: XIX.19), the emperor Marcus Aurelius had left him behind in 169 to look after the health of his heir, Commodus, while he campaigned against the German invaders in the North. The unexpected prolongation of the war allowed Galen even more free time in which to write. Commodus, though rude and recalcitrant, was not a permanent invalid, and apart from the occasional temperature (XIV.662f.) and the irritation of moving from one royal residence to another at the prince's whim, he may not have troubled Galen much. Indeed, we know that he paid one brief visit to the front in the early 170s, leaving Galen behind in Italy, and that he left to join his father in May 175 (CMG V I,1, 212, 224). The bibliographies of Ilberg and Bardong show just how much use Galen made of his relative leisure.[17] The books that he wrote then included, as well as the first part of the *Method of healing* and the first group of Hippocratic commentaries, *On the use of parts*, *On the opinion of Hippocrates and Plato*, 7-9, *Anatomical procedures* 1-5, and *On crises*, to say nothing of smaller tracts like *On medical terminology*, of c. 172.[18] Galen must have been writing at a furious speed, rather like a newspaper columnist. In addition, he carried out some medical work—many of his remarks to Hiero can only be understood on the assumption that Hiero had accompanied him on visits to patients—, performed his private anatomies, and continued his discussions, both in public and in private, with the

---

[16] K. Deichgräber, Die griechische Empirikerschule, ed. 2, Berlin, Weidmann, 1965, pp. 75-79, unfortunately not known to Kudlien, op. cit. (above, n. 15).

[17] J. Ilberg, 'Über die Schriftstellerei des Klaudios Galenos, III', *Rheinisches Museum* 51 (1896) 194 f.; Bardong, art. cit., above, n. 4, pp. 633-637.

[18] In my edition of *On prognosis*, CMG V 8,1, p. 48, n. 1, I suggested a later date for *On medical terminology* of c. 176, but the evidence of X.42, 89f., dates it some years earlier.

Aristotelians. It is unfortunate that we have few medical cases that can be dated to this period of Galen's life—the man with the intermittent pulse (CMG V 8,1, 228), and plague sufferers (IX.341, 359; X.360)—but given the fact that patients sought him out even in the backwoods or consulted him by letter from all over the Roman Empire, it seems unwise to assume that he lived the life of a tranquil scholar, seated in his study, writing away at his books. Far from it, *The Method of healing* 1-6 gives the impression of a doctor battling, if not always against disease, at least against his fellow doctors. Reading the first books of the *Method of healing*, one is constantly reminded of the polemical prefaces of A. E. Housman, which, he said, found purchasers among the unlearned who had heard that Manilius, I, contained a scurrilous preface and hoped to extract from it a low enjoyment.[19]

But, however much one might admire Galen's rhetorical skills, which at their worst enliven the Fachprosa of his technical arguments, it must be admitted that they do not immediately enhance his stature as a doctor or as a man, and that at times they only serve to complicate an already complex issue. There is an argument running through the first two books to which Galen constantly returns after digressions—ring-composition is an apt description—, and in this the Methodists are Galen's chief opponents. At the same time, he feels the need to defend himself on all fronts, against the Empirics and against the semidogmatists. The result is often confusion, with Galen's own method defined as much by what it is not as by what it is. The later books, where he has less to do with the fundamental bases of his opponents' therapy and can dole out praise or blame on the simpler grounds of the adoption or rejection of a Galenic cure, are both clearer to follow and less obstreperous in their polemic. Although Galen repeats his denunciation of mindless Methodists (910, 928), and continues to call them 'Thessalian asses' (915; a pun on the famous broodmares of Thessaly), there is nothing to compare with Book 1 for sustained ferocity. One might be tempted to ascribe this to the greater tranquillity that old age brings along with forgetfulness (456), yet Galen obviously still regards the Methodists as his chief foes, and his story of the death of Theagenes (909-916) is as bitter and sarcastic as anything he ever wrote. It was obviously a cause célèbre, for Theagenes was a famous man, not least as the devoted pupil of Lucian's Peregrinus, and the doctor, Attalus, is almost certainly to be identified with the royal physician, Statilius Attalus of Heraclea.[20] In this story, Galen's malice and sense of timing are equally as evident as the unwillingness of Attalus

---

[19] A. E. Housman, Manilius V, London, The Richards Press, 1930, p. i (= A. E. Housman, Selected prose, Cambridge University Press, 1961, p. xi).

[20] J. Benedum, 'Statilios Attalos', *Med. hist. J.* 6 (1971) 264-277.

to listen to Galen, and, to be fair, we cannot be certain that Theagenes would not have died even with Galen's own treatment. But the impression Galen intends us to take away is of his own abilities as contrasted with Attalus' stupidity and boorishness, and in its characterisation of the Methodists as ignorant fools, it may be more effective than the more conventional jibes at Thessalus the woolworker, the teacher of half-trained slaves.

But before we turn to look in detail at this rhetoric of hate, we must be clear as to what Galen himself meant by a method of healing. It was, I think, a series of general practical rules for treatment based on a sound knowledge of humoral physiology, from which a competent practitioner could devise the appropriate treatment for an individual case.[21] It comprised, too, an understanding of the various indications of diseases, both chronic and acute, the principles of therapy, and a basic armamentarium. Galen's method stood in opposition to the more famous one of Thessalus of Tralles, fl. 40 A.D., who sought, on the basis of a physiology of atoms and pores, to reduce all diseases to a form of constriction, dilation or both: recognition of these states would automatically lead the doctor to a knowledge of the proper treatment.[22] But Thessalus was not the only one to have a method. One could talk of an Empiric method or of the method of Erasistratus and Herophilus (309f.), to say nothing of that of Hippocrates. Indeed, I should like to argue that there were variant methods within Methodism, and that the Asclepiadeans, or, as Plutarch called them, 'Democriteans', should not be assumed to have followed Thessalus in everything.[23] M. Modius Asiaticus of Smyrna, 'champion of medical method', 'a Methodist doctor', may have produced his own refinements on Thessalus and Asclepiades, just as later Soranus did.[24] The parallel with the Renaissance, when competing medical methods were two a penny, although most were ultimately based on Hippocrates and Galen, may not be far-fetched, for Galen seems to suggest at 346 and 628 the existence of a great variety of methods.

But for Galen the only true method was that of Hippocrates, the great leader (309, 346) who had first found out the true way (117, 633) and

---

[21] It is important to note that Galen, while accepting humours and elements as the basis of his physiology, places far more emphasis in his diagnosis and treatment on qualitative changes within the body, and individual humours as such play only a restricted part.

[22] A recent defence of the Methodists has been made by M. Frede, 'The method of the so-called Methodical school of medicine', in J. Barnes, et al., Science and speculation, Cambridge University Press, 1982, pp. 1-23. But his article depends on there being a total consistency between Methodist authors over a period of centuries.

[23] Plutarch, Symposiaca VI.2; VIII.9.

[24] CIG 3283; J. Benedum, 'Markos Modios Asiatikos', *Med. hist. J.* 13 (1978) 307-309.

who had provided the seed for others to sow and reap (459), although far from garnering the harvest, most had simply destroyed the precious seed (459). Hippocrates had not hesitated to teach all that had been most neglected before, all that was essential for healing (686). Galen's role was, like the emperor Trajan, to broaden, improve or clear away misunderstandings from a road whose line had already been settled in general by Hippocrates (632f.). That it was Hippocrates who had laid the foundation of a true medical method had been acknowledged by philosophers as well as doctors, although they had failed to take up the task unfinished by Hippocrates. It was left to Galen to fill in the gaps, to the surprise of his teachers and the envy of his fellow students (561), and to bring out fully all the implications of the scattered and often obscure aphorisms of the great man. Indeed, Galen's own book on method could be recommended as a most suitable introduction to the writings of Hippocrates (420), although Galen had no intention thereby of consigning the works of the master to the great unread. Two points should be noticed in all this. Galen, unlike some modern interpreters of Hippocrates, does not view him as simply the provider of the data of experience, from which one can then create one's own system. Hippocrates has a system of doctrine of his own, which is confirmed by the cases in the 'Epidemics' and briefly and succinctly expressed in the 'Aphorisms', and it is no surprise that Galen draws most of his examples from these two works. The Hippocratic method is open to correction by logic and the light of experience (just like Galen's, 375), and such obscurities as exist are not due to any incompatibility between the various texts, but to Hippocrates' own failure to express himself clearly or to deal thoroughly with everything.[25]

Secondly, it is remarkable how little attention Galen pays to that prime document of Hippocratic method in modern eyes, the testimony of Plato in his 'Phaedrus', 270C.[26] Not that this was unknown to Galen, for he quotes it very early on in Book 1 (13) as part of his more general thesis that all authorities, if asked, would confess the superiority of Hippocrates over Thessalus, the boastful charlatan. But apart from that, Plato's description of Hippocratic method, and particularly the importance of *diairesis*, logical subdivision, is very much subordinated to Galen's more broadly medical conception of method. I find a hint of it only at 194, where Galen stresses the importance of understanding the simple components first, before going on to consider the more complex.

---

[25] W. D. Smith, The Hippocratic tradition, Ithaca and London, Cornell University Press, 1979, pp. 61-176.
[26] Cf. G. E. R. Lloyd, 'The Hippocratic question', *Class. Quart.*, n.s. 25 (1975) 171-192.

Galen's idea of method encompasses a wider range of practical guidelines than this, in his attempt to circumscribe as far as possible the individuality of each particular clinical case, which, as he admits, is in the last resort ineffable and indefinable (206, 659).

Galenic (or Hippocratic) method, then, contrasts, in Galen's eyes, with that of Thessalus and the Methodists in being verifiable by reason and experience. Like that of the Empirics, it aims to take into account as far as possible the patient's individual condition, but unlike theirs, it provides a series of options for treatment, should the first one fail, and a means whereby general rules can be applied to individual cases. It is founded, above all, on a knowledge of the elements, on physiology, and on an understanding of the anatomy of the human body (349, 409, 421), backed up by the power of logic (469) and apodeictic (62). It is not enough simply to be a great anatomist, like Erasistratus (461); one must go further, otherwise one would be like a sculptor who made a beautiful statue and left out its eyes (379). What is needed above all is a knowledge of physiology, which should not be greeted with raised eyebrows or condemned as philosophically irrelevant (170, 180). The Methodists fail on every count, and the result is the wholesale slaughter of patients with even simple injuries and ailments (390). They are like pilots who wreck the ship and then graciously hand over the planking for the passengers to cling to (377). Half-trained, often uneducated, they are content to tyrannise their patients in an effort to gain power, glory, and influence (114).

How much of this abuse was actually true is far more difficult to determine. That the Methodists gave as good as they got is clear from Galen's complaints of medical debates ending in disorder, with the language of bargees and Billingsgate (109,112), and there can be no doubt of their professional and social successes. Statilius Attalus was an imperial doctor; the unnamed Methodist of XIV.663 served the imperial family; and although Methodist doctrine was gradually filtered out in the later Greek medical compendia in favour of more and more of Galen, it enjoyed a long survival in the Latin West, and Soranus' 'Gynaecology' remained pre-eminent among Greek texts on the diseases of women and childbirth.[27] It is also hard to discover how far Galen was indeed attacking his own Methodist contemporaries in Rome, rather than using the century-old doctrines of Thessalus as a stalking-horse. With the exception of Julianus (who may never have visited Rome and who may have died before the 170s) there is no contemporary Methodist named in

---

[27] For an example of a piece of Methodist doctrine surviving outside strictly medical authors, see V. Nutton, 'The seeds of disease', *Med. Hist.* 27 (1983) 1-34.

Books 1-6, and Attalus stands alone in Books 7-14. I am reminded of the
scholarly debate as to whether Juvenal was satirising his contemporaries
or merely attacking the dead, and it may be that we have to reckon with
certain conventions in abuse at least as much as with a historical situation. Thessalus, whose boastfulness and self-confidence (to say nothing
of his success) were known to his contemporary, Pliny,[28] is a convenient
object for attack because all Methodists could by implication be seen in
some way as his disciples, and because his failings could by implication
be attributed to them all. For the purposes of polemic, it mattered little
that Soranus had modified Methodist doctrine and reinstated aetiology
and physiology, if only to give an impression of sound learning for the
purposes of advertising (CMG IV 4,6-7), and that Attalus had been his
pupil (910); that other Methodists had changed for the better and been
converted to truer, Hippocratic, opinions on certain points; or that the
disciples of Olympicus held a, to Galen, correct belief about what a
symptom was (74). In attacking Methodism, a social as well as a medical
rival, all insinuations were valid to Galen. Argument and contradiction
are either muddle-headed or frivolous (109,113), and there is even the
suggestion that some doctors are prevented from openly confessing their
mistakes (though they are prepared to do so in private) by the fear of los-
ing their reputation (114, cf. 760). Others are said to go so far as to add
various coloured earths to their drugs in order to disguise the fact that
they had learned about them from Galen (396), New terminology,
which, to my mind, implies a renewed and vigorous interest at least in
some areas of medicine, is condemned as 'late-learning' (44), or quibbling (109), and its inventors set among the dreadful sophists, χριομύξαι
ἄνδρες (406).[29] What more can be expected of a man who was brought
up among women and later, as he sat alongside his father, made a mess
of carding wool (10), and who was willing to accept as pupils immature
slaves, shoemakers, dyers, carpenters, smiths and the like (4, 5, 22)? But
one should pause a moment before accepting this abuse as true
biographical data. The list of despised trades may be as much the product
of convention as of reality. Woolworkers, cobblers and dyers all appear
as the typical illiterate supporters of Christianity, according to Galen's
contemporary, Celsus, and the Galenic Christian heretic, Theodotus of
Byzantium, is called a cobbler.[30] Both Themison of Laodicea and
Thessalus of Tralles came from towns in Asia Minor long famous for

---

[28] Pliny, Nat. hist. 29.9; cf. L. Edelstein, Ancient medicine, Baltimore, Johns
Hopkins University Press, 1967, pp. 173-191.
[29] The emendation is owed to C. G. Cobet, 'Ad Galenum', *Mnemosyne*, n.s. 12 (1884)
445.
[30] Origen, Contra Celsum III.44; Eusebius, Hist. V.28.

their woollen goods, and this fact would have easily given Galen, and presumably others, an opportunity to blacken their memory by associating them with the lowest of the low, female weavers. It is far more likely that they both came from a higher stratum of society, the owners of the land over which the sheep grazed.

A similar obfuscation can be found in Galen's account of the various types of ulcers and their treatment in Books 3-6. His bitter complaints about the novelty of his opponents' terminology (423ff.), far from reflecting their perversity, demonstrate instead a heightened interest in practical wound surgery, with new discoveries being made, new techniques tried out, and new instruments devised. Leaving aside the 'arteriotome', invented by one unfortunate surgeon to cut out at one stroke a whole section of artery (II.643f.), we can find references in Galen to a variety of new instruments, some made out of specially tempered Norican steel (II.682), others with grooves to channel the blood away from the operator's fingers, and others devised for specific purposes, like the 'scolopomachaerion' (a pointed knife, 1011, cf. II.682). This lively interest in surgery is only to be expected in an age that saw the revival of anatomy with Marinus, Satyrus and their pupils,[31] and for which we have independent confirmation in both medical and epigraphic texts. At Ephesus, during Galen's lifetime, the doctors engaged in open competitions in ὄργανα and χειρουργία. Although what these words mean exactly, is unknown, it is very likely that they concerned surgical instruments (possibly a competition for new instruments) and some aspect of surgery (perhaps involving a public display of expertise on an animal).[32] From a generation or so before Galen we possess a tract, the pseudo-Galenic *Introduction* (XIV.674-797), which contains a substantial amount of information on surgical techniques, and which has recently been singled out for high praise, albeit by an author writing under the misapprehension that the book was genuinely Galenic.[33] Discoveries and new techniques were not confined to intellectuals. In Book 14 Galen reports favourably, if somewhat patronisingly, on the tricks of a surgeon who removed warts and verrucas by sucking them upwards and then biting them off at their roots (1011), and of the oculist Justus (1019), who

---

[31] Cf. XV.136; CMG V 10.1, 312.

[32] Die Inschriften von Ephesos, Bonn, Habelt, 1980, nos. 1160-1169, there assigned to a date c. 155 A.D.

[33] L. H. Toledo-Pereyra, 'Galen's contribution to surgery', *J. Hist. Med.* 28 (1973) 357-375, all of whose references to Galen after p. 366 are to pseudo-Galen. Cf. also, for the writings of a near-contemporary, R. L. Grant, 'Antyllus and his medical works', *Bull. Hist. Med.* 34 (1960) 154-174. Cf. also for surgery, Galen's own comments in *On examining physicians* ch. 14, CMG Suppl. Or. 4, pp. 134-137.

managed to displace the suffusion that was blocking a patient's vision simply by vigorous shaking. These men showed what native wit and experience could do by themselves: the man who had both *logos* and *peira*, the Galenic physician, could, of course, do even better.

The contrast in Part I with the empiric practitioner and, in particular, with the methodless Methodists, is further exaggerated by some of Galen's literary techniques, his use of choice words and phrases, e.g. ὀριγνωμένου (5, 122; cf. also ἐκβόσκονται 505, 730; ἐντυλίσσειν 541; ἐγκυρίων 914), his literary allusions and quotes from Homer, Hesiod and Euripides (6, 7, 11, 17) and his learned references to Salmoneus and Zoilus Homeromastix (18f.). The piling up of lists, be they of slaves (4), doctors (6), philosophers (12), or mere humble tradesmen (19), immediately suggests that Galen is a man of great erudition—an opinion that Galen held with massive, and not unjustified, self-confidence from his student days (254). Further conviction is given to Galen's attack by his vigorous style, which avoids long and complex sentences (contrast 244, 305), and instead poses brisk rhetorical questions (13, cf. 198), with, if the text is right, unusual asyndeton (90). The dullest of passages can be enlivened with a sneer (cf. 113, 264, ἐταρίχευσεν), by examples from the animal world (133f., 138f.) and even by an occasional joke (114, and, if τιτρώσκονται is right, 95). The result is a sense of life and vigour, which helps to convince the reader that Galen must be right.

Many of these features recur in Books 7-14 (e.g. 779, a reference to Thucydides; 732, an animal story; 627, a joke), but the attack on the Methodists, though never entirely broken off, is not so sustained in intensity as it is in the first two books. In part this is due to the type of subject and material with which Galen is dealing, since he can often claim agreement on some fundamentals of treatment between all the sects. Indeed, at one point he may even be adopting the famous slogan of Asclepiades, 'Swiftly, safely and pleasantly' (989), although in Galenic fashion, his paraphrase is more wordy and more sententious. But he still complains about ridiculous terminology, the worthlessness of reputation (457), still extols the blessings of philosophy, still emphasises his own superiority to his teachers and to all and sundry (465. 560f.). Galenic common sense is still far superior to any of the pompous pronouncements of the sophists (581f.), the *logiatroi*, who are ignorant of good manners (609), let alone of the ideas of that most philosophically minded of men, Hippocrates (561). There are no major changes of doctrine, such as Galen had experienced in his younger days over the order in which the organs of the foetus were formed (IV.663f.), and Galen's hesitation over the exact site, and indeed existence, of the vital spirit is an isolated example even of doubt.[34] This consistency between the two halves of the work adds strength to Galen's practical advice and to the hints to his friends and pupils in which he sums up a lifetime of medicine, from his employment as doctor to the gladiators in the late 150s to cases he had recently attended with Eugenianus in the 190s.

What Books 7-14 offer above all is a wide range of information on Galen's own position at Rome, and from it I choose only three topics for comment, the reactions of some of his fellow-practitioners to him, his attack upon the rich, and the changes in his perspective from Asia Minor to Rome. Together, they preach the same message: that over the twenty or so years that separate the earlier from the later books, Galen had become more and more convinced of his own success, and had a greater variety of evidence to prove it.

At times his ebullient rhetoric, most notably in *On prognosis* and in Book 1, with its vigorous denunciations of others and its picture of Galen as a saint, a genius and a social celebrity, at home with both peasant and prince, at once arouses suspicion, and any inconsistencies that are found there rightly create doubts. How far is Galen being sincere, how far is he being carried away by his winged words into wildly exaggerated statements?[35] One answer to these questions can be found in an examination of the assumptions that govern his writings and of some of the incidents he mentions almost insouciantly, which, by the way in which they are introduced, may provide a better guide than his open rhetoric to the place he occupied in Roman society. If, as I shall show, the assumptions and incidents retailed in the last books of the *Method of healing* reveal a consistently strong conviction in Galen of his own social and professional success, we must either accept this as true, or regard him as the victim of a massive self-delusion. Egocentric, bombastic and self-assertive he may have been, but, to my mind, he was no fool.

I have already referred to Galen's conviction in Books 1-7 that his opponents, even though they might believe him to be right, were unwilling for various reasons to adopt his ideas publicly, some out of shame, others out of spite. In the later books, he talks in passing of another, and, I suggest, a new, hazard, immoderate respect. His therapy for sufferers from fever—feeding them, and even making them bathe—brought him the reputation of a miracle-worker, and his careful and detailed explanations of why this treatment worked, far from dispelling this air of magic

---

[34] 839f. Cf. O. Temkin, The double face of Janus, Baltimore, Johns Hopkins University Press, 1977, pp. 154-161.

[35] J. Scarborough, 'The Galenic question', *Sudhoffs Arch.* 65 (1981) 1-31, in a very confusedly organised paper, himself exaggerates the extent of the difficulty of penetrating behind the Galenic facade.

and miracle, only succeeded in labelling him further as a 'wonderteller' (684, cf. XIV.641, and the testimonia at CMG V 8,1, 110). Not that Galen was not occasionally prepared to accept this sort of flattery (cf. 859, 869), but this particularly annoyed him, precisely because what he had intended to do was to show that, far from being a miracle, his cure was based on good sense and sound experience. There were other practitioners too who, in ignorant imitation, had followed his treatment in cases where death was already certain, and their apparent failure thereby cast doubt on the treatment's (and hence Galen's) efficacy (761). It was, of course, a familiar precept of ancient medicine that one should distinguish carefully between those patients who were likely to die and those who would recover, and Galen went out of his way to stress that his treatment would not work in hopeless cases. To use it then would be stupid, for failure would reflect badly on the doctor, however undeservedly, and perhaps indirectly on his teacher (cf. 560; CMG V 10,2,1, 401f.). Hence Galen's anger and concern at his incompetent imitators, even among the Methodists (928; cf. Sudhoffs Arch. 1929, 83). Yet, if Galen had not some evidence for this imitation—and his relations with the Erasistrateans on the subject of bloodletting provide a close parallel—[36] there would be no point in mentioning them, and he could label those who hailed him as a miracle healer his detractors, not his encomiasts.

A second indication of the increased stability of his position in Roman society may be found in the reactions he expresses towards some of his wealthy patients. It is true that in Books 1-6 and in *On prognosis*, he had denounced the manifold evils of contemporary society, a decline in culture and rampant ambition allied to a gluttonous materialism, but they are given in very broad terms. In Books 7-14, however, his attack on the failings of the wealthy becomes stronger and more orientated towards medicine. Galen holds up to ridicule the delicate women who demand dressings of soft scarlet Tyrian wool, and who may, through their life of luxury, be unable to bear even the weight of such a light bandage (574f.), or who prefer anything to being given a purgative to remove bile (1007). They are not confined to Rome (942), but can be found in the larger cities all over the world. Men are hardly better. Some are frightened off venesection by their servants (620, 865), others through cowardice refuse to submit to scarification (863), still others perish through the servility of their doctors in providing them with excessive painkilling drugs (816f.). Galen tells with a mixture of glee and

---

[36] P. Brain, Galen on venesection, Diss., Durban, 1978 (now in print, 1986, Cambridge University Press).

revulsion a story of a rich man who got so drunk at a banquet that he had to be led home staggering all over the road (581). Indeed, such Roman luxury is, in Galen's eyes, a positive danger to health, not just because the rich are more likely to suffer from diseases of plethora more than the poor, but because in such a condition, their treatment is likely to be worse even than that which they give their slaves (783f.). Their delicate sensibilities do not allow them to be bled, the best and swiftest cure, and they are convinced that least done, soonest mended. Hence all they want is for a little something to be done each day to their tummy. Since their physicians equally want to be seen to be doing something— and naturally they expect that they will thereby gain a larger fee—, they rub their patients with olive oil and relaxants, with disastrous results, for this leads to the settlement of humours in the body and to the inflammation of the liver or stomach, shortness of breath and even death. Although this disdain for Roman luxury is by no means confined to this treatise (cf. IX. 218f., *On examining the physician*, and *On prognosis*), Galen's attack on a group from which would come some of his most important patients may represent his own confidence in his position at Rome, not to speak of a useful advertising ploy.

This supposition might appear somewhat forced, but it would agree with a third change that I detect between the earlier and the later books of the *Method of healing*. In the first part, Galen sometimes speaks of himself as a provincial coming to Rome: in deference to Roman custom he leaves cranial surgery to the surgeons (454), and three times in passing he refers to his home province of Asia as 'with us' (334, 370, 404, cf. *Hermes* 1917, 107ff.). By contrast, the phrase παρ' ἡμῖν or καθ' ἡμᾶς is absent from part II, and the three instances in which he uses καθ' ἡμῶν (916, 941, 1019) are best taken in a chronological sense ('my contemporaries') or, with less plausibility, relate to Rome. With the exception of the long description of Stabiae and Vesuvius (363-365),[37] which Galen may well have visited while with Commodus on a tour of imperial estates around the bay of Naples, there are few snippets of information about life in Rome and Italy in Books 1-6, but several in Books 7-14. Leaving aside his criticisms of Roman luxury, Galen remarks on the activities of slavetraders (998), the alum springs of Albula (536), the tricks of punters to discover a horse's condition (478), a type of cord from Gaul on sale in the shops along the Via Sacra (942), and the poor quality of Italian or Neapolitan nard as compared with that of Laodicea in Phrygia (791). His perspective has subtly altered, so that while still writing for a Greek

---

[37] The emendation, passim, to Στάβιαι was made by Cobet, loc. cit., above n. 29, who also emended 364.6 to ἄκλυστον.

audience, he is conscious both of being in Rome and of having to explain
to his Greek readers some of his findings. The lists of wines at 468, 483,
501, 831, are headed by Italian wines, not those of Asia Minor, and his
sympathies extend at times even to the Celts (877). His vocabulary
includes Latin words, which he interprets for the Greeks: *cestiana* (911,
cf. 469, where the word is not glossed), *sapo* (569), *foliata* and *spicata* (574)
and possibly *cocta* (815,12), if Darderius' emendation is right.[38] He can
even report a Latin joke (582), for the word in question, *diatritarius*, is a
Latin formation based on a Greek root word. What are we also to make
of his references to snow-cooled refreshments, *decocta* (467) and *melka*
(468), a sort of yogurt, which enjoyed a great vogue in Rome? Still more
remarkable in a Greek author is the comparison of Galen's own
achievements with the emperor Trajan's road-building in Italy, and for
two reasons. The first is that, while Greek authors often refer several
times in the beneficent activities of their Roman overlords, they never,
as far as I know, use them as a yardstick by which to compare their own
successes and activities, even in a rhetorical simile. Secondly, in such
panegyrics as survive to us from the Greek world, the emperor's
achievements are described always as affecting either the whole empire
or a specific area of the Greek-speaking half, be it a province or an
individual city. Galen's praise of Trajan, which relates to his roads in
Italy, and not to anything he did in the Greek East, is thus isolated even
in the context of Greek encomia of emperors.[39]

These small details cumulatively suggest a change of Galenic perspective. He has arrived in Roman society, and feels it. He has moved from
being a Greek medical author with Roman patients to a resident of Rome
writing for Greeks. He no longer has to hide behind the skirts of the
emperor (or a senatorial patron) to escape his detractors, although these
still exist, but he believes he has an assured position from which he can
look down upon the ignorant and stupid, the powerhungry and the
plutocratic. He still fights his battles against the Methodists, the
Erasistrateans and the rest, but his victory is certain, and even at times,
with his unsuccessful followers, embarrassing. This conclusion is neither
new nor surprising. A man who, so he tells us (CMG V 10,2,2, 494),
gave advice to senators who lived in fear of being poisoned on the orders
of the emperor, must have been a man of great ability, tact and social
eminence. Galen despised in others the passion for power and glory, and

---

[38] Samuel Darderius, M. D., apud H. Mercurialis, Variae lectiones, Venice, G. Per-
chacinus, 1570, Ch. I.4.

[39] X.632f. In general, see my article, 'The beneficial ideology', in P. Garnsey, C. R.
Whittaker, eds., Imperialism in the ancient world, Cambridge University Press, 1978,
pp. 209-221, 338-343.

liked to believe that it was by his obvious medical abilities and his philosophical bearing that he had climbed to the top of the physicians' greasy pole. Yet, paradoxically, despite all its case histories, despite all its wise saws and adages, all its recommendations drawn from a long and full medical life, the *Method of healing* throughout displays Galen's mastery of another art essential for success in Rome, the art of rhetoric. The author of *On the nature of man* and Plato in the 'Gorgias' had long ago bewailed the fact that the best doctor might have to yield in public esteem to a worse physician but a better speaker.[40] The finer the rhetoric of Galen, the more entertaining and convincing the polemic, the more attractive the case-histories, the more the suspicion grows that it was not by simple medicine alone that Galen rose to eminence at Rome, the imperial city.[41]

---

[40] Hippocrates, On the nature of man 1: CMG 1,3, pp. 164-166; Plato, Gorgias 456B.

[41] I am grateful to Jonathan Barnes and Fridolf Kudlien for their comments on the paper presented to the conference, and, in particular, to Andrew Wear, for his advice and criticism of a later draft.

NIKOLAUS MANI

DIE WISSENSCHAFTLICHEN GRUNDLAGEN DER CHIRURGIE BEI GALEN (MIT BESONDERER BERÜCKSICHTIGUNG DER *MM*)

Galens eigenständige Leistungen in der Anatomie, Physiologie, Pathologie, Diagnose, Therapie etc. sind von der historischen Forschung immer anerkannt worden. Anders verhält es sich mit der Chirurgie. Es ist schon bemerkenswert, daß Galen der Chirurgie als bedeutender ärztlicher Disziplin kein geschlossenes monographisches Werk gewidmet hat, obwohl er über die Anatomie, Physiologie, Pathologie, Diagnose, Hygiene, Therapie etc. ausführliche Spezialwerke verfaßt hat.

E. Gurlt stellt in seiner monumentalen, auf strengen Quellenstudien beruhenden Geschichte der Chirurgie fest: "Dieselbe (= Chirurgie) fehlt in seinen Werken nicht, aber sie bildet keinen hervorragenden Theil derselben. Er hatte sie, wie wir gesehen haben, in seinen jungen Jahren in Pergamon bei der Behandlung der Gladiatoren ausgeübt; in Rom aber beschränkte er sich auf die innere Heilkunde."[1] M. Michler, der gegenwärtig wohl beste Kenner antiker Chirurgie, läßt in einer brillanten Analyse Galen höchstens als Wundarzt gelten.[2] Michler führt aus: "Nur selten und offensichtlich unwillig hat er (= Galen) von der Chirurgie als eigenem Fachgebiet Kenntnis genommen: Im Rahmen seiner Einheitsbestrebungen mußte er sie als integrierenden Bestandteil der Therapeutik auffassen ..."[3] Aber selbst in der Wundarznei, so stellt Michler fest, war Galen nicht auf voller Höhe seiner Zeit; dies zeige sich z.B. in der zögernden Anwendung der Ligatur bei Behandlung der Blutungen.

Zu einer positiveren Einschätzung von Galen als Chirurgen kommt L. H. Toledo-Pereyra: "He (= Galen) did surgery extensively while he was physician to the gladiators at Pergamon and was proud of his surgical techniques and dressings for wounds".[4]

In diesem Beitrag möchte ich an den Beispielen der Blutstillung, der Thoraxchirurgie und der Behandlung von Bauchwunden folgende Merkmale galenischer Chirurgie herausarbeiten:

---

[1] E. Gurlt, Geschichte der Chirurgie, Bd. 1, Berlin 1898, S. 431.
[2] M. Michler, Das Spezialisierungsproblem und die antike Chirurgie, Bern/Stuttgart 1969, S. 50-62.
[3] op. cit., S. 53.
[4] L. H. Toledo-Pereyra, Galen's contribution to surgery, *J. Hist. Med.* 28 (1973) 357-375.

1) Für Galen ist die Chirurgie integraler Bestandteil der Heilkunde; deshalb muß auch die Chirurgie auf eine wissenschaftliche Basis gestellt werden. Sie stützt sich auf Erfahrung und Theorie. Die Theorie befaßt sich mit der gesamten Physis des Menschen. Sie berücksichtigt den stofflich-energetischen Zustand des Körpers, sein Temperament, das sich aus der Mischung der Elemente und Qualitäten ergibt, und sie befaßt sich mit dem baulichen Gefüge, der Tätigkeit und der vitalen Bedeutung der einzelnen Organe.

2) Galens eigene chirurgische Erfahrung liegt vornehmlich in der Wundbehandlung. Bei der Blutstillung und der Behandlung von Bauchwunden verbindet er in glücklicher Weise sein differenziertes Wissen im Bereich der Anatomie, Physiologie und Pathologie mit eigener praktischer chirurgischer Tätigkeit.

3) Punktuell stößt Galen auch in die "große Chirurgie", etwa der Brustwand vor. Voraussetzung dieses Eingriffs sind die Ergebnisse experimenteller Untersuchungen am lebenden Tier. Nicht aus genuinem chirurgischem Temperament, sondern als experimenteller Physiologe, der sich mit der Tätigkeit der Brustorgane befaßt hat, wagt Galen Eingriffe an der Brustwand des Menschen.

Wissenschaftliche Begründung der Heilkunde

In der Schrift *Quod optimus medicus sit quoque philosophus* führt Galen folgendes aus. Der Arzt mit wissenschaftlicher Denk- und Arbeitsweise (λογικὴ μέθοδος) berücksichtigt drei Ebenen therapeutischer Überlegungen:[5] 1) Er beachtet die Physis auf der Ebene der primären Elemente und deren Mischung (πρῶτα στοιχεῖα). 2) Er muß mit der Physis der sekundären und sichtbaren Elemente, d.h. der homoiomeren Körperteile oder Gewebe, vertraut sein (τὴν (φύσιν) ἐκ τῶν δευτέρων [= στοιχείων] τῶν αἰσθητῶν, ἃ δὴ καὶ ὁμοιομερῆ προσαγορεύεται).[6] 3) Schließlich muß der wissenschaftliche Arzt auch die Natur der organischen Teile (μόρια ὀργανικά) kennen, d.h. die instrumentale Struktur der Organe, die sich aus den homoiomeren Teilen oder Geweben zusammensetzen. Kurz, der Arzt muß mit der Natur des menschlichen Körpers (φύσις τῶν σωμάτων), mit der Tätigkeit (ἐνέργεια) und dem Nutzen (χρεία μορίων) der Organe vertraut sein, er muß die Unterschiede der Krankheiten (διαφοραὶ νοσημάτων) und die therapeutischen Indikationen (θεραπειῶν ἐνδείξεις) kennen.[7]

Im *Methodus medendi* führt Galen im einzelnen Folgendes aus.[8] Eine

---

[5] I 59f. K.
[6] I 60.
[7] I 62.
[8] X 309-310, 313, 324-329, 359, 421.

wissenschaftliche Therapie (θεραπεία λογική)[9] muß ihre Indikationen aus einer doppelten Quelle schöpfen:

1) Einmal aus der Kenntnis der zusammengesetzten oder organischen Körperteile (μόρια σύνθετα, ὀργανικά).[10] Das ärztliche Handeln beruht auf dem Wissen um die organische Struktur (ὀργανικὴ κατασκευή)[11] (διάπλασις),[12] die funktionelle Dignität (κυριότης),[13] die Lage (θέσις) und die Tätigkeit (ἐνέργεια) der Organe.[14] Diesen topisch-organischen Gesichtspunkt hat Galen in seinem pathologischen Werk *De locis affectis* auf eindrückliche und originelle Weise vertreten. Es handelt sich hier nicht um eine pathologische Anatomie, die auf der Sektion menschlicher Leichen beruht, sondern um eine Pathologie und Physiopathologie, die aus der tierischen Anatomie und experimentellen Physiologie indirekt erschlossen wird. Stellt sich z.B. nach einer Halsoperation Heiserkeit ein, so kann der die Kehlkopfmuskeln versorgende Nervus recurrens beschädigt sein.[15] Diese Erklärung fließt aus zwei Bereichen. Die tierische Anatomie zeigt den Verlauf der Nervi recurrentes am Hals und in der Brust, und die experimentelle Physiologie demonstriert den Stimmverlust nach Durchschneiden oder Unterbindung der Nervi recurrentes, die Galen deshalb auch phonetische Nerven nennt.

2) Der wissenschaftlich denkende Arzt muß aber auch die Natur der einfachen oder homogenen Teile (Gewebe) des Körpers kennen (ὁμοιομερῆ μόρια;[16] οὐσία ὁμοιομερῶν).[17] Ferner muß er die Mischung der Elemente (στοιχείων κρᾶσις)[18] kennen, und aus der Konstellation der Qualitäten warm, kalt, trocken und feucht in Gesundheit und Krankheit leitet er die therapeutische Indikation ab.[19] Die Kenntnis der Diathesis, d.h. der elementaren Beschaffenheit, des Temperaments und der humoralen Disposition,[20] ist auch für den Chirurgen unerläßlich. Bei einem Fäulnisprozeß muß man die zugrundeliegende Diathesis kennen, um rationell zu behandeln.[21] Am schlimmsten ist es um die wissenschaftliche Grundlage der methodischen Sekte bestellt, die sich weder um den Bau

---

[9] X 421.
[10] X 310.
[11] X 410.
[12] X 310.
[13] ibid.
[14] II 228 (*De anat. administrat.*).
[15] VIII 52-57 (*De loc. aff.*); III 567-585 (*De usu part.*).
[16] X 309.
[17] X 359.
[18] X 410.
[19] X 310 ὅσα μεν ἀπὸ τοῦ θερμοῦ καὶ φυχροῦ καὶ ξηροῦ καὶ ὑγροῦ σώματος ἢ πάθους εἰς τὴν ἔνδειξιν λαμβάνεται.
[20] X 309f., 313, 324-326, 329.
[21] X 324f.

und die Funktion der Organe noch um das Temperament der homogenen Gewebe kümmert.[22]

Definition der Chirurgie. Verhältnis der Chirurgie zur Gesamtmedizin

In der Schrift an *Thrasybulos*[23] über die Frage, ob die Hygiene der Heilkunde oder der Gymnastik zuzuordnen sei, zählt Galen drei Grundpfeiler der Heilkunde auf: Die διαιτητική, die φαρμακευτική und die χειρουργική.[24] Galen unterstreicht nachdrücklich, daß diese drei Untergruppen nicht untereinander wesensverschiedene τέχναι seien wie etwa die Rhetorik und die Baukunst. Was die Techne iatrike als Ganzes bestimmt, ist der gemeinsame Zweck (κοινὸς σκοπός)[25] aller ihrer Teile oder Gattungen. Und dieser Zweck ist die Erreichung von Gesundheit (ὑγίεια). Wegen dieses gemeinsamen Zieles werden sowohl die Chirurgen wie auch die Pharmakotherapeuten Ärzte genannt.[26] Unterscheidende Kriterien liegen in der Tätigkeit (Chirurgie), im benutzten therapeutischen Stoff (Pharmakotherapie) und in der Organspezialisierung (Augenheilkunde).[27]

Die Chirurgie läßt sich in zahlreiche Bereiche gliedern. Man unterscheidet blutige Operationen von unblutigen Verfahren. Operationen mit dem Messer sind z.B. das Raffen der Augenlider nach oben, die Staroperation, die Exzision eines gebrochenen Schädelknochens, die Bruchoperation, der Steinschnitt etc. Unblutige Eingriffe sind das Schröpfen, die Reponierung einer Luxation, das Katheterisieren etc. Es gibt unzählige chirurgische Operationen und Verfahren (μύριαι χειρουργίαι). Die Unterteilung der Heilkunde in verschiedene Disziplinen ist zulässig, aber nur unter der Bedingung, daß alle Teilgebiete der einen Heilkunde untergeordnet sind. Die Zerstückelung der Medizin betrachtet Galen als unheilvoll. Dies geschehe, wenn die Ärzte aus mangelnder Begabung die Heilkunde in viele Einzelgebiete aufteilten.[28] Der Chirurg muß auch die anderen Gebiete der Medizin, die Diätetik und die Pharmakotherapie beherrschen.[29]

Wie viele bedeutende Ärzte vor und nach ihm betrachtet Galen die Spezialisierung als Bedrohung der Heilkunde. Galen ist in überwältigen-

---

[22] X 421.
[23] Galen, Scripta minora, ed. G. Helmreich, Vol. 3, Leipzig 1893, S. 60-65.
[24] op. cit., S. 63.
[25] ibid.
[26] op. cit., S. 64.
[27] op. cit., S. 61-62.
[28] op. cit., S. 65 "... μοχθηρόν, ἢ διὰ τὴν ἀφυΐαν τῶν τεχνιτῶν εἰς πολλὰς κατακερματίζειν τὴν μίαν" [= τέχνην ἰατρικήν].
[29] Galen: *De composit. medicamentor. sec. gen.* (XIII 604).

der Weise Vollarzt. Jeder Arzt muß sich um die Physis, die Diathesis, die Krasis seiner Patienten kümmern, und er muß das Temperament der homogenen Körperteile erkennen. Er soll aber auch über den Bau, die Tätigkeit, die vitale Dignität und die gegenseitige sympathische Verknüpfung der Organe Bescheid wissen. Der Chirurg darf sich nicht mit spezialisierter operativer Technik zufriedengeben. Es zeigt sich hier allerdings auch das Überlegenheitsgefühl des "wissenschaftlichen" Mediziners, des philosophischen Kopfes gegenüber dem "einfachen Praktiker", dem handwerklichen Chirurgen, eine Einstellung, die in späteren Zeiten erst mit voller Macht einsetzte.

Die anatomischen, physiologischen und physiopathologischen Grundlagen der Chirurgie

Kriegschirurgie

Der Nutzen der Anatomie für die Kriegschirurgie (τὰ κατὰ πόλεμον τραύματα) ist beträchtlich. Um Geschosse zu extrahieren, Abszesse zu eröffnen oder Luxationen zu reponieren, sind anatomische Kenntnisse erforderlich. Wenn der Chirurg nicht weiß, wo wichtige Nerven, Arterien oder große Venen liegen, trägt er mehr zum Tode als zur Rettung des Lebens bei.[30]

Tierische und menschliche Anatomie

Zergliederung von Tieren gibt eine ausgezeichnete Einführung in die humane Anatomie. Wer z.B. beim Affen die Lage und Größe der Sehnen und Nerven gesehen hat, wird sich auch beim Menschen schnell zurechtfinden, wenn eine Gelegenheit zu humaner Anatomie da ist. Ohne anatomische Vorübung am Tier kann man eine solche Gelegenheit kaum nutzen. Dies zeigte sich im Germanischen Krieg (κατὰ τὸν Γερμανικὸν πόλεμον), wo die Ärzte freie Hand zur Zergliederung der Leichen von Barbaren hatten und doch daraus nicht mehr lernten als es Köche und Metzger bei ihrer Arbeit tun. Selbst bei anatomischen Demonstrationen durch den Lehrer sind mehrere Wiederholungen erforderlich, bis das Wissen sicher sitzt; um so weniger kann Anatomie allein aus Büchern gelernt werden.[31]

---

[30] *De anat. administrat.* (II 283-284).
[31] s. Anm. 29, S. 604f.

Chirurgie der Ligamente, Sehnen, Nerven

Ligamente, Sehnen und Nerven werden heillos miteinander verwechselt. Der anatomisch ausgebildete Chirurg aber weiß, daß die Nerven aus Gehirn und Rückenmark entspringen, die Sehnen aus Muskeln hervorgehen und die Bänder knöchernen Ursprungs und empfindungslos sind: deshalb sind die Bänder für chirurgische Eingriffe auch am unbedenklichsten.[32]

Grundlagen der Muskelchirurgie

Übungen in tierischer Anatomie sind gerade für die Muskelchirurgie von großem Nutzen. Die Zergliederung des toten Tieres wird durch vivisektorische Untersuchungen ergänzt. Dabei erkennt man Ursprung (ἀρχή) und Ende (τελευτή) eines jeden Muskels. Man beobachtet den Faserverlauf und erkennt die homogene oder heterogene Faserschichtung. Dies alles bildet die Grundlage der Muskelchirurgie und gibt zudem noch Aufschluß über die Funktionen der Muskeln.[33] Die Kenntnis der Muskelfunktion ist auch für die chirurgische Prognose von Bedeutung. Bei schweren Verletzungen mit querer Durchtrennung eines ganzen Muskels kann man gleich voraussagen, welche Muskeltätigkeit ausfällt (ἀπολλυμένη ἐνέργεια). Wenn man dies prognostiziert, so machen einem die zum Tadel geneigten Menschen keine Vorwürfe, obwohl diese Leute es gewohnt sind, die gelähmte Funktion eher der ärztlichen Behandlung zuzuschreiben als auf die ursprüngliche Verletzung zurückzuführen.[34] Die Vertrautheit mit der Muskeltätigkeit verleiht der Chirurgie erst Präzision πρὸς τὴν ἐν ταῖς χειρουργίαις ἀκρίβειαν.[35] Einige Muskeln sind von kapitaler funktioneller Bedeutung, andere sind weniger wichtig. Die ersteren muß der Chirurg mit größter Sorgfalt präparieren, während er bei den letzteren mit etwas weniger Schonung operieren kann.

Präparation der Brusthöhle und Freilegen des Herzens am lebenden Tier[36]

Es ist vorteilhaft, die Thorakotomie zunächst am toten Tier einzuüben und dann erst zur Vivisektion überzugehen. Am besten wird ein kleineres Tier viviseziert, wo nur kleine Instrumente benötigt werden. Das Versuchstier wird rücklings auf ein Brett festgebunden. Dann führt man

---

[32] XIII 604; X 391-410.
[33] Galen: *De anat. administrat.* (II 228) ἃ σύμπαντά σοι χρήσιμα πρός τε τὰς χειρουργίας ἔσται, ἔτι τε καὶ πρὸς τὴν τῶν ἐνεργειῶν εὕρεσιν.
[34] II 228f.
[35] II 229.
[36] II 626-631.

mit einem Skalpell auf einer Seite längs des Brustbeins von oben nach unten einen Einschnitt aus und durchtrennt dann die Gegend des Schwertfortsatzes quer. Anschließend nimmt man die parasternale Inzision auch auf der anderen Seite vor und klappt dann das Brustbein hoch. Nun präpariert man den Herzbeutel weg und legt das Herz frei. Auch wenn das Herz bloßgelegt ist, bewahrt das Tier alle Funktionen unversehrt. Es atmet weiter, und wenn man es von den Fesseln befreit, läuft es schreiend umher.[37]

Zwei Dinge müssen bei diesem vivisektorischen Eingriff streng beachtet werden:

1) Das Mittelfell darf nicht durchbohrt und die Pleurahöhlen dürfen nicht eröffnet werden.[38] Wenn man nämlich das Rippenfell durchschneidet, tritt beim Einatmen von außen Luft durch die Schnittstelle ein und setzt sich zwischen Lunge und Brustkorb fest, und beim Ausatmen strömt die Luft wieder aus.[39]

2) Eine zweite Gefahr bildet die bei diesem Eingriff unvermeidliche Durchschneidung der beiden Arterien, die rechts und links seitlich unter dem Brustbein bis zum Schwertfortsatz hinabziehen. Der tödlichen Verblutung kann man nur vorbeugen, indem man die Arterien durch Fingerdruck abdichtet.[40] Nichts stört die Chirurgie am lebenden Tier so sehr wie Blutungen.[41]

Resektion des Sternum beim Menschen[42]

Ein junger Sklave wurde in der Ringschule durch einen Schlag auf das Brustbein getroffen.[43] Zunächst schenkte man dieser Verletzung keine Beachtung; aber nach vier Monaten bildete sich im verletzten Organ Eiter. Der Abszeß wurde eröffnet, aber die Wunde heilte und vernarbte nicht. Der Besitzer des Sklaven ließ ein Ärztekollegium zusammenrufen, darunter auch Galen, um über den Fall zu beraten. Alle Ärzte waren sich einig, daß es sich um eine Nekrose des Brustbeins handle. Da auf der linken Seite die Bewegung des Herzens erkennbar war, wagten die Ärzte

---

[37] II 631 ἐπὶ δὲ τῆς γυμνουμένης καρδίας ἀπαθεῖς φυλάττειν πρόκειταί σοι τὰς ἐνεργείας ἁπάσας.

[38] ἀτρώτους δὲ φυλάξας τοῦ θώρακος τὰς κοιλότητας.

[39] II 664 τμηθέντος γὰρ αὐτοῦ [ὁ τὰς πλευρὰς ὑπεζωκὼς ὑμήν] διὰ τῆς τομῆς ἐν μὲν τῷ διαστέλλεσθαι τὸν θώρακα τοῦ περιέχοντος ἔξωθεν ἀέρος οὐκ ὀλίγον εἰς τὴν μεταξὺ θώρακός τε καὶ πνεύμονος ἕλκεται χώραν.

[40] II 628f.

[41] II 628 οὐδὲν δ' οὕτως χειρουργίαν ἅπασαν ἐν ζῴου σώματι ταράττειν εἴωθεν ὡς αἱμορραγία.

[42] II 632f.

[43] II 632 πληγεὶς ἐκεῖνος ὁ παῖς ἐν παλαίστρᾳ κατὰ τὸ στέρνον.

nicht, den erkrankten Knochen zu entfernen.[44] Sie befürchteten, daß durch diesen Eingriff eine Öffnung der Pleurahöhle (σύντρησις) entstehe. Galen aber versprach, das Sternum ohne eine solche Verletzung der Brusthöhle auszuschneiden.[45] Als Galen die sternale Region freipräpariert hatte, schien vom Brustbein kein größerer Anteil gelitten zu haben als schon vorher sichtbar gewesen war. Galen wagte nun die Operation, und zwar vor allem deshalb, weil der Knochenfraß das Gebiet der großen Brustarterien und -venen (Arteriae thoracicae int.) nicht ergriffen hatte.[46] Galen schnitt den erkrankten Knochen heraus, und zwar den Abschnitt des Brustbeins, an den sich der obere Teil des Herzbeutels anlegt. Das Herz lag nun bloß da, weil das Perikard an Fäulnis zugrunde gegangen war. Aus diesem Grunde schöpfte man wenig Hoffnung auf einen glücklichen Ausgang. Aber der Knabe genas in kurzer Zeit.[47] Galen führte aus: Die Heilung wäre nicht gelungen, wenn niemand gewagt hätte, den erkrankten Knochen zu entfernen. Niemand aber hätte dies ohne vorherige Übung und Erfahrung in der Anatomie und Vivisektion zu tun gewagt.[48]

In der Schrift *De placitis Hippocratis et Platonis* schildert Galen ebenfalls diesen Fall auf ähnliche Weise, wobei der Heilungsprozeß noch etwas ausführlicher beschrieben wird.[49]

Experimentelle Neurophysiologie und Schädelchirurgie

Um den Ursprung von Bewegung und Empfindung evident zu machen, greift Galen zur Methode der experimentellen Neurophysiologie. Wenn man über den Hirnhöhlen auf das Gehirn einen Druck ausübt, verliert das Versuchstier Bewegung, Empfindung und Stimme.[50] Bei der Trepanation des Menschen beobachtet man dasselbe Phänomen. Wenn man die gebrochenen Knochenstücke herausschneidet, schiebt man die sogenannten "Hirnhautschützer" (μηνιγγοφύλακες) unter den Knochen.

---

[44] ibid. ἐφαίνετο δὲ καὶ ἡ τῆς καρδίας κίνησις ἐκ τῶν ἀριστερῶν αὐτοῦ μερῶν, οὐδεὶς ἐκκόπτειν ἐτόλμα τὸ πεπονθὸς ὀστοῦν.

[45] II 633 ἐγὼ δ᾽ ἐκκόψειν μὲν ἔφην αὐτὸ [= στέρνοιν] χωρὶς τοῦ τὴν καλουμένην ἰδίως ὑπὸ τῶν ἰατρῶν σύντρησιν ἐργάσασθαι.

[46] ibid.

[47] ibid. ἐκκοπέντος δὲ τοῦ πεπονθότος ὀστοῦ κατ᾽ἐκεῖνον μάλιστα τὸν τόπον, ἐν ᾧ ἐμπέφυκεν ἡ τοιαύτη κορυφὴ τοῦ περικαρδίου, καὶ φανείσης γυμνῆς τῆς καρδίας, ἐσέσηπτο γὰρ ὁ περικάρδιος κατὰ τοῦτο, παραχρῆμα μὲν οὐκ ἀγαθὴν ἐλπίδα περὶ τοῦ παιδὸς εἴχομεν, ὑγιάσθη δὲ εἰς τὸ παντελὲς οὐκ ἐν πολλῷ χρόνῳ.

[48] ibid. ἐτόλμησε δ᾽ ἂν οὐδεὶς ἄνευ τοῦ προγεγυμνάσθαι κατὰ τὰς ἀνατομικὰς ἐγχειρήσεις.

[49] Galen on the doctrines of Hippocrates and Plato. Ed., transl. and comment. by Phillip de Lacy, first pt., books I-V, sec. ed. Berlin: Akad. Verl. 1981 (CMG V 4,1,2) S. 70-77.

[50] op. cit. 78-79.

Drückt man nun mit diesem Instrument etwas zu kräftig auf das Gehirn,
wird der Patient empfindungslos (ἀναίσθητος) und verliert das Vermögen
zu willkürlicher Bewegung.[51] Dies geschieht aber nicht beim Zusammen-
drücken des Herzens.

Überzeugend weist Galen nach, wie wichtig anatomische und physio-
logische Kenntnisse für den Chirurgen sind. Ein herausragendes Beispiel
einer chirurgischen Intervention, die unmittelbar aus der anatomisch-
physiologischen Grundlagenforschung hervorgeht, ist die Resektion
eines vereiterten und nekrotisierten Brustbeins durch Galen selbst. Un-
bedingte Voraussetzung für das operative Gelingen sind hier

1) Kenntnis der topographischen Anatomie,
2) das Wissen um die Gefahr massiver Blutungen aus den Arteriae
   thoracicae (mammariae) internae,
3) die Vermeidung des gefährlichen Pneumothorax, der bei Verletzungen des Rippenfells entsteht,
4) die experimentelle Beobachtung, daß auch das entblößte Herz weiter pulsiert.

Alle diese Voraussetzungen entspringen der anatomischen Untersuchung und dem Tierexperiment. Galen wagt den keineswegs selbstver-
ständlichen Schritt vom Tierversuch zum chirurgischen Eingriff am
Menschen. Hier zeigt Galen — der wohl im ganzen eher internistisch di-
sponiert ist — ein wahrhaft chirurgisches Temperament.

Blutung und Blutstillung

I. Allgemeines

Blutungen gehören zur pathologischen Kategorie der Trennung des Zu-
sammenhängenden, solutio continui, λύσις ἑνώσεως (oder) συνεχείας.[52]
Hämorrhagien treten an einfachen oder homogenen Körperteilen
(ὁμοιομερῆ μόρια, ἁπλᾶ μόρια) auf oder sie erfolgen an zusammengesetzten
oder organischen Teilen (μόρια σύνθετα, μόρια ὀργανικά).[53] Die therapeutische Indikation (ἔνδειξις τῶν βοηθημάτων) ist verschieden, je nachdem
man es mit organischen Strukturen oder mit einfachen Geweben zu tun
hat.[54]

---

[51] op. cit. 80, 1-3 εἰ βραχεῖ βιαιότερον ἐπιθλίψει τις αὐτοῖς τὸν ἐγκέφαλον, ἀναίσθητός τε καὶ
ἀκίνητος ἁπασῶν τῶν καθ᾽ ὁρμὴν κινήσεων ὁ ἄνθρωπος ἀποτελεῖται.
[52] X 309; zur Blutung und Blutstillung bei Galen s.a. Gurlt (Anm. 1), S. 452-454.
[53] X 309.
[54] ibid.

Die aus der hippokratischen Tradition schöpfenden Ärzte berücksichtigen für ihre therapeutische Indikation die Beschaffenheit beider Körperteile: das Temperament bei den homogenen Geweben, die strukturellen Änderungen bei organischen Läsionen. Die Herophileer und Erasistrateer kümmern sich nicht um das Temperament, aber sie berücksichtigen bei den therapeutischen Indikationen die Struktur (διάπλασις), die Lage (θέσις), die funktionelle Dignität (κυριότης) und die sensorische Integrität (εὐαισθησία) der zusammengesetzten Teile oder Organe.[55] Bei Verletzung eines großen Gefäßes, besonders einer Arterie, entsteht sofort eine starke Blutung. Diese ist schwer zu stillen, weil die Wunde fast nicht zur Verleimung (κολλᾶσθαι) kommt.[56]

II. Pathophysiologische Mechanismen der Blutung

Die minutiöse Analyse der pathophysiologischen Mechanismen der Blutung ist für die wissenschaftliche Denkweise Galens ungemein charakteristisch. Gewiß ist diese Denkweise in der hellenistischen Pathologie[57] entstanden, aber nirgends tritt uns eine so detaillierte Beschreibung der verschiedenartigen Blutungsmechanismen entgegen wie bei Galen. Galen unterscheidet Blutungen mit qualitativer und quantitativer Veränderung des Blutes und Hämorrhagien durch vaskuläre Verletzungen oder Erkrankungen.

1) *Blutung durch Anastomosis*

Die Hämorrhagie durch Anastomosis erfolgt an den Enden der Blutgefäße, wobei sich die winzigen peripheren Gefäßmünder erweitern und Blut austreten lassen (κατὰ τὸ πέρας ἀνεστομωμένων τῶν ἀγγείων).[58] Ursache der "anastomotischen Blutung" ist Schwäche der Gefäße oder Blutplethora (διά τε ἀτονίαν ἀγγείου καὶ πλῆθος αἵματος).[59]

2) *Blutung durch Diapedese*

Der Durchtritt von Blut durch die Gefäßwand erfolgt aus zwei Gründen: bei dünnflüssigem Blut und bei verdünnter Gefäßwand.[60] Diapedese er-

---

[55] X 309f.

[56] X 310.

[57] s.u. den Abschnitt: Einteilung der Blutungen bei hellenistischen Ärzten.

[58] X 311; s. auch Schema der "Anastomosen" zwischen Venen und Arterien bei G. Majno, The healing hand. Man and wound in the ancient world. Harvard Univ. Press 1975, S. 335.

[59] X 311.

[60] ibid.: ἡ δὲ διαπήδησις ἀραιωθέντος μὲν τοῦ χιτῶνος, λεπτυνθέντος δὲ τοῦ αἵματος ἀποτελεῖται.

folgt durch Filtrierung (διηθεῖσθαι) oder Ausschwitzung (διϊδροῦσθαι) von Blut durch die Gefäßwand. Diapedese erfolgt auch bei Eröffnung kleiner Gefäße (ἀναστόμωσις ἀγγείων μικρῶν).[61]

3) *Durchtrennung der Blutgefäße* (διαίρεσις)[62]

Die Durchtrennung eines Blutgefäßes erfolgt durch Verletzung (τρῶσις) mit schneidenden spitzen Gegenständen (τὰ ὀξέα), durch Quetschung (θλᾶσις) und bei Einwirkung schwerer und harter Gegenstände. Die Ruptur (ῥῆξις) von Blutgefäßen geschieht auch durch übermäßige Spannung (τάσις) bei heftigen Tätigkeiten oder großer Saftmenge. Eine Ruptur von Blutgefäßen erfolgt beim Aufprall schwerer Gegenstände auf den menschlichen Körper sowie beim Sturz des menschlichen Körpers aus größerer Höhe. Fällt dabei ein harter Gegenstand gegen prall gefüllte Blutgefäße, so bersten diese, bevor sie gequetscht werden; sind die Gefäße wenig gefüllt oder leer, dann werden sie gequetscht. Dasselbe Phänomen beobachtet man bei folgendem Versuch. Wenn man einen Schlauch oder eine Tierblase mit Flüssigkeit füllt und darauf einen Stein wirft, oder wenn man den Schlauch auf einen Stein schlägt, dann birst der Schlauch. Ein ähnlicher Mechanismus ist beim Sturz aus größerer Höhe anzunehmen. Der Mensch fällt dann zu Boden analog dem Schlauch, der gegen einen Stein geschlagen wird.[63] Durch Schreien zerreißen Lungengefäße, dasselbe geschieht beim Heben schwerer Lasten. Auch bei schnellem Lauf, beim Springen, können Blutgefäße reißen. Der Mechanismus ist in all diese Fällen derselbe: Übermäßige Anspannung, ähnlich wie beim Strecken eines Seiles oder Lederriemens.[64] Ruptur eines Gefäßes kann auch dann erfolgen, wenn die Gefäßwand einem Blute von schäumend-spirituöser Beschaffenheit nachgibt und reißt, vergleichbar dem Riß eines Fasses, das mit jungen Wein angefüllt ist.[65] Eine ähnliche Klassifikation der Blutungsmechanismen, wenn auch nicht so detailliert beschrieben wie bei Galen, findet sich in einem Aetius-Abschnitt, der Rufus zugeschrieben wird (ex Ruffo). In der lateinischen Übersetzung heißt es dort: ''Ab arteria igitur vel vena sanguis emanat, aut osculis earum reclusis, aut discissis tunicis, aut quod extra, tamquam per colum, ut ita dixerim, traiiciatur''.[66] Dies entspricht ziemlich genau dem galeni-

---

[61] ibid.
[62] X 312.
[63] ibid.
[64] X 313.
[65] ibid.
[66] Aetius. Aetii Amideni de re medica, Tomus tertius, Basel Froben 1535, Liber XIV, cp. 52, S. 46.

schen Text in MM, ἐχχεῖται τοίνυν αἷμα φλεβὸς καὶ ἀρτηρίας ἤτοι κατὰ τὸ πέρας ἀνεστομωμένων τῶν ἀγγείων, ἢ τοῦ χιτῶνος αὐτῶν διαιρεθέντος, ἢ ὡς ἄν τις εἴποι διηθούμενον, ἢ διϊδρούμενον.[67] Die Beschreibung von physiopathologischen Mechanismen (und noch viel weniger von physikalischen Modellen) sind sonst in der postgalenischen Literatur nicht mehr zu finden, auch bei Paulus von Aegina nicht, der sonst die ausführlichste Einteilung der Blutungen gibt und sich wesentlich, in Passagen sogar wörtlich, an Galen hält.

Außer dem eben besprochenen Abschnitt aus dem *Methodus medendi* hat Galen eine zweite ausführliche Schilderung der hämorrhagischen Mechanismen geliefert. Sie findet sich im Werk *De symptomatum causis*[68] und enthält wertvolle Präzisierungen.

Mit Ausnahme der Menses, so hält Galen fest, sind alle Blutungen παρὰ φύσιν,[69] pathologisch. Die Klassifikation ist hier folgende:

1) Es gibt traumatische Blutungen durch Schneiden, Reißen, Anspannung und Schlag.[70]

2) Daneben treten spontane Blutungen auf (ἀπὸ ταὐτομάτου).[71] Solche Blutungen finden sich häufig in der Nase, in Darm, Lunge, Uterus etc. Ursache der spontanen Blutungen sind

   a) schlechte Säftequalität des Blutes (αἷμα κακόχυμον). Dieses Blut zerfrißt (διαβιβρώσκειν) die umgebende Gefäßwand (τὰ περιέχοντα).[72]

   b) Ist die Blutmenge zu groß, so vermag das Blut die Gefäße zu eröffnen und zu zerreißen (ἀναστομοῦν, ῥήσσειν).[73]

   c) Krankhafte Beschaffenheit der Gefäße (ἀγγείων ἡ κάκωσις) kann ebenfalls zu spontanen Blutungen führen.[74] Weiche, d.h. übermäßig flüssige Gefäße reißen durch Schwäche (ἀσθένεια), die verhärteten, d.h. trockenen Gefäße bersten durch mangelnde Dehnbarkeit (τῷ μὴ ῥᾳδίως ἐπὶ πλέον ἐκτείνεσθαι).[75] Die Arrosion (διάβρωσις) erfolgt mit Vorliebe bei schlaffen, weichen Wänden, sie verschont eher die gespannten, dicken, harten Gefäße (εὔτονον, παχύ, σκληρόν).[76]

---

[67] X 311.
[68] Galen: *De symptomatum causis* (VII 231-234).
[69] VII 232.
[70] ibid.
[71] VII 233.
[72] ibid.
[73] ibid.
[74] VII 234.
[75] ibid.
[76] ibid.

d) Galen beschreibt ferner blutig-seröse (ὁρ(ρ)ὸς αἱματώδης) Ausscheidungen in Stuhl und Harn, die bei Schwäche (ἀτονία) von Leber und Niere vorkommen.[77]

e) Die anastomotische Blutung kommt unter folgenden Bedingungen vor: bei Überfülle an Blut (πλῆθος) und durch Irritation der Gefäßmünder.[78]

Einteilung der Blutungen bei hellenistischen Ärzten

Die differenzierte Klassifikation der Blutungen durch Galen wurzelt in den Vorstellungen der hellenistischen Ärzte über die Pathogenese der Hämorrhagie. Einen guten Einblick in die Einteilung der Blutungen durch die hellenistischen Ärzte gibt Caelius Aurelianus bzw. Soran im historischen Vorspann seines Kapitels über die differentiae fluoris sanguinis.[79]

Asklepiades beschrieb zwei Blutungsarten, die eruptio, Ruptur des Gefässes und die putredo oder entzündliche Arrosion der Gefäßwand.[80] Erasistratos unterschied drei Blutungsmechanismen:[81]

1) eruptio, Ruptur und traumatische Durchtrennung der Gefäßwand (bei Galen διαίρεσις)

2) putredo, d.h. Zerstörung der Gefäßwand durch einen Fäulnisprozeß (bei Galen ἀνάβρωσις σηπεδονώδης)

3) Osculatio quam Graeci anastomosin vocant, d.h. die Blutung aus den winzigen peripheren Gefäßmündern (bei Galen ἀναστόμωσις)

Baccius (Bakcheios), 3.Jh. v.Chr.,[82] fügte diesen von Erasistratos aufgezählten Blutungsarten noch eine vierte hinzu, die ohne jede Verletzung durch Auspressung oder Ausschwitzung, expressio sive sudatio (bei Galen διαπήδησις, διηθεῖσθαι, δι̇ιδροῦσθαι). Auf dies Weise blute z.B. das Zahnfleisch.

Demetrius von Apamea (2.Jh. v.Chr.)[83] unterschied zwei Hauptgruppen von Blutungen:

---

[77] ibid.
[78] ibid. ὑπό τε τῶν ἐρεθιζόντων τὰ στόματα τῶν ἀγγείων.
[79] Caelius Aurelianus: On acute diseases and on chronic diseases, Ed. and transl. by I. E. Drabkin, Univ. of Chicago Press 1950, S. 642-646 (Chron. dis. lib. 2 cp. 10) (Quot vel quae sunt differentiae fluoris sanguinis).
[80] op.cit., S. 642.
[81] ibid.
[82] ibid.; M. Michler, Die alexandrinische Chirurgie. Eine Sammlung und Auswertung ihrer Fragmente, Wiesbaden 1968, S. 46, 97-98.
[83] Caelius Aurelianus (Anm. 79), S. 642-643; Michler (Anm. 82), S. 49-55.

I) Traumatische Blutungen durch Schnittverletzungen (incisura)
II) Spontane, nicht durch Traumata entstehende Blutungen (sine ulla incisura)

Diese spontanen Blutungen lassen sich in vier Gruppen unterteilen:

1) Blutungen durch "raritas", d.h. bei Verdünnung oder poröser Beschaffenheit der Gefäßwand (bei Galen ἀραιωθέντος μὲν τοῦ χιτῶνος τοῦ ἀγγείου)
2) Blutung durch expressio sive sudatio, d.h. durch Auspressung oder Ausschwitzung (bei Galen διηθεῖσθαι, διϊδροῦσθαι)
3) Defectio vel debilitas corporis quam atonian Graeci vocant, d.h. Schwäche der Gewebe und Gefäße (bei Galen ἀτονία τοῦ ἀγγείου)
4) Osculatio, d.h. eine anastomotische Blutung (bei Galen ἀναστόμωσις)
   a) bei übermäßiger Blutfülle (Galen πλῆθος)
   b) durch eröffnende Pharmaka
   c) Praedilektion der osculatio sind die letzten Gefäßenden, venarum ultimi fines (Galen κατὰ τὸ πέρας ἀνεστομωμένων ἀγγείων)
   d) Blutaustritt aus den Seiten der Gefäße, per venarum latera

Bemerkenswert ist Galens Einteilung der Blutungen und zur Hämorrhagie führenden Mechanismen, die in großen Zügen auch heute noch, zum Teil bis ins terminologische Detail, gültig sind. Es sind dies:

1) Blutungen aus fehlerhafter Blutbeschaffenheit (αἷμα κακόχυμον). Dies entspricht den heutigen Koagulopathien (Hämophilie, Thrombopenie etc.).
2) Blutungen durch Schädigung der Gefäßwand. Hier ist die galenische Terminologie in groben Umrissen bis heute erhalten geblieben.
   a) Der heutige Terminus der Blutung per diabrosin, der Arrosionsblutung, geht auf Galens Vorstellung der διάβρωσις und ἀνάβρωσις zurück.
   b) Die Blutung per diapedesin (vaskuläre hämorrhagische Diathesen durch Hypovitaminosen, allergische Reaktionen, Dysproteinämien etc.) geht auf Galens Konzept der Diapedese, d.h. des Blutaustritts durch die pathologisch veränderte Gefäßwand, zurück.
   c) Die Blutung per rhexin durch Einreißen der Gefäßwand entsprich der galenischen Vorstellung der ῥῆξις.

Galens anastomotische Blutung (ἀναστόμωσις) bildet einen Sonderfall. Sie beruht auf der von Erasistratos entworfenen Lehre der Blutgefäße.[84]

---

[84] C. R. S. Harris, The heart and vascular system in ancient Greek medicine, Oxford 1973, S. 196; s.a. Majno (Anm. 58), S. 335.

Alle Gefäße enden mit feinsten Mündern (ἔσχατα στόματα). Wenn nun das Blut in Menge und Macht zur terminalen Gefäßöffnung hinströmt, tritt es dort aus. Dieser Blutaustritt ist ein pathologischer Vorgang. Im gesunden Zustand gibt es keine anastomotische Blutung.

III. Therapie der Blutung

1) *Allgemeine Überlegungen*

Bei der traumatischen Ruptur wirkt die verursachende Schädigung nach der Verletzung nicht mehr ein. Der Arzt kann sich dann auf die Behebung des lokalen Schadens beschränken. Wenn hingegen das Blutgefäß durch eine zu große Blutmenge (πλῆθος) reißt, dann bleibt die verursachende Bedingung weiter bestehen. Hier muß zunächst die Plethora durch Entleerung behandelt werden (ἐκκενωτέον τὸ πλῆθος);[85] dann erst soll die spezielle Therapie einsetzen. An erster Stelle des Behandlungsplans steht die Blutstillung. Erst wenn die Gefahr der Verblutung behoben ist, kann an die Behandlung der Wunde gedacht werden. Die Blutstillung umfaßt eine allgemeine und eine lokale Therapie. Die allgemeine Therapie ist bestrebt, das Blut aus dem Wundgebiet durch Säfteableitung (Derivation und Revulsion) in andere Körpergegenden zu lenken.[86] Zur allgemeinen Therapie gehören auch die innere oder lokale Kälteapplikation, sodann adstringierende Mittel, z.B. herber Wein. Die Gefässverletzung selbst wird durch Verschluß oder Verstopfung behoben.[87] Der Verschluß geschieht durch kältende und adstringierende Mittel, durch den Druck des Verbandes und durch Anlegen der Ligatur. Die Verstopfung der Gefäßwunde erfolgt von innen oder von außen: im Innern durch das Blutgerinnsel, von außen durch Leinentampons, durch Schwämme, durch Schorfbildung und durch verstopfende Pharmaka sowie durch Druck von überlagertem Gewebe.[88]

2) *Technik der lokalen Blutstillung*

a) *Lagerung der blutenden Wunde*[89]

Die zweckmäßigste Stellung (ἐπιτήδειον σχῆμα) der blutenden Wunde besteht in der schmerzlosen Hochlagerung (ἀναρροπία, ἀνωδυνία) der blutenden Gliedmaßen. Diese Anweisung findet sich auch bei Oribasius.[90]

---

[85] X 313.
[86] X 315, 326, 332.
[87] X 327 στεγνοῦται δὲ ἡ διαίρεσις ἢ μύσαντος ἢ φραχθέντος τοῦ διῃρημένου.
[88] X 327.
[89] X 318.
[90] Oribasius: Synopsis ad Eustathium. Libri ad Eunapium. Ed. J. Raeder, Leipzig/Berlin 1926 (CMG VI,3), Synopsis VII,20,1 (S. 223), libri ad Eunap. III 36,1 (S. 416) αἱμορραγίαις βοήθημά ἐστι τὸ ἐπιτήδειον σχῆμα τοῦ τετρωμένου μορίου · τοιοῦτον δ' ἐστὶ τὸ ἀνάρροπον μετ' ἀνωδυνίας.

b) *Fingerdruck, Ligatur, Verband*

Die lokale Behandlung erfolgt durch Fingerdruck,[91] durch Ligatur des blutenden Gefäßes[92] und durch einen Verband.

Der abdichtende Finger soll einen sanften schmerzlosen Druck auf die Gefäßöffnung ausüben. So wird die Blutung zum Stillstand gebracht, und über der Wunde bildet sich ein Gerinnsel.[93] Der aufgelegte Finger zeigt zugleich die Lage (θέσις) und Größe (μέγεθος) sowie die Art des blutenden Gefäßes, der Arterie oder Vene.[94] Derselbe Abschnitt findet sich wörtlich bei Paulus von Aegina.[95] Eine weitere Methode der Blutstillung ist die Torsion des blutenden Gefäßes mit einem durch die Arterienwand gestochenen Haken, der maßvoll gedreht wird.[96]

Die mit dem Namen Galens verbundene Torsion hat bis zur Mitte des 19.Jahrhunderts noch vereinzelte Liebhaber gefunden, die auch Torsionspinzetten entwickelten.[97]

Auch Paulus von Aegina beschreibt die Torsion auf ähnliche Weise: Ein großes blutendes Gefäß soll mit einem Haken durchbohrt, dann angehoben und maßvoll gedreht werden.[98] Wenn die Blutung, insbesondere die arterielle Hämorrhagie, mit Fingerdruck, Torsion oder Wundbehandlung nicht gestillt werden kann, muß man zur Ligatur schreiten.[99] Die Erfahrung zeigt, daß arterielle Wunden nicht leicht zusammenwachsen, und einige Ärzte glauben sogar, dies sei ganz unmöglich.[100] Ursache davon ist die harte, fast knorpelige Natur der Arterienwand. Bei Kindern und Frauen hat Galen erfahren und beobachtet (πεῖρα, ὁρᾶν), wie die Arterienwunde sich verlötete und ringsum Fleisch gebildet wurde (κολλάω, περισαρκόω).[101] Hier zeugt die Erfahrung für die Theorie (ἡ πεῖρα τῷ λόγῳ μαρτυρεῖ).[102] Die Theorie erklärt die Heilungstendenz: Wegen der weichen und feuchten Beschaffenheit des kindlichen und weiblichen Körpers kann die Arterienwunde wieder zusammenwachsen

---

[91] X 317 δάκτυλοι συνάγοντές τε καὶ σφίγγοντες αὐτὰ [= ἀγγεῖα αἱμορραγοῦντα]; s.a. Majno (Anm. 58), S. 404.
[92] X 317 ὁ βρόχος ὁ περιτιθέμενος αὐτοῖς τοῖς αἱμορραγοῦσιν ἀγγείοις.
[93] X 318 αὐτίκα μὲν ἐπιβαλλέτω τὸν δάκτυλον ἐπὶ τὸ στόμιον τοῦ κατὰ τὸ ἀγγεῖον ἕλκους, ἐρείδων πραέως καὶ πιέζων ἀνωδύνως, ἅμα τε γὰρ ἐφέξει τὸ αἷμα καὶ θρόμβον ἐπιπήξει τῇ τρώσει.
[94] X 318.
[95] Paulus Aegineta, ed. J. L. Heiberg, pars prior, libri I-IV, Leipzig 1921 (CMG IX,1) lib. IV,53,1 (S. 373f.); s.a. Oribasius (Anm. 90) Synopsis VII,20,2 (S. 223).
[96] X 318; s.a. Majno (Anm. 58), S. 404.
[97] Handbuch der allgemeinen und speciellen Chirurgie, red. von Pitha und Billroth, Bd. 1 (O. Weber, Die Gewebserkrankungen), S. 165.
[98] Paulus Aegineta (Anm. 95), S. 374.
[99] X 318f.; s.a. Majno (Anm. 58), S. 404.
[100] X 333.
[101] X 334.
[102] X 336.

(συμφῦναι τὴν διαίρεσιν ἐθεασάμην).[103] Wenn die Ligatur nicht ausführbar ist, etwa bei tiefliegenden Gefäßen, sollen diese durchschnitten werden (διακόπτειν, διατέμνειν).[104] Die Gefäße ziehen sich dann von der Schnittstelle zurück und die Blutung hört auf.

Eine solche spontane Blutstillung durch Einrollung der zentralen Gefäßstümpfe wird auch von modernen Chirurgen beobachtet.[105] Am zweckmäßigsten ist nach Galen die doppelte Sicherung: Anlegen einer Ligatur an der Wurzel des blutenden Gefäßes, dann Durchschneiden des Gefäßes peripher davon. Die Wurzel des Gefäßes ist bei den Venen leberwärts, bei den Arterien herzwärts gerichtet.[106]

Eingehend beschreibt Galen die Ligatur und Resektion[107] der Schläfen- und Stirnarterien bei Arteriotomie. Die Arteriotomie ist eine mit chirurgischer Technik vollzogene humoraltherapeutische Maßnahme. Wenn zuviel warmes, mit Dämpfen gefülltes Blut zum Kopfe strömt, kann mit dem Arterienschnitt den Kopf- und Augenleiden abgeholfen werden. Die hinter den Ohren gelegenen Arterien sowie Schläfen- und Stirnarterien sind das Operationsfeld der Arteriotomie, insbesondere trifft dies für die Schläfenarterien zu.[108]

Die beim Befühlen am wärmsten empfundenen und am stärksten pulsierenden Arterien sollen durchschnitten werden. Bei kleineren Arterien ziehen sich die beiden Teile der durchschnittenen Arterie voneinander zurück. Wenn die Arterien groß sind und stark pulsieren, ist es sicherer, eine Doppelligatur anzulegen und das dazwischenliegende Stück herauszuschneiden (ἐκκόπτειν).[109] Das beste Nahtmaterial ist Seide, die in größeren Städten bei reichen Römerfrauen zu finden ist. Bekommt man keine Seide, so kann man auch dünne Darmsaiten gebrauchen. Das Nahtmaterial darf sich nicht zu schnell zersetzen, es muß "aseptisch" (ἄσηπτος) sein, d.h. nicht leicht in Fäulnis übergehen. Sonst blutet es von neuem nach zu raschem Abfallen der Ligatur. Bei den Venen braucht die Ligatur nicht so lange zu haften, denn hier ist kein steter heftiger Puls vorhanden, der die Gefäßwunden wieder öffnet, so wie dies bei den Arterien geschieht.[110]

Klarer als Galen beschreibt Celsus die Doppelligatur eines stark blutenden Gefäßes. Celsus legt zu beiden Seiten der blutenden Gefäßwunde

---

[103] ibid.
[104] X 319.
[105] A. Kappert, Lehrbuch und Atlas der Angiologie, Stuttgart 1976, S. 371.
[106] X 319.
[107] X 941-943.
[108] X 941.
[109] X 941f. εἰ δ'ἐν τῷ γυμνοῦν φαίνοιτό σοι μέγα τὸ ἀγγεῖον ἢ μεγάλως σφύζοι, ἀσφαλέστερον αὐτῷ βρόχον περιβάλλοντα πρότερον, οὕτως ἐκκόπτειν τὸ μεταξύ.
[110] X 943.

eine Ligatur an und durchschneidet hierauf den dazwischenliegenden Teil des Gefäßes. Diese Methode gibt Celsus als allgemeine Behandlungstechnik starker Blutungen an. Auch Celsus beschreibt das Auseinanderweichen der beiden Gefäßabschnitte nach Durchtrennung der Gefäße: "Venae quae sanguinem fundunt adprehendendae circa id quod ictum est duobus locis deligandae intercidendaeque sunt, ut et in se ipsae coeant, et nihilominus ora praeclusa habeant".[111]

Paulus von Aegina beschreibt die Blutstillung, insbesondere auch die Torsion und Ligatur, in engster Anlehnung an Galen, aber in strafferer und übersichtlicherer therapeutischer Indikation.[112] Er empfiehlt ein schrittweise Vorgehen:

1) Zuerst stillt man die Blutung durch Fingerdruck, worauf sich bald ein "Thrombos" bildet. Dabei kann zugleich die Diagnose arterielle oder venöse Blutung gesichert werden.
2) Wenn die Gefäße klein sind, genügen blutstillende Pharmaka.
3) Bei großen Gefäßen ist die Torsion mit dem Haken erforderlich.
4) Fruchtet auch dies nichts, dann muß man die Arterien und großen Venen unterbinden. Das blutende Gefäß kann auch durchschnitten werden; am besten gelingt dies, wenn vorher in Richtung der Gefäßwurzel eine Ligatur angebracht worden ist.

c) Schorfbildung[113]

Gewisse Blutungen bedürfen der verschorfenden Therapie (ἐσχαρόω). Die Verschorfung geschieht durch verschorfende Pharmaka (ἐσχαρωτικά) oder mit dem Brenneisen (καυτηρίοις διαπύροις). Die Verschorfung ist an dringende Indikationen gebunden, z.B. bei Blutungen aus faulendem Fraß.[114] Wenn man faulendes Gewebe herausschneidet, ist es ratsam, die Wurzel der Wunde anzubrennen oder mit verschorfenden Mitteln (z.B. ungelöschtem Kalk) zu behandeln. Der Schorf darf nicht zu frisch entfernt werden, weil dann Blutungsgefahr besteht.[115] Die Bildung des Schorfes geht auf Kosten des verschorften Gewebes, und nach Wegfall des Schorfes bleibt ein Hohlraum zurück.

---

[111] Celsus: De Medicina, ed. F. Marx, Leipzig 1915 (Corp. Med. Latinor. Vol. 1) S. 220, 11-14 (lib. V,26, 21).
[112] Paulus Aegineta (Anm. 95), S. 373f.
[113] X 315, 324-326.
[114] X 325.
[115] X 320.

d) *Auffüllen der Wunde*[116]

Nach der Blutstillung muß die Wunde aufgefüllt werden. Besonders schwierig ist dies bei verschorften Wunden, deshalb sind stopfende Blutstillungsmittel besser als verschorfende. Ein hervorragendes, auch noch im 17.Jahrhundert als Standardmittel gepriesenes Pharmakon besteht aus Aloe mit Weihrauch gemischt, dann mit Eiweiß zu honigartiger Konsistenz gebracht und mit feinem Hasenhaar versetzt. Dieses Mittel wird auf das verletzte Gefäß und die Wunde gelegt.[117]

3) *Das Aneurysma*

Eine gefährliche und häufige Komplikation der arteriellen Verletzung ist nach Galen das Aneurysma. In der Schrift über die widernatürlichen Geschwülste (*De tumoribus*) befaßt sich Galen vor allem mit der Pathologie und der Diagnose des Aneurysmas.[118]
Ein Aneurysma entsteht, wenn die über der Arterienwunde liegende Haut vernarbt ist, die arterielle Wunde aber nicht zusammengewachsen, nicht vernarbt ist und nicht mit Granulationen (Fleisch) gestopft wurde. Die Diagnose stellt man aus folgenden Erscheinungen: Eine mit dem Arterienpuls synchron wechselnde Schwellung, die sich mit der Hand eindrücken läßt, wobei das Blut in die Arterie zurückweicht. Das Blut im Aneurysma ist gelb, warm, dünnflüssig und mit feinem Pneuma vermischt. Wird das Aneurysma eröffnet, spritzt das Blut im Strahl heraus.

Damit hat Galen die Pathogenese des traumatischen Aneurysmas erfaßt: Arterienverletzung mit herausgetretener pulsierender Blutmasse, die von Gewebe sackartig überdeckt ist. Morphologische, funktionelle und pathophysiologische Kenntnisse und Überlegungen liefern die Elemente zur ärztlichen Diagnose und zur Beschreibung der pathogenetischen Mechanismen.

4) *Blutungen verschiedener Körperregionen*

Blutungen der Halsvenen[119]

Die Blutungen aus den Halsvenen brauchen nicht unterbunden zu werden, ein fester Verband genügt. Man komprimiert den unterhalb der

---

[116] ibid.
[117] ibid.
[118] VII 725f. (*De tumoribus praeter naturam*); Deutsche Übers. von P. Richter, Galenos über die krankhaften Geschwülste, Leipzig 1913 (Klassiker der Medizin, hg. v. K. Sudhoff, Bd. 21), Aneurysma S. 20-21; J. Reedy, Galen on cancer and related diseases (engl. Übers. der Schrift *De tum. praet. nat.*), *Clio Med.* 10 (1975) 227-238 (Aneurysma S. 236).
[119] X 323.

Wunde liegenden Venenabschnitt mit der einen Hand, mit der anderen wird das Wundpflaster direkt auf die Wunde aufgelegt; dann legt man in Richtung der venösen Gefäßwurzel, d.h. nach unten, einen festen Verband an. Bei den Gliedmaßen muß der Verband nach oben geführt werden, also herz- und leberwärts, wo die Wurzeln der Gefäße liegen, für die Venen die Leber, für die Arterien das linke Herz. Auch hier begegnen wir einer physiologisch orientierten Chirurgie, die auf der galenischen Lehre des Blutflusses fußt.

Blutungen der Blase, des Uterus, der Därme[120]

In diesen Fällen werden blutstillende Medikamente mit Instrumenten verabreicht, die dem jeweiligen Organ angepaßt sind, dem Katheter für die Blase, dem Metrenchytes für die Gebärmutter, der Klistierspritze für den Darm. Im Sinne einer rationellen Therapie muß außer der Berücksichtigung von Physis und Diathesis des Körpers auch die Quantität des Blutverlustes in Rechnung gestellt werden.

Lungenblutungen[121]

Lungenblutungen sind schwer heilbar. Dafür spricht die Erfahrung (πεῖρα) und die Theorie (λόγος).[122] Die Erfahrung zeigt unmittelbar die schlechte Heilungstendenz der Lungenblutung. Die Theorie besagt, daß die atmende Lunge ständig in Bewegung ist; aus diesem Grunde ist die für den Heilungsprozeß so wichtige Bedingung der Ruhe nicht gegeben.[123] Bei der Lunge ist zudem der Husten das einzige Mittel zur unmittelbaren Reinigung (κάθαρσις) der Lungen.[124] Beim Husten ist aber wiederum die so nötige Ruhe (ἡσυχία) nicht gewährleistet.
Heftiges Schreien oder auch ein Sturz kann eine Lungenblutung auslösen.[125] Wenn viel warmes florides Blut ohne Schmerzen ausgehustet wird, darf man als Quelle der Blutung die Lunge selbst betrachten.[126]
Die sofort einsetzende Behandlung eines Blutsturzes hat Aussicht auf Erfolg. Die frische und blutige Wunde in der Lunge kann dann zur Verklebung gebracht werden, bevor sie eitert.[127]
Der Behandlungsplan der Lungenblutung sieht so aus:[128]

---

[120] X 328f.
[121] X 338-342.
[122] X 338.
[123] X 338.
[124] X 343.
[125] X 338.
[126] X 341.
[127] X 343.
[128] X 341f.

1) Anhalten des Patienten zu oberflächlicher Atmung
2) Sprechverbot
3) Phlebotomie in der Ellenbeuge
4) Bandagen der Gliedmaßen, um den Blutfluß von den Extremitäten in die Brust zu vermeiden.[129]
5) Essigwasser wird lauwarm zum Trinken gegeben. So löst sich das Gerinnsel und kann ausgehustet werden. Schließlich muß man noch stopfende und adstringierende Mittel anwenden.

5) *Allgemeine Therapie der Blutung*

Galen mißt der allgemeinen Therapie bei Blutungen große Bedeutung bei.[130] Sie reguliert das Temperament, die ganze Verfassung des Körpers, sie hält durch die ableitenden Verfahren der Derivation (παροχέτευσις) und der Revulsion (ἀντίσπασις) das Blut von der Wunde fern. Die Derivation leitet die Säfte in nahe gelegene Körperteile ab (Reinigung des Gaumens durch die Nase, der Gebärmutter durch den Darm), während die Revulsion eine Säfteableitung in entfernte oder gegenüberliegende Regionen bewirkt. Die Natur selbst bedient sich der Revulsion: Nasenblutung bringt die Menstruation zum Stillstand. Der Arzt wendet die Revulsion an, wenn er z.B. bei Uterusblutungen große Schröpfköpfe auf die Brust legt. Auch die Diät muß der Blutungsneigung entgegenwirken. Wenn Diapedese aus einer Blutverdünnung entsteht, soll man eine verdickende Diät anwenden (ὑπὸ τῆς παχυνούσης διαίτης).[131] Immer muß die gesamte krasische und humorale Konstitution in den therapeutischen Plan einbezogen werden.

Galens Darstellung der Blutung fußt auf einer für die Antike unvergleichlich detaillierten anatomischen Kenntnis, physiopathologischen Denkweise und klinischer Erfahrung. Galen interessiert sich insbesondere für die pathogenetischen Mechanismen der Blutung. Er unterscheidet zwei große Gruppen:

1) Blutungen wegen fehlerhafter Qualität oder übermäßiger Quantität des Blutes (heute Koagulopathien, z.B. Hämophilie, Thrombopenie etc.).
2) Vaskuläre Blutungen durch Verletzungen oder krankhafte Schäden der Blutgefäßwand (per diabrosin) und bei Durchtritt von Blut ohne vorherige Verletzung der Gefäßwand (Diapedese).

---

[129] X 341; vgl. Majno (Anm. 58), S. 336.
[130] X 315, 328, 332.
[131] X 332.

Galen geht auch auf die Mechanik der Blutung ein. So beschreibt er Rupturen der Blutgefäße durch stumpfe Verletzungen, z.B. heftigen mechanischen Aufprall (Sturz aus großer Höhe), ähnlich wie ein Schlauch beim Aufschlag auf einen Stein birst. Hier verwendet Galen sogar das mechanische Modell zur Erklärung des hämorrhagischen Mechanismus. Auch die moderne Chirurgie kennt z.B. das Einreißen der Aorta bei schwerem Aufprall (crushing injuries) und Sturz aus großer Höhe.[132] Daneben beschreibt Galen Blutungen durch mechanische Überdehnung, Überstreckung (Tasis) und durch Kontusion (Thlasis). Beide stumpfe Arterienschäden werden auch von der modernen Gefäßchirurgie beschrieben.[133]

Galen unterscheidet die heftige pulsierende arterielle Blutung von der profusen venösen Hämorrhagie. Er beschreibt die lokale Blutstillung durch Fingerdruck, Verband, Torsion, Ligatur und Verschorfung. Daneben unterstreicht er die Wichtigkeit der allgemeinen Therapie.

Die Bauchwunden. Gastrorrhaphie

Die Wichtigkeit morphologischer und funktioneller Kenntnisse zeigt sich auch bei der Behandlung von Bauchwunden, wo Struktur und Beschaffenheit der Organe von Galen selbst erforscht wurden: δι' ἀνατομῆς ἐμάθομεν ἁπάντων τῶν τῇδε μορίων τὴν φύσιν.[134] Die anatomischen Verhältnisse präsentieren sich so:[135] Außen wird das Abdomen von der Haut bedeckt. Unter der Haut folgt in der mittleren ventralen Region eine doppelte Muskelaponeurose (ἀπονεύρωσις τῶν μυῶν). Zu beiden Seiten davon liegen die zwei geraden fleischigen Baummuskeln (δύο μύες ὄρθιοι σαρκώδεις), die vom Sternum bis zum Schambein reichen. Weiter innen folgt das Bauchfell. Es besteht aus dem eigentlichen spinnwebenartigen Bauchfell und der von den queren Bauchmuskeln (μύες ἐγχάρσιοι) ausgehenden Aponeurose. Die seitliche Bauchwand besteht aus drei Muskelschichten, zwei äußeren schrägen Muskeln, die sich kreuzweise überschneiden, und dem inneren queren Muskel. An der seitlichen fest überdeckten Bauchdecke besteht weniger Verletzungsgefahr als im mittleren Teil mit aponeurotischem Überzug und einfacher Muskellage. Die Bauchnaht ist in der medianen Region am schwierigsten auszuführen. Hier fallen die Baucheingeweide wie Därme und Netz am leichtesten heraus und sind hier auch am schwierigsten zurückzuhalten. Die gera-

---

[132] W. H. Edwards, Vascular surgery, Baltimore 1976, S. 157. Hier wird Aortenruptur bei Fall aus großer Höhe und schweren Aufprall-Unfällen beschrieben.
[133] Kappert (Anm. 105), S. 370.
[134] X 411.
[135] X 411f.

den beidseits der Mittellinie verlaufenden Bauchmuskeln festigen die
Bauchdecken. Sind sie verletzt, wird der Bauchinhalt nach außen gesto-
ßen, wobei die starken seitlichen Bauchmuskeln die abdominalen Viscera
gegen die Wundöffnung auspressen. Die mittlere Bauchregion ist also
besonders anfällig für den Vorfall von Bauchinhalt (ἐπιτήδειός τε χώρα εἰς
πρόπτωσιν).[136] Bei großen Wunden ist die Reposition der Baucheingeweide schwierig. Kleinere Wunden stellen aber auch besondere Probleme;
wenn hier die vorgefallenen Därme nicht sogleich reponiert werden, blä-
hen sie auf und sind nur unter großen Schwierigkeiten an ihren gewohn-
ten Ort zurückzubringen.

Das therapeutische Vorgehen besteht aus vier Schritten, Reposition,
Bauchnaht, Anlegen von Wundarznei und Wundverband. Die Aufblä-
hung des vorgefallenen Darms mit Luft (προπεσὸν ἔντερον ἐμφυσηθέν) geschieht durch die Kälte der umgebenden Luft, daher muß Wärme zuge-
führt werden. Ein in warmem Wasser angefeuchteter Schwamm wird
über den Därmen ausgepreßt, noch besser wirkt warmer Wein.[137] Wenn
die Darmblähung auch jetzt nicht nachläßt, muß die peritoneale Wunde
erweitert werden. Dabei sollen zweischneidige oder spitze Messer ver-
mieden werden.[138] Bei Reposition großer Wunden bedarf der Chirurg
eines Helfers.

Die Bauchnaht (Gastrorrhaphie)[139]

Die Bauchnaht wird laufend von außen nach innen und dann auf der gegenüberliegenden Seite von innen nach außen geführt. Zuerst werden
auf einer Seite Haut und Muskeln durchstochen, dann wird die Nadel
auf der gegenüberliegenden Seite in umgekehrter Reihenfolge von innen
nach außen durch die Bauchdecke geführt, wobei sie den Bauchfellrand
dieser Seite in die Naht einbezieht.[140] Eine andere Technik vereinigt
gleichartige Gewebe, Haut zu Haut, Muskel zu Muskel, Bauchfell zu
Bauchfell. Zunächst wird die Nadel auf einer Seite von außen nach innen
durch die Bauchdecke gezogen; dann kehrt man die Nadel um und vereinigt die beiden Wundlippen des Bauchfells. Dann wendet man die Nadel
wiederum und durchsticht die Bauchdecken auf der gegenüberliegenden
Seite von innen nach außen. So wird die Nadel in einem Zuge durch vier
Wundlippen geführt.[141]

---

[136] X 413.
[137] X 414.
[138] X 415.
[139] X 416-418; s.a. Gurlt (Anm. 1), S. 454f.; J. Walsh, Galen's writings and influ-
ences inspiring them, *Annals Med. Hist.*, N.S. 9 (1937) 34-61 (Bauchwunden s. 40-42);
Toledo-Pereyra (Anm. 4), S. 364.
[140] X 416.
[141] X 418.

Wenn das Bauchfell verletzt ist, fällt oft das große Netz heraus. Ist es schwärzlich verfärbt, muß man eine Ligatur anlegen und den nekrotischen Abschnitt resezieren.[142] Auch in diesem Fall muß sich der Arzt über zwei Dinge klar sein: die Lebenswichtigkeit des Organs und die Blutgefäßversorgung. Die Methodiker vor allem lassen hier jede Einsicht vermissen. Galen aber überlegt in diesem Falle so: Das Netz ist kein lebenswichtiges Organ. Es besteht vornehmlich aus einer dünnen Haut und einem Geflecht aus Venen und Arterien. Bei partieller Entfernung des großen Netzes ist nicht der Funktionsausfall, sondern die Blutung zu befürchten.

Die Beschreibung der Bauchwunden und der Gastrorrhaphie beruht sicherlich auf persönlicher Beobachtung und Erfahrung. Viele treffende Einzelheiten anatomischer, pathologischer und chirurgischer Natur sprechen dafür. Auch hier zieht sich wie ein roter Faden die Forderung nach einem wissenschaftlichen Überbau chirurgischen Handelns.

---

[142] X 421-423.

JONATHAN BARNES

GALEN ON LOGIC AND THERAPY*

1. *Philosophical Physicians*

The best doctors, according to Galen, are also philosophers; and he wrote a pamphlet to show how a competent physician 'possesses all the parts of philosophy—logic, natural science, ethics'[1] (*opt. med.* I 60-61).[2] Philosophy and medicine are constantly conjoined in Galen's writings.[3] Galen counts himself among 'those who teach the greatest and finest of human achievements—the theorems which philosophy and medicine impart' (*lib. propr.* XIX 9). The emperor Marcus Aurelius used to refer to Galen—so Galen himself tells us—as 'first among physicians, unique among philosophers' (*praecogn.* XIV 660).[4]

---

* This is a revised and augmented version of a paper presented to the Kiel Conference. I am grateful to my fellow participants at the Conference for many helpful suggestions. In addition, I thank Myles Burnyeat and Vivian Nutton for advice and comments. I am particularly indebted to Jim Hankinson and Geoffrey Lloyd, both of whom generously supplemented my ignorance by their knowledge and did much to make this paper at least moderately competent.—References to Galen's works cite the volume- and page-number of Kühn's edition whenever that is possible; since later and better editions always print Kühn references in the margins, that practice will cause no annoyance. (Conversely, it is annoying to be given a naked CMG reference, since the passage cannot then be readily found in Kühn). When a work does not appear in Kühn (e.g. *inst. log.* or *caus. procat.*) references are to the standard editions. I have abbreviated the Latin titles of Galen's writings. The abbreviations are mostly obvious; but I should note that I refer to the lost treatise *On Demonstration* by the name *dem.*, i.e. *de demonstratione*.

[1] The tripartite division of philosophy is usually associated with the Stoics, and it was certainly accepted by Zeno, Chrysippus and their followers (see e.g. Diogenes Laertius VII 39; Plutarch, *stoic. rep.* 1035B). But it was a commonplace in Hellenistic and later writers (cf. Sextus, *M* VII 2-19)—and its origins are probably to be found in the Old Academy (Xenocrates: Sextus, *M* VII 16). Galen's readers are constantly reminded of texts and opinions of the philosophers, and it is easy to imagine that those texts are Galen's 'source'. Galen was a profoundly learned man. He often quotes or paraphrases or alludes to philosophical texts. There we may properly speak of sources. But Galen was also a member of a long scientifico-philosophical tradition: many of the parallels we observe—*opt. med.* I 61 is an evident example—exhibit not Galen's individual genius but the richness of that common tradition. In the following notes I shall occasionally cite philosophical parallels to Galen's remarks: those citations should be construed in the light of this footnote.

[2] For the text of *opt. med.* see E. Wenkebach, 'Der hippokratische Arzt als das Ideal Galens', *Quellen und Studien zur Geschichte der Naturwissenschaften und der Medizin* 3 (1932/33) 363-383.

[3] Note the frequent conjunction of φιλοσοφία τε καὶ ἰατρική—e.g. *nat. fac.* II 5, 8, 27, 38, 116, 132, 150; *lib. prop.* XIX 9, 50, 51, 52. The phrase is characteristic of Galen but not by any means peculiar to him. Athenaeus, *Deipnosoph.* 1e, uses it of Galen's writings.

[4] Philoponus later described Galen as 'the most scientific of men, no less versed in the theorems of philosophy than in his own discipline' (*aet. mund.* 599.24-26).

A modern physician might scout the suggestion that he should study philosophy. But Galen's notion of philosophy, 'the greatest of divine goods' (*protr.* I 3), is generous. It includes anatomy and physiology, biology and physics, the pertinence of which to medicine no doctor will deny. Again philosophy embraces astronomy and geography,[5] and those disciplines have an evident connexion with a medicine that pays serious attention to the physiological effects of 'times and places'. Finally, a thoroughly modern doctor might countenance the proposal that he should be acquainted with moral philosophy: he might make a bow in the direction of medical ethics.[6]

Nor did Galen himself regard the message of *opt. med.* as innovatory: on the contrary, he meant to enunciate an antique commonplace, a platitude of the Hippocratic tradition.[7] The platitude required reaffirma-

---

[5] See e.g. *meth. med.* X 5, which lists geometry, astronomy, dialectic, music, 'and the other disciplines'; cf. ib. 17. The physician must gain first-hand geographical knowledge: *ord. lib. prop.* XIX 58-59 (for Galen's travels in search of medically relevant knowledge see e.g. *simp. med. temp.* XII 171-172, 203, 226-227); *antid.* XIV 708; there is a brief account of Galen's medical peregrinations in Kühn (I xliii-xlv).

[6] For moral philosophy see esp. *ord. lib. prop.* XIX 59. Note that the constraints of medical science itself require that doctors be moral men: medicine is essentially a philanthropical art and doctors must be lovers of humanity (*opt. med.* I 56-57), and the practice of medicine demands industry and dedication which in turn demand the virtue of temperance (ibid. I 59).

[7] Galen imagines a unified philosophico-medical tradition, beginning with Hippocrates and passing through Plato, Aristotle and Chrysippus to Galen himself: see esp. *adv. Iul.* XVIIIA 257-264. Galen generally has little time for Epicurus, whose views he associates with such doctors as Erasistratus and Asclepiades, men who left the true Hippocratic path. But see below, nn. 86 and 101, and note that at *Thras.* V 837-838 it is possible that Galen adverts, with approval, to the celebrated Epicurean distinction between necessary and unnecessary desires). Of course, Galen's interpretation of this tradition was not universally shared, and the exegesis of Hippocrates in particular (as Galen's own commentaries show with abundant illustrations) was highly controversial: the 'Hippocratic tradition' to which I refer in the text is the tradition as seen through Galen's eyes.—On the connexions between Greek medicine and Greek philosophy see the classic papers by L. Edelstein, collected in his Ancient Medicine (Baltimore, 1967)—see esp. pp. 349-366; and compare, for the later history of the connexion, L. G. Westerink, 'Philosophy and Medicine in Late Antiquity', *Janus* 51 (1964) 169-177, and E. Lieber, 'Galen: Physician as Philosopher; Maimonides: Philosopher as Physician', *Bull. Hist. Med.* 53 (1979) 268-285; add the references on p. 174 of V. Nutton (ed.), Galen: On Prognosis, CMG V 8,1 (Berlin, 1979)—Nutton's commentary is a treasury of information from which I have liberally borrowed.—On Galen's philosophical debts see L. Garcia Ballester, 'La Utilizacion de Platon y Aristoteles en los escritos tardios de Galeno', *Episteme* 5 (1971) 112-120; P. de Lacey, 'Galen's Platonism', *American Journal of Philology* 93 (1972) 27-39; H. Diller, 'Empirie und Logos: Galens Stellung zu Hippokrates und Platon', in K. Döring and W. Kullmann (eds.), Studia Platonica (Amsterdam, 1974); P. Moraux, 'Galien et Aristotle', in F. Bossier et al. (eds.), Images of Man in Ancient and Medieval Thought (Louvain, 1976); id., 'Galien comme philosophe—la philosophie de la nature', in V. Nutton (ed.), Galen: Problems and Prospects (London, 1981); P. Donini, 'Motivi filosofici in Galeno', *La Parola del Passato* 194 (1980) 333-370; id., Le scuole, l'anima, l'impero—la filosofia antica da Antioco a Plotino (Turin, 1982), pp. 124-132; and, briefly, J. Scarborough, 'The Galenic Question', *Sudhoffs Arch.* 65 (1981) 1-31, at pp. 13-17.

tion. Such was the degeneracy of the times that many of Galen's contemporaries, whether from ambition, indolence or inability, ignored or denied the Hippocratic truth.[8] Against such men Galen inveighed with a passionate intensity, summoning up all his logical and rhetorical resources. But in doing so he was raising no revolutionary banner: he saw himself rather as a champion of ancient orthodoxy, and his method as one 'which men of old introduced and their successors attempted to perfect' (*meth. med.* X 5).[9] Galen was heir to Hippocrates, his method 'the method of Hippocrates' (ibid. X 309; cf. 346).

Yet there remains something both remarkable and novel in Galen's notion that the good doctor is also a philosopher. For philosophy includes logic, and Galen insists—expressly and repeatedly—that physicians must study logic. He is not merely insisting that doctors, if they argue at all, should argue logically: that would be true but banal. Nor yet is he simply insisting that medicine depends upon reasoning and theory no less than upon observation and experience: that would have been controversial in his own time[10] but a commonplace in ours. Rather, he is asserting that a good doctor must be trained in the science of logic, that he must be, in the technical sense, a logician.[11]

That assertion is remarkable: I do not imagine that many doctors would regard a grounding in logic as a prerequisite for clinical practice.

---

[8] See e.g. *meth. med.* X 5 for Thessalus, who denied that the doctor needed any of the arts and sciences; cf. Plutarch, *san. tuend.* 122BE on the antiphilosophical doctor Glaucon.

[9] Galen says that 'most doctors who have attempted to discover the method have failed' (*meth. med.* X 30; cf. 117-118); but he is thinking here of the Rationalist doctors, not of the great men of old; cf. *Hipp. elem.* I 457-458.

[10] I am thinking of the debate between the ancient 'schools' of medicine, wherein the Empiricists claimed that observation and experience were alone sufficient to ground the art of medicine.—The ancient division of medicine into three schools or sects, Empiricist, Rationalist, Methodist, is crude but serviceable. Galen has sometimes been presented as a quasi-Rationalist. It is true that he will occasionally prefer a Rationalist to an Empiricist stance (he is unrelentingly hostile to the Methodists). But that means little: whereas his contemporaries are eager to enroll themselves in the books of a half-understood sect (*nat. fac.* II 52-53), Galen rejects all three schools (see esp. R. Walzer, Galen on Jews and Christians (Oxford, 1949), pp. 37-45), which he regards as having deviated from the old Hippocratic tradition, the uniquely estimable method of medicine. (Not that Galen will even be called a Hippocratic, for membership of any school is a sort of slavery: *lib. prop.* XIX 13). On Galen's attitude to Rationalism and Empiricism see esp. Michael Frede, 'On Galen's Methodology', in Nutton, o.c. n.7: I owe much to Frede's excellent paper, which was not available to me when I produced the first draft of this essay.

[11] It is not only doctors who must be logicians: doctors need logic because they are scientists, and all the other sciences depend upon the science of logic—see e.g. *const. med.* I 226; *pecc. dign.* V 61; *Thras.* V 810. Cf. Vitruvius, I 1: the architect ,,ut litteratus sit, peritus graphidos, eruditus geometria, historias complures noverit, philosophos diligenter audierit, musicam scierit, medicinae non sit ignarus, responsa iurisconsultorum noverit, astrologiam caelique rationes cognitas habeat''.

It is also peculiarly Galenian. Galen, it is true, fathers his view upon Hippocrates, who, he claims, 'exhorts us to practise logical studies' (*opt. med.* I 54);[12] and a few other medical men may have indulged in dialectic.[13] But Galen's reference to Hippocrates evinces piety rather than historical scholarship, and there is no reason to think that logic played a significant part in the studies of any doctor before Galen.[14]

---

[12] Galen was thinking of such passages as Hippocrates, *off. med.* III 272L. (cf. *Hipp. Plat.* V 724). See e.g. *corp. temp.* IV 805 ('I do not place my trust in the man [i.e. Hippocrates] in the way in which most do: it is because I see his firm demonstrations that I too praise Hippocrates'); *nat. fac.* II 5 (Hippocrates 'was the first of the doctors and philosophers we know to have attempted to demonstrate' the theory of the four qualities, and 'the first principles of demonstrations, which Aristotle later adopted, are to be found first in his writings'); ib. 141. Hippocrates 'exhorts us to logical studies' by his practice, not by precept. Not even Hippocrates was punctilious in his logical practice; indeed, a main aim of Galen's work is to provide proofs when Hippocrates omitted them: *meth. med.* X 420, 425, 632-633; cf. *nat. fac.* II 117, 178-179 (for a good example of this see *in Hipp. acut. morb.* XV 549-551).

[13] 'Surely', it may be said, 'the Rationalist doctors—λογικοί—were keen students of logic?' The case is not clear. Certainly, the nomenclature of the sect does not itself refer to any logical studies. The Rationalists are also called δογματικοί. They are δογματικοί because they advance δόγματα, i.e. propositions about τὰ φύσει ἄδηλα or items not open to direct inspection (see e.g. Sextus, *PH* I 13); they are λογικοί because such items are apprehensible only by λόγος or reason. (See esp. *sect. ingred.* I 65). Since the Rationalists rely upon λόγος they will surely lace their medicine with argument: that does not, however, imply that they have studied logic or that they required probationer physicians to become proficient in the science of logic. At *ars med.* I 305-306 Galen allows that 'the Herophileans, and some of the Erasistrateans, and Athenaeus, have attempted the method of synthesis'. He does not say that they succeeded in their attempt—still less that they theorized about the method. And his usual complaint against the Rationalists is that they produce unsound proofs because they are ignorant of logic (see below, n. 26). The only passage I have come across in which the Rationalists are said to be devotees of logic is *sect. ingred.* I 77: The Empiricists say that 'no art needs διαλεκτική', whereas the Rationalists 'praise διαλεκτικὴ θεωρία' (Cf. ib. I 96). There, I think, Galen means just what he says: the Rationalists praise logic—but, as he frequently remarks elsewhere, they do not practise it. Epigenes, the addressee of *praecogn.*, is described as 'trained from boyhood in geometry and dialectic' (*praecogn.* XIV 651). It is not certain that Epigenes was a doctor—and if he was he may have been a pupil of Galen's. See Nutton, o.c. n.7, pp. 147-148. Of course, our information about all this comes almost exclusively from Galen himself, and he was not an impartial source. Nonetheless, I incline to believe that in his insistence on logical training he was unique among ancient doctors.

[14] According to Galen, his contemporaries did not hold logic in high regard: the rich and powerful think that logic is 'as useless as drilling holes in millet seeds' (*praecogn.* XIV 605); 'even some of those who profess to philosophize admit that they shy away from training in logical studies' (*pecc. dign.* V 71). As for the doctors, Galen was disillusioned at an early age. When he was 19 he chopped logic with one of his teachers who tried to explain the theories of Athenaeus; the teacher eventually exploded: "This fellow has been fed on dialectic and filled with the rubbish that it produces ... he is overthrowing and distorting and confounding everything!" (*elem. Hipp.* I 464—the whole of the Socratic dialogue at ib. I 460-465, which Galen swears is historically accurate, repays study); cf. e.g. *art. sang.* IV 727 (the Erasistrateans say that 'medical theory should not be subject to the superfluities of logic'); *foet. form.* IV 695; *Hipp. Plat* V. 654-655; *meth. med.* X 76. Many doctors and philosophers, when chastised for their logical ignorance, would say

Galen earned the admiration of some of his Christian contemporaries. There were some Christians who 'do not inquire what the holy scriptures say but sedulously endeavour to discover a form of argument to support their own ungodliness. If anyone propounds a passage of holy scripture to them they try to see whether it can produce a conditional or a disjunctive form of argument; and abandoning the sacred scriptures of god, they study geometry'. Those heretics read Euclid, they admire Aristotle and Theophrastus—and 'Galen, I suppose, by some of them is actually worshipped' (Eusebius, *HE* V xxviii 13-14).[15] There survive surprisingly few references to Galen by his near contemporaries. It is significant that his Christian worshippers should have revered him for his insistence on the use of logical techniques. The striking fact about Galen, in the eyes of at least some observers, was his devotion to logic.

2. Galen's Logic

Galen studied logic from an early age. 'I was educated by my father who, being versed in the study of arithmetic and calculation and grammar, brought me up in these and the other disciplines of education; and when I was fourteen, he introduced me to the study of dialectic, for I was intended to apply myself to philosophy alone' (*ord. lib. prop.* XIX 59). So he was 'put into the hands of someone who taught the logical theory of Chrysippus and of the celebrated Stoics' (*lib. prop.* XIX 43). His Stoic teacher was a pupil of Philopator (*anim. aff.* V 41). Galen's father, determined to ensure breadth and independence in his son's intellectual outlook, took him also to hear a Platonist pupil of Gaius, a Peripatetic pupil of Aspasius, and an itinerant Epicurean (ibid. V 41-42). If Philopator's pupil taught Galen Stoic logic, his Platonist and Peripatetic teachers will have given him instruction in Aristotelian syllogistic, and he will have received a rounded logical education. When Galen was sixteen, his father, moved by a dream, made Galen take up medicine;[16] but he continued with his philosophical studies and never abandoned logic. 'Throughout the whole of my life there has been nothing to which I have devoted more attention than the learning of demonstrative science and

---

either 'There's no such thing as proof' or else 'Proof comes naturally to everyone' (*ord. lib. prop.* XIX 52; cf. *const. med.* I 254). Throughout his life Galen found that his audiences fought shy of mathematical reasoning; hence 'God knows that not only here but in many places in my writings I have omitted proofs which belong to astronomy or geometry or music or some other logical discipline, lest my books should be thoroughly hated by the doctors' (*us. part.* III 837).

[15] Eusebius is probably quoting Hippolytus; on this passage see Walzer, o.c. n. 10, pp. 75-86.

[16] See *meth. med.* X 609; *praecogn.* XIV 608; *ord. lib. prop.* XIX 59.

the practising of it with every attention' (*adv. Iul.* XVIIIA 274-275).[17]
We know something of Galen's logical studies from his autobibliography. His writings included commentaries—on Aristotle's *Analytics*, on Theophrastus, on Chrysippus' various books, on the logic of Plato, nineteen titles and fifty-eight books in all (*lib. prop.* XIX 46-47; cf. 41-43). He also composed logical treatises of his own. The centrepiece was the massive work *On Demonstration*, in fifteen books (*lib. prop.* XIX 41), written in about the year 160. Around that work, and composed in a more expansive style, Galen wrote some forty shorter treatises amounting to almost fifty books (*lib. prop.* XIX 43-45).[18] The list is impressive: if it does not compare in quantity to the Chrysippean canon, it rivals the production of any other ancient logician.

From that library only three short tracts survive:[19] the *de sophismatis*, a juvenile essay on ambiguity; the *de optima doctrina*, a polemical pamphlet attacking Favorinus' version of scepticism and saying a little about Galen's own views on epistemology; and the *institutio logica*, a brief introductory handbook on formal logic.[20] It is difficult to form any estimate of Galen's standing as a logician.[21] Certainly, some of the items

---

[17] Cf. *meth. med.* X 609 ('throughout my life I have laboured at both disciplines [i.e. medicine and philosophy] in deeds rather than in words'); *ord. lib. prop.* XIX 59. Eudemus, the Peripatetic philosopher, took Galen for a member of his own profession: he believed that Galen 'had a reputable standing simply in philosophy and that he studied medicine as a hobby' (*praecogn.* XIV 608).

[18] The text of *lib. prop.* is badly corrupt in these pages and a precise tally of Galen's output escapes us.

[19] The loss of *On Demonstration* deprives us of one of Galen's key writings. Fragments of, and references to, *dem.* were collected by I. von Müller, Ueber Galens Werk vom wissenschaftlichen Beweis, Abh. Bayer. Akad. 1895, 2 (Munich, 1897); see also W. Jaeger, Nemesios von Emesa (Berlin, 1914), part I (esp. pp. 16-19, 36-47). More material is available in Arabic manuscripts (see S. Pines, 'Razi critique de Galien', in Actes du VIIᵉ Congrès International d'Histoire des Sciences (Paris, 1953), pp. 485-487; G. Strohmaier, 'Galen in Arabic: prospects and projects', in Nutton, o.c. n. 7; but it is so far unpublished (except for a short fragment, probably from *dem.*, printed by G. Strohmaier, 'Demokrit über die Sonnenstäubchen', *Philologus* 112 (1968) 1-19, at pp. 1-6). Note that the Arabs did not have a complete text of *dem.*: Hunain, after a prolonged and exhaustive search, could discover less than half of the work (see G. Bergsträsser, Ḥunain ibn Ishaq über die syrischen und arabischen Galen-Uebersetzungen, Abh. f.d. Kunde d. Morgenlandes 17 (2) (1925), pp. 38-39).

[20] *Soph.* and *inst. log.* are not mentioned in our text of *lib. prop.* (but see n. 18); their authenticity, however, is not seriously questioned by scholars. Note also the page from Galen's *de possibilitate* preserved in an Arabic manuscript of Alexander's attack on the work: N. Rescher and M. E. Marmura, The Refutation by Alexander of Aphrodisias of Galen's Treatise on the Theory of Motion (Islamabad, n.d.), pp. 69-70.

[21] On Galen's logic see C. Prantl, Geschichte der Logik im Abendlande, vol. I (Leipzig, 1855), pp. 559-577, 591-610 [Prantl thought that *inst. log.* was spurious]; E. Chauvet, La philosophie des médecins grecs (Paris, 1886), pp. 109-169; J. W. Stakelum, Galen and the Logic of Proposition, Logicalia 2 (Rome, 1940); J. Mau, Galens Einführung in die Logik—kritisch-exegetischer Kommentar (Berlin, 1960); W. and M. Kneale, The Development of Logic (Oxford, 1962), pp. 182-185; J. Kieffer, Galen's

he lists were "juvenilia" (*lib. prop.* XIX 43), and others were notes made by Galen for his private use (ib. 41).[22] Many of the other items may have been trifling, polemical, or derivative.

Yet there is reason to believe that Galen made at least one serious contribution to logical studies.[23] He says that he found the logic of the Schools, both Stoic and Peripatetic, unsatisfactory, and that their deficiencies could be made good by studying the practice of the mathematicians (*lib. prop.* XIX 40-41). In the *institutio*, having discussed the Aristotelian categorical syllogism and the Stoic hypothetical syllogism, he remarks that there is a 'third kind' of syllogism—the syllogism of relations; and this 'third kind' is to be found especially in the works of the arithmeticians and the calculators (*inst. log.* xvi 1,5). There can be little doubt that the *institutio* here gives substance to the abstract observation of *lib. prop.* His attention to the logic of relations is Galen's original gift to the science of reasoning. Admittedly, Galen was not the first logician to mention relational arguments; and his treatment of relations in the *institutio* is jejune.[24] Nonetheless, he was the only ancient logician to recognize that, from a scientific point of view, the study of relations is a vital part of formal logic; and he was the only ancient logician to see that relational arguments could not be subsumed under either of the existing School logics. Those facts are enough to secure Galen an honourable place in the history of logical science.

3. *Medical Vices*

Galen studied logic. His fellow physicians, whatever school of thought they adhered to, did not. The Empiricists, who rejected the use of reason in medicine, at least had the intelligence (or so Galen said) to realize that they were thereby debarred from employing proofs and must be content

---

Institutio Logica (Baltimore, 1964); N. Rescher, Galen and the Syllogism (Pittsburgh, 1966); U. Egli, Zur stoischen Dialektik (Basel, 1967), pp. 73-85; I. Garofalo and M. Vegetti, Opere Scelte di Galeno (Turin, 1978), pp. 1083-1091.

[22] Galen describes *inst. log.* (xi 2) as 'an outline of logical theory, not a detailed treatment'.

[23] Some would find originality in Galen's eclecticism, pointing in particular to the fact that he saw through the foolish rivalry between Stoics and Peripatetics and recognized that the schools were complementary to one another (see *inst. log.* vii 2-3). Galen was certainly an eclectic, even a syncretist, in logic; but I am not convinced that his attitude to the Stoic-Peripatetic quarrels is correct—the quarrels, I suspect, reflect not a trivial competitiveness between the schools but a deep-seated division of opinion about the fundamental structure of logic.—The *inst. log.* contains some points not found elsewhere in ancient logic texts: it is possible that some of them may be original to Galen (e.g. the account of the 'conversion' of syllogisms at vi 5-6).

[24] But he discussed relational syllogisms, at greater length and perhaps with more subtlety, in *dem.* (*inst. log.* xvii 1).

with an unmethodical procedure (*meth. med.* X 37). The Rationalists professed an appetite for proof; but they (according to Galen's opinion) did not understand what a proof was, since they had no logical training. Consequently, their attempts at proof misfired (*meth. med.* X 32),[25] and often they too abjured proper method: 'You will not—for it is perhaps better to say you will not than you cannot—use demonstrations, and you do not follow those who both will and can' (*meth. med.* X 109).[26]

Galen reserved his deepest scorn for the Methodists, and especially for the Thessalians.[27] Thessalus himself, who boasted that he had discovered the one true method of medicine, was in fact 'the most unmethodical of men' who 'produced his assertions in a way wholly opposed to the noble name with which he titled himself' (*meth. med.* X 27).[28] 'He wrote so many vast books and babbled so many thousands of words, yet did not attempt to state a single demonstration anywhere in his writings' (ibid. X 20).[29] Thessalus' followers 'try indeed to offer demonstrations; but what the principles of demonstrations are—of what sort and how many—they do not know and will not inquire; nor will they stand and listen to anyone else who might teach them' (ibid. X 37; cf. *adv. Iul.* XVIIIA 275).[30]

How did those men suffer, professionally speaking, from their logical inexpertise? Galen's attacks upon them are marked more by vehemence than by system—he nowhere sets out the charges against them in a calm and orderly fashion. Nonetheless, from his writings it emerges that there were three vices for which the logicless doctors were to be especially condemned.

---

[25] The Empiricists 'say something about the unsound modes of proof which the Rationalists are accustomed to use' (*sect. ingred.* I 77)—but that does not imply that the Empiricists recognized sound proofs.

[26] Cf. *meth. med.* X 122; *diff. puls.* VIII 578 (Archigenes will not give proofs for his dogmatic assertions about the types of pulse). Galen insists that such men argue badly because they do not understand what a proof is: *temp.* I 590-591; *pecc. dign.* V 61; *meth. med.* X 28-30, 32.

[27] For Methodism see Edelstein, o.c. n. 7, pp. 173-191; M. Vegetti, 'La polemica di Galeno contro la medicina metodica', in F. Romano (ed.), Democrito e l'Atomismo antico (Catania, 1980); M. Frede, 'The Method of the so-called Methodical School of Medicine', in J. Barnes, J. Brunschwig, M. F. Burnyeat, M. Schofield (eds.), Science and Speculation (Cambridge, 1982); Nutton, o.c. n. 7, pp. 223-224 (with references).

[28] Cf. *meth. med.* X 421 ('those from the sect which has adorned itself with the proud name of "methodical" but which in fact is most unmethodical'); ibid. X 169, 204; *adv. Iul.* XVIIIA 270.

[29] Cf. *meth. med.* X 28; there is just one syllogism which, by chance, Thessalus validly propounded: medicine is the best of arts; Thessalus is the first of doctors; therefore Thessalus is the first of men (*meth. med.* X 11).

[30] Compare Galen's sarcastic comment on the 'new logic' of the Methodist Julianus: *adv. Iul.* XVIIIA 295.

First, they became intellectual despots. 'They give us commands like tyrants' (*meth. med.* X 105); 'they simply furrow their brows and castigate us in a high-handed fashion' (ibid. X 107); 'their words are nothing but quarrels and boastings and challenges to insults and squabbles' (ibid. X 109). 'We hate Dionysius and Phalaris and the other tyrants because they give commands and orders, and do not persuade and teach' (ibid. X 105). And if the unlogical doctors are like the bogeymen of the Greek past, they are also to be compared to another group of irrationalists among Galen's contemporaries: they are like 'the followers of Moses and Christ' who 'order their pupils to accept everything on faith' and refuse to offer reasons or arguments for their dogmas.[31] Lack of logic leads to professional bad manners: doctors are heard shouting at one another instead of reasoning, making ex cathedra pronouncements instead of constructing arguments—the profession gets a bad name.[32]

Secondly, ignorance of logic induces professional misconduct and moral depravity. Tyrants to their pupils and colleagues, the unlogical doctors become slaves to their patients. Rich patients want servile doctors 'who will give them cold water if they are asked, who will wash them if they are commanded, who will offer snow and wine, and who will obey every order like slaves—the reverse of those old sons of Asclepius who thought fit to rule their patients as generals rule their soldiers and monarchs their subjects'. Thessalus took careful note of this demand for medical toadies—hence his 'method' (*meth. med.* X 4-5). For the 'method', which could be learned in six months—it might as well be six minutes, Galen tartly observes[33]—, gave the doctors time to cultivate rich patrons—and to wallow in the follies of the Roman aristocracy.[34] Galen records 'how great is the power of the therapeutic method, and how much harm has been done by those who have abandoned the old medicine and established the new schools. ... They are now governed by a contempt for what is noble and a desire for wealth and reputation and political power' (ibid. X 172). 'Unless there is a great and miraculous

---

[31] The quotation, preserved in Arabic, is from Galen's treatise *On the Prime Mover* (text in Walzer, o.c. n. 10, p. 15); cf. the Arabic citation from *On Hippocrates' Anatomy* (Walzer, p. 11); *diff. puls.* VIII 579.—Galen's Christian admirers (above, p. 54) evidently took these strictures to heart.

[32] The tyrants here are the Rationalists—cf. *meth. med.* X 116; for the tyranny of the Thessalians see ibid. X 20, 28, 29, 71, 76; for their λοιδορία, ibid. X 18. Galen explains at length (ibid. X 109-114) how ignorance of logic inevitably leads to unseemly and futile bickering.

[33] *meth. med.* X 781; for the Methodists' πολυθρύλητοι ἓξ μῆνες see e.g. *sect. intr.* I 83; *dign. puls.* VIII 770; *meth. med.* X 5; 927.

[34] And of course those lecherous leeches aren't really enjoying themselves as much as sober old Galen is: logic is a lot more fun than the crude pleasures the Methodist pursues: *pecc. dign.* V 87.

change in human affairs, everything noble is lost, confounded, destroyed, since no-one cares for the truth but only for its semblance. For you know very well that we have not come across five men in all who desire to be wise rather than to seem so—and even if one of them were to desire wisdom for its own sake, he would not have the time to train in logical method but, in his care for wealth and reputation and political power, he would spend his whole life busying about such things' (ibid. X 114-115).[35]

The third consequence of logical nescience is the greatest damnation. Thessalus knew no logic. Were he to defend his medical views before judges who were 'dialecticians, scientists, practised in discriminating truth and falsehood, skilled in distinguishing what is consistent and what inconsistent, experienced from youth in demonstrative method', he would receive short shrift (*meth. med.* X 9; cf. *pecc. dign.* V 103; *adv. Iul.* XVIIIA 272). Knowing no logic, he advanced medical theories that were vacuous, confused, contradictory. And for that reason he was a bad physician in the most damning sense: he killed his patients. 'An egregious Thessalian', treating a patient whose hand had been punctured by a dagger, 'killed him within six days' (ibid. X 390). 'One of them, using a powerful drug which would effect a splendid cure (as he himself thought) for sufferers from dysentery, cured many inside a day—but he killed some' (ibid. X 815). 'You can see many people every day being destroyed by the ignorance of their doctors' (ibid. X 820). In the most barbed and brilliant of the many digressions in *meth. med.*, Galen tells the story of Attalus the Thessalian and Theagenes the Cynic philosopher.[36]

---

[35] Cf. the splendid jeremiad which opens *meth. med.* (X 2-7); the treatise contains many similar passages: e.g. X 609 (most doctors care for δοξοσοφία rather than ἀλήθεια, and 'while they were running round the whole city and escorting and dining with the rich and powerful, I was working hard ...'); 76-77; 172. Cf. e.g. *const. med.* I 244; *nat. fac.* II 179-180; *pecc. dign.* V 69; *diff. puls.* VIII 656; *dign. puls.* VIII 773; *praecogn.* XIV 599-600. Such passages are highly coloured: Galen writes with gusto: he employs the figures and tropes of rhetoric: he takes over the stock accusations of polemic and satire (see e.g. Nutton, o.c. n. 7, pp. 146-147). The denunciations were not written, and should not be read, as documentary history. But if a text is rhetorical it does not follow that it is fictional. When allowance is made for exaggeration and rodomontade, there remains the fact that, in Galen's view, contemporary physicians were, many of them, rude, corrupt and incompetent. We should not doubt that that was indeed how Galen saw matters; and there is reason to think that Galen was not wholly mistaken in his perceptions. (Note the remarks in Pliny, *nh* XXIX i 1 - ix 28: his jaundiced view of the history of medicine, and of the aims and practices of doctors, makes Galen's rhetoric seem mild). See also Nutton, o.c. n. 7, pp. 179-180.

[36] Attalus is probably Statilius Attalus, the ἀρχιατρὸς Σεβαστῶν, see J. Benedum, 'Statilios Attalos', RE Suppt. XIV, 63-66. For Theagenes see A. Modrze, 'Theagenes (11)', RE VA 1348-1349.—Joint consultations of the type Galen describes here were common—and perhaps partly explain the agonistic aspect of much of Galen's therapeutic writings. They were a Hippocratic tradition: see G. E. R. Lloyd, Magic, Reason and Experience (Cambridge, 1979), p. 91, n. 174.

Theagenes was ill and Attalus attended him. Galen, who was also at the bedside, heard Attalus' Methodist prescription with horror. He gave a long and helpful lecture. Attalus, not unnaturally, interrupted, saying (according to Galen) that 'I would not have put up with any of that if I did not hold you in such esteem'. He promised Galen that Theagenes would be perfectly recovered in three or four days. Galen kept his peace. Three days later, to Galen's evident satisfaction, Theagenes was dead.[37] 'And the other Methodists kill a thousand patients every day, yet even now they do not dare to change their mode of therapy nor will they try even once the therapy that has been described by other doctors who genuinely care for the effects of the art: so stubborn a thing is ignorance' (ibid. X 909-916).

Those doctors who abjure logical studies are therefore ignorant of the methods of medicine; being ignorant, they therefore kill their patients. Professional boorishness and unscientific appetites might perhaps be overlooked were the physician a successful practitioner. But doctors who know no logic do not succeed in their practice. If your doctor has not studied formal logic, beware—he will probably poison you. 'In the past they put such people to menial trades. God knows where it will all end' (nat. fac. II 53).

4. Logic and Virtue

Doctors must diagnose their patients' maladies, they must predict the likely course of their conditions, they must prescribe a remedy. In all three aspects of medical practice—diagnostics, prognostics, therapy—a knowledge of logic is, according to Galen, essential. We need not believe every word of his diatribes against his contemporaries, for they are doubtless biassed both by Galen's personal antipathies and by his evident love of rhetorical hyperbole. But I assume that Galen means at least most of what he says—and I suppose that his accusations are not wholly baseless.

However that may be, we may still wonder exactly how logical science can save the doctors from the mire in which they allegedly flounder.

---

[37] Just as the Thessalians offered a short-cut to medicine, so the Cynics offered an 'easy road to wisdom' and a 'short path to virtue' (pecc. dign. V 71; cf. 89). No doubt Galen thought that Attalus and Theagenes were well-matched. Galen also criticizes the Stoics for being content with 'the short and level road' instead of the 'long and rough' one (Hipp. Plat. V 233). In Galen's view, the acquisition of knowledge is arduous (below, n. 43); but, once acquired, knowledge may be easily applied by way of brief proofs (see Hipp. Plat. V 655-660 [see below, pp. 69-72]; opt. doct. I 51)—here Galen is at one with Zeno the Stoic (Diog. Laert. VII 20).

How, after all, can logic prevent medical malpractices and avert professional turpitude?

At bottom, Galen's answer is simple. Logic is the science of discerning truth and falsity (*meth. med.* X 18);[38] and logicians are thereby technically equipped to detect falsehoods and to discover truths.

The ability to detect falsehoods is of no small moment; for medicine, in Galen's opinion, had become corrupted by sophisms and charlatanry. 'The men of old spoke well on these subjects but they did not defend their views by argument, never suspecting that there would be sophists so shameless as to try to contradict the evident facts. And more recent men sometimes have been conquered by the sophistries and persuaded by their authors, and sometimes have tried to contradict them with what seems to me far less force than that of the men of old' (*nat. fac.* II 178; cf. *caus. procat.* i 1-3, x 132-133). Those who are conquered suffer defeat because they are ignorant of logic—indeed, the sophistical doctors positively encourage such ignorance: 'they do not draw their pupils towards reason or allow them to approach dialectic, in order, I suppose, that they may convince them by trivial sophisms; and the pupils, not being trained in solving sophisms, admire their teachers as gods' (*caus. procat.* xi 142).

Much of Galen's energy was consumed in polemic against those sophists; 'for the sophists do not let you engage in any worthwhile studies (of which there is no lack) but compel you to waste your time in solving the sophisms they propound' (*nat. fac.* II 44).[39] Thus the art 'which, as Hippocrates so rightly said, is long, has been made yet longer, I think, by these remarkable sophisms' (*caus. procat.* i 5).

Victory over the sophists is ensured by logical skill. 'As I have continually said, no-one can remain entirely undeceived unless he has been trained in dialectical theory' (*caus. procat.* xiii 170; cf. 172, viii 106). If you have a robust sense of reality you may, it is true, dismiss the sophists with a Johnsonian disdain, as Diogenes the Cynic dismissed the sophistical arguments against the possibility of motion: 'If there is no such thing as motion I wonder why the sailors ask each morning "Anyone for Rhodes? Cnidos? Cos?"' (ibid. ix 116).[40] But such

---

[38] Cf. e.g. ibid. X 9; *const. med.* I 245; *pecc. dign.* V 72; *adv. Lyc.* XVIIIA 245; *ord. lib. prop.* XIX 50. Galen is here adopting the Stoic definition: e.g. Sextus, *PH* II 94; Diog. Laert. VII 62 (ascribing it to Posidonius).

[39] Cf. *nat. fac.* II 56-57 (Galen was obliged to spend many pages on 'the blatherings of Asclepiades' and 'as the proverb has it, I was compelled to run mad with the madmen'), 67-68, 141-142; *in Hipp. morb. acut.* XV 450; *caus. procat.* vii 95, xii 160 (the whole of *caus. procat.* is pertinent). Jim Hankinson kindly drew these passages to my attention and made me see the importance of Galen's remarks on sophisms.

[40] See *Med. Exp.* xxii 2 Walzer—a different version of the story at Sextus, *PH* III 66 (cf. II 244); Diog. Laert. VI 39.

realism—at any rate in the face of medical sophisms— is rare; and unless you can resolve a paradox, by the application of logical techniques, you are likely to be deceived by it (ibid. xi 141).[41]

The 'logical methods' are thus indispensable for the unmasking of falsehood. More importantly, they are also indispensable for the discovering of truths.[42] 'If a man not only learns the methods of proof but also trains in them,[43] then he will discover the truth on every kind of subject' (ord. lib. prop. XIX 53); in particular, 'the man who has been trained in the therapeutic method will discover drugs and will be able to use correctly what he has discovered' (meth. med. X 386). Logic provides a method of scientific discovery. What is more, it is the unique provider; for 'apart from the study of logic, it is not possible to establish any doctrine with precision' (elem. Hipp. I 460).

Admittedly, logic is not an infallible guide to truth. In the case of some speculative questions (those concerning matters 'outside the cosmos', say) we must rest content with a 'maybe' or a 'plausibly' (e.g. pecc. dign. V 93, 100, 102; cf. subst. nat. fac. IV 759-760)[44]—but such speculative questions are in any case of no utility (Hipp. Plat. V 780-782). More important is the fact that on other, less remote, issues we may find ourselves at a stand: on the subject of the artificer of the animal kingdom Galen confessed himself reduced to perplexity; he had not proceeded 'as far as an opinion, let alone certain knowledge' (foet. form. IV 696). And

---

[41] Contrast Sextus' attitude to sophisms (PH II 229-259): 'those who praise dialectic [e.g. Galen] say that it is necessary for the solution of sophisms' (II 229); in fact, it is wholly useless. Trivial sophisms may perhaps be unmasked by the application of logical technique, but serious puzzles require serious professional solutions—in particular, medical sophisms are resolved not by dialecticians but by medical scientists (II 237-240).

[42] Galen is clear that logic is a tool for discovering truths: e.g. meth. med. X 28-29 ('the logical methods have the power to discover what is being sought'); Hipp. Plat. V 721; inst. log. i 2. This is a Stoic view (see J. Barnes, 'Proof Destroyed', in M. Schofield, M. F. Burnyeat, J. Barnes (eds.), Doubt and Dogmatism (Oxford, 1980), at pp. 176-180); it is not Aristotelian (see J. Barnes, 'Aristotle's Theory of Demonstration', in J. Barnes, M. Schofield, R. Sorabji (eds.), Articles on Aristotle, vol. I (London, 1975).

[43] The reference to training is not an idle addition: Galen constantly insists that, in addition to learning the logical methods, a medical student must train and practise in them—see e.g. opt. med. I 59; const. med. I 244; nat. fac. II 179-180; Hipp. Plat. V 222; 732-733, 783 (where the same insistence is ascribed to Plato and to Hippocrates); meth. med. X 39-40; and esp. pecc. dign. V 61ff (the student must (i) discover that there is such a thing as proof; (ii) investigate 'for a long time' and with the help of gifted and highly trained teachers, the nature of the demonstrative method; (iii) practise the method 'for a long time' in simple, empirically testable (V 66-68, 101) cases—e.g. in the task of constructing and calibrating a sun-dial (V 80-86); then (iv), he may use the method for serious scientific study). Few are prepared to undertake that long training: simp. med. temp. XI 403-404.

[44] For Galen's explanation of where and why he is content to 'proceed as far as what is plausible' see the fragmentary subst. nat. fac. (IV 757-766); cf. an. mor. IV 773.

he reached the same nonplus over the nature of the soul (ibid. IV 700, 701-702).[45] Sometimes we shall be able to form an opinion but not to proceed beyond what is plausible (e.g. *Hipp. Plat.* V 715)—and that may be true even in matters of anatomy (e.g. *meth. med.* X 839). Again, not all problems of therapy are soluble by demonstration: sometimes we can get no further than conjecture or 'stochastic' proof (ibid. X 860),[46] sometimes Galen will confess outright defeat—'logical method is no use for therapy on this topic for certain affections' (ibid. X 1018). But such cases, in Galen's view, are exceptional; for he was charmingly optimistic about the possible scope of human knowledge. In any event, Galen's occasional admissions of ignorance do not derogate from the authority of logic: it remains true, in Galen's mind, that whatever can be known with certainty can only be known with the aid of logic.

Here an objection will raise itself. "I grant you, Galen", the objector will say, "that certain knowledge is available only with the aid of logic and only to students of logic. And no doubt certain knowledge is a

---

[45] Cf. *us. part.* III 542; *resp. us.* IV 472; *an. mor.* IV 776; *in. Hipp. epid.* XVIIB 247-248. Those questions about God and the soul, however, are deemed to have a plausible (πιθανόν) answer at *Hipp. Plat.* V 793, where Galen is explicitly following Plato (*Tim.* 29CD, 72D); cf. *subst. nat. fac.* IV 758-759; *an. mor.* IV 787-788.—See also Nemesius, *nat. hom.* 86-87 M (with a reference to *dem.*) and the Arabic text quoted in F. W. Zimmermann, Al-Farabi's Commentary and Short Treatise on Aristotle's *de Interpretatione* (Oxford, 1981), p. lxxxi n. 2.

[46] Cf. *opt. sect.* I 114-115: medicine is a τέχνη στοχαστική, not because its theorems are στοχαστικά (they are all βέβαιά τε καὶ ἑστηκότα), but because 'the activity of physicians is not certain of success'; see also *loc. aff.* VIII 145; [*introd.*] XIV 684-685 (where a similar view is ascribed to Erasistratus, and then rejected); Celsus, *prooem.* 48 ("est enim haec ars coniecturalis"), II vi 16. At *san. tuend.* VI 365 Galen says that 'most diseases have a conjectural diagnosis' and elsewhere he suggests that diagnostics 'is the only thing in the art which generally involves conjecture' (*plen.* VII 581). But see *meth. med.* X 206: 'since the peculiarities of every individual's nature are ineffable and cannot be grasped with the most accurate knowledge, the best doctor for all individual diseases is the man who had provided himself with a method by which he can diagnose their natures and conjecture the cures peculiar to each' (on individual peculiarities, which escape rational discussion, see e.g. *ars med.* I 353; *loc. aff.* VIII 117, 339-340; *meth. med.* X 169, 181, 209; and cf. K. Deichgräber, Galen als Erforscher des menschlichen Pulses, *Sitz. Berl. Akad.* 1956. 3 (Berlin, 1957); *cur. rat.* XI 285: 'nothing shows the art of medicine to be conjectural in its practice so much as the question of the quantity of each remedy' (cf. *in. Hipp. acut. morb.* XV 585); note also the limits set to ἀκρίβεια by the very nature of the bodily parts (e.g. *anat. admin.* II 609). Conjecture is not uninformed guesswork: for στοχασμὸς ἀκριβής see esp. *loc. aff.* VIII 14; also *const. med.* I 291; *ars med.* I 353 (where Galen refers to our evidence for the state of an individual patient's internal organs); cf. *san. tuend.* VI 129, on 'accurate conjecture'; also e.g. *comp. med. gen.* XIII 887; *praesag. puls.* IX 278; *meth. med.* X 653. The distinction between 'certain' and 'conjectural' arts has a very long history in the philosophical tradition, beginning with Plato (see *Phlb* 55 DE; Philodemus, *rhet.* B II 15-24, VI 3-8 (medicine is στοχαστική) [for the text of *rhet.* see the edition by Longo Aurrichio in vol. 3 of F. Sbordone (ed.), Ricerche sui Papiri Ercolanesi (Naples, 1977)]; Sextus, *M* I 72, II 13; Alexander, *quaest.* 61.4-28). See M. Isnardi, 'Techne', *La Parola del Passato* 16 (1961) 257-296, at pp. 262-268.

desirable possession. But is it a possession indispensable to the busy doctor? May he not content himself with a lower grade of cognition—with something adequate to his practical ends and yet not dependent upon an exhausting propaedeutic study of logical theory?

"The Empiricists, after all, claim to have discovered many things; and you yourself appear to grant their claim (e.g. *meth. med.* X 122, 127)[47]—even though, as you say, 'they rightly agree that for them there is no necessary order either in discovery or in teaching; for trial and error is something apart from science and from reason, requiring good fortune if it is to discover what it is looking for' (ib. X 31-32). You allow that Empiricists are doctors, but you insist that they know no logic. Or again, consider your own pupils. Surely many of them—the less gifted or the less industrious—decide to follow your practice rather than your method. Do they not then cure their patients while knowing no logic? You concede that if a student has observed you closely and come to trust you, then 'such a man will benefit from my treatises even apart from demonstrative theory—not by gaining precise knowledge (for that belongs only to those who produce demonstrations) but by obtaining right opinion, of which the ancients[48] plausibly said that it is no worse than knowledge with regard to action, though it does not possess permanence and reliability' (*ord. lib. prop.* XIX 54). Does not experience (aided by good luck) or right opinion (instilled by a good teacher) suffice for the practical physician?[49] does he really need logical theory?"

Galen would have conceded something to that objection: he allows that Empiricists may, after a fashion, become good doctors (e.g. *meth. med.* X 122); and one of his purposes in writing medical textbooks was presumably to instill 'right opinion' into his students. But the concession would have been severely limited. 'Anyone who has adequately practised the discipline which philosophers call logic will be able to undertake any inquiry with equal facility; but to read books of cases without knowing logic is merely a waste of time—for you do not know how to judge what in them has been said truly and what falsely, and you cannot remember everything that has been written' (*Thras.* V 810).[50]

---

[47] In *meth. med.* Galen urges that it is important not to confuse nor even to discuss in a single tract, the two procedures of λόγος and πεῖρα (X 31, 123, 127, 159). Here, he says, 'it is now our project to discuss not all ways of discovering remedies' (ibid. 31; cf. 123-124): that allows that there are modes of discovery not covered by the method.

[48] I.e. Plato, *Meno* 97AD.

[49] Cf. *subf. emp.* 67.3-5: Galen has argued "quomodo possibile sit ei qui permittet substantiam totam invenire constituere medicativam artem emperice absque quod coadsit usus rationis".

[50] Cf. *comp. med. gen.* XIII 605, where doctors who rely on 'learning by way of the anatomical handbooks' are likened to 'the proverbial helmsman who steers from the book' (Galen illustrates their shortcomings with graphic anecdotes)—cf. *libr. propr.* XIX 33.

There are two points here. One is practical, and applies both to the slavish student and to the Empiricist (cf. *meth med.* X 169): without a method or a system, the doctor cannot retain in his memory the myriad disconnected details he has learned—his 'right opinion' lacks 'permanence and reliability'. The second point applies to the slavish student and is theoretical in nature: if the student has not learned logic, case-studies will be of no use to him—for, lacking logic, he will lack the ability to discriminate truth and falsity in what he reads or what he hears.

A further two points can be added. First, against the Empiricists Galen can urge that numerous therapies are not available to them: if they abjure logical method, then they must rest content not merely with 'right opinion' but with 'right opinion' on a restricted number of issues. (This point will be taken up later). Secondly, both the Empiricist and the slavish imitator will be perpetually foxed by new cases. If an Empiricist comes upon a case outside his experience, all he can do is experiment at random and trust to luck. If an imitator comes upon a case not treated by Galen, he can do nothing at all—except call in his master. When a Galenian comes upon a novelty, he will able, by virtue of his methodical technique, to diagnose the condition, offer a prognosis, and discover the appropriate treatment.[51]

Logic, in short, bestows the capacity to discover. Without that capacity a physician may, if he is sensible, achieve some diagnostic and therapeutic success; but his successes will be haphazard and in the lap of the gods.

5. *The Logical Methods*

To say that all knowledge depends upon logic may be true; but it is vague and unilluminating. Exactly how does logic provide us with knowledge? What is the content of logic and what are the 'logical methods'? What, in other words, do the logicless doctors lack? 'Most doctors, without first training in the logical methods, either attempt to demonstrate something and deceive themselves by fallacy, or else attempt to divide something into its species and differentia and then, like bad cooks,[52] do not cut at the joints' (*meth. med.* X 123). The two main failings of non-logicians are

---

[51] A man trained in method need only know the universal form of therapy—the particular applications he can work out for himself (e.g. *meth. med.* X 486; cf. Alexander, *in APr.* 340.13-21). More precisely: you must learn the method, which consists of universal truths; you must practise the method in individual cases; and then you will be equipped to use the method yourself and to make appropriate discoveries. Cf. *meth. med.* X 608, 628, 901, 944; *Thras.* V 842.

[52] 'Bad cooks': from Plato, *Phaedr.* 265E.

in proofs and in divisions.[53] The two main parts of the logical method are division and proof.

Common to both division and proof is the generic notion of method. 'To investigate something by method ... is to do so with some direction and order, so that there is something first in the investigation, and something second and third and fourth, and so on through all the rest in order until you arrive at what was originally proposed' (*meth. med.* X 31). That is hardly enlightening: it is difficult to see how any investigation, however unmethodical, could fail to include a first step, a second step, and so on. But Galen means, of course, that the 'first' thing must be a genuinely or naturally first thing—not simply the first item you chance to hit upon.

In 'division', the first item will be 'what is common and universal'. The successive steps will be 'cuts', dividing the common genus into species and subspecies. The final step will be the cut which produces infimae species, species which themselves have no subspecies (e.g. *ad Glauc.* XI 3-4; *cur. rat.* XI 258; *diff. puls.* VIII 601).

In proof or demonstration (apodeixis), the first items will be the appropriate archai—first principles or axioms; the successive steps will be intermediate deductions; and the final step will be taken when the desired theorem has been proved. For 'it had been written in *On Demonstration* how, by starting from the elements and principles in each case, a man may best demonstrate whatever can be demonstrated' (*opt. doct.* I 52). The 'demonstrative' method is thus the axiomatic method. The truths of medicine, as of any other science, consist of two sorts: there are primary truths—first principles or axioms; and there are derivative truths—theorems. The theorems depend upon the axioms insofar as they are deducible from them; and knowledge of the theorems is attained precisely by deducing them from the appropriate axioms. The axiomatic method had been known five hundred years before Galen wrote: Euclid's *Elements* provided its most celebrated exemplification, Aristotle's *Posterior Analytics* its most refined exposition. Yet Galen's appeal to demonstrative method is no mere commonplace. For he is intent on applying the method not to such 'hard' sciences as geometry and astronomy nor yet to empirical disciplines such as biology or botany but to an empirical art. The mathematical sciences yield to axiomatisation without great strain; and it was permissible to imagine (as Aristotle had done) that the axiomatic method could be extended to the other theoretical sciences. The theorems of medicine, on the other hand, contain not only empirical but also prac-

---

[53] At *ad Glauc.* XI 4 Galen says that the 'first and greatest' error of his contemporaries is their failure to produce proper divisions.

tical matter, and it was a bold thought that demonstrative procedure might be followed in such cases too.

There is a third type of logical method. A scientist will usually start his investigations from some particular problem—for example, from the question: What is the 'regent' part of the body (i.e. what part is causally responsible for perceptions and voluntary motion)? (cf. *Hipp. Plat.* V 227). He must endeavour to proceed towards the appropriate first principles from which he can then derive a proof. The method of 'upward' procedure is taken by Galen from the mathematicians—it is their celebrated notion of 'analysis'.[54] By that procedure you will first uncover propositions from which the problem in question can be directly solved, but which themselves are not axioms; 'these need certain other propositions for their proof, and those again need others—until you ascend to the primary propositions' (*meth. med.* X 33; cf. *pecc. dign.* V 80-81).[55]

Methodical division will enable you to articulate any problem, and its solution, in the appropriate scientific terms; methodical analysis will lead you to the apposite first principles on which the solution depends; methodical deduction, finally, will yield a demonstrative proof of the appropriate theorem and a definitive solution to the problem.[56] Those 'logical methods' are entirely general in their scope. They apply to all scientific problems, and hence in particular to medical problems—and ultimately to detailed therapeutic problems of the form: What is the cure for this disease?

The logical methods were described in detail in Galen's treatise *On Demonstration*. 'You Eugenianus, and those of you who are concerned with medicine alone, will find my *On Demonstration* sufficient; for others

---

[54] The texts on geometrical 'analysis' are scattered and puzzling. Scholars have reached no consensus. The best paper is still that by R. Robinson, 'Analysis in Greek Geometry', in his Essays in Greek Philosophy (Oxford, 1969). See also K. J. J. Hintikka and U. Remes, The Method of Analysis (Dordrecht, 1974), with my review in *Mind* 86 (1977) 133-136.

[55] For analysis see also *ars med.* I 305; *pecc. dign.* V 80, 84; *diff. puls.* VIII 601-602, 609 ('anyone who claims to be a logician must have the ability to analyse into its primary and simple conceptual elements whatever complex item may be proposed'—but here analysis and division are very close).

[56] Galen frequently uses the phrases 'logical methods' (or 'logical method'), 'demonstrative method', 'method of division'; he speaks far less often, in *meth. med.* at least, of 'analytical method'. I am assuming that demonstrative method and the method of division are the two main logical methods, analytics being—in *meth. med.*—a minor partner. I assume, too, that most of the content of λογικὴ θεωρία will fall under one or other of these methods. As for the relationship among the different methods, the suggestion in the text is only one of several possible accounts: I have found no passage in which Galen explicitly discusses the question. (The three μέθοδοι are identical with—or at least intimately related to—the three διδασκαλίαι of *ars med.* I 305; see also the preface to *ars med.*, preserved in Latin and Arabic: J. S. Wilkie and G. E. R. Lloyd, 'The Arabic Version of Galen's *Ars Parva*', *JHS* 101 (1981) 145-148).

who are busy in philosophy, there are the rest ⟨of my logical treatises⟩—
which should also be read by anyone who is to pursue correctly both
disciplines, medicine and philosophy' (*ord. lib. prop.* XIX 58). *On Demonstration* is lost, but we can make a plausible guess at much of its contents.

'I hold', Galen says, 'that the best writings on ⟨demonstrative
method⟩ are those of the old philosophers, Theophrastus and Aristotle,
in their books of *Posterior Analytics*' (*Hipp. Plat.* V 213).[57] The Peripatetic
Analytics will have served Galen as a model for his *dem*. *Dem.* certainly
included, first, a reasonably extensive account of formal deduction[58]—a
description of the various kinds of syllogisms with which Galen was
acquainted. (That answers to Aristotle's *APr.*: in *dem.* Galen follows the
Analytics as a whole, and not just the *Posterior Analytics*[59]). Secondly, *dem.*
contained a discussion of the axioms of the sciences or the first principles
of demonstration: what are their general characteristics? what are their
main varieties? (That answers roughly to the first book of Aristotle's
APst.) Thirdly, *dem.* provided a theory of definition and of 'essence'.
(That will have corresponded to the second part of *APst*; but Galen's
theory of definitions was closely connected with 'division'—and there
Plato was his master).[60] Finally, *dem.* dealt with questions of
epistemology: how can we acquire knowledge of the axioms? what is the
scope of human knowledge? (The last chapter of *APst.* engages very
briefly with such issues).

Galen's *dem.* was perhaps four times the length of Aristotle's *Analytics*.
Galen included some account of post-Aristotelian logic; he surely devoted
more space to division than Aristotle had done; no doubt he indulged,
characteristically enough, in illustrative anecdote, learned quotation,
vituperative polemic. The details almost all escape us and we have no

---

[57] The dismissive remarks about Stoic and Peripatetic logic at *lib. prop.* XIX 39-40 are
an impatient exaggeration. But Galen is often less than complimentary about the Stoics'
scientific use of their logic: 'Chrysippus and his followers have not written anything
worthwhile on the subject, nor do they appear to make any use of it' (*Hipp. Plat.* V 224;
cf. 220-221; 225-226). Moraux ('Galien et Aristote' [o.c. n. 7], p. 130) says that 'tout
ce que Galien dit de la méthode ... découle de l'enseignement d'Aristote'; but that judg-
ment ignores the Stoic elements in his thought—and also his own contribution to the
issue.

[58] See e.g. *inst. log.* xii 1: *dem.* established technical metatheorems for categorical
syllogistic (there can be only three figures; there can be no valid categorical syllogisms
apart from those in the Aristotelian-Theophrastean canon).

[59] 'Galen's main logical work *On Demonstration* is entirely based on Aristotle's *Analytica
Posteriora*' (Walzer, o.c. n. 10, p. 40, n. 3); cf. Garofalo and Vegetti, o.c. n. 21, p. 1083.

[60] For division you need to read Aristotle's *Parts of Animals* and Theophrastus, but
especially Plato—*Philebus, Sophist, Politicus* (*meth. med.* X 26; cf. e.g. ibid. X 659, and esp.
Hipp. Plat. V 753-760). At *adv. Lyc.* XVIIIA 209 Galen adds Chrysippus, and also
Mnesitheos, the fourth century doctor; and *ad Glauc.* XI 3 singles Mnesitheos out as a
master of medical divisions; see H. Hohenstein, Der Arzt Mnesitheos aus Athen (Jena,
1935); J. Bertier, Mnésithée et Dieuchès (Leiden, 1972).

idea of the general flavour of the work; but its scope and content, in the most general terms, can be conjectured with some assurance.[61]

6. *The Elements of Proof*

Of the three logical methods the demonstrative is perhaps the most important, at least as far as Galen's medicine goes; certainly it is the most prominent of the methods in *meth. med.*. Accordingly, in the following sections I shall attend almost exclusively to the demonstrative method, leaving analysis and division—large subjects in themselves—for independent treatment.

Of the deductions by which theorems are derived from axioms there is not much to be said. Galen's logic was eclectic: it included the categorical syllogisms of the Peripatetics as well as the 'hypothetical' syllogisms which were associated primarily with the Stoics.[62] In addition, and as an important novelty, the deductive machinery of *On Demonstration* included relational syllogisms. The logic of demonstration is not, however, a complete formal logic. Galen notes explicitly that certain types of hypothetical syllogism are useless for demonstrative purposes (*inst. log.* xiv 3,8);[63] he is reported to have disparaged, on the same grounds, certain categorical syllogisms;[64] and in general he will have disregarded any parts of orthodox formal logic which did not, in his view, serve a demonstrative function. The deductive sections of *On Demonstration* will have

---

[61] This rough sketch of the contents of *dem.* is based on the evidence collected by von Müller, o.c. n. 19. *Dem.* certainly contained some surprising material: an account of the physiology of perception; a critical discussion of Aristotle's theory of time; a demolition of Asclepiades' views on atoms. But von Müller, I think, pays too much attention to those odd items. For he in effect crams all the subject matter of the *Analytics* into Books I-III of *dem.* Book IV, he suggests, dealt with some areas of thought where scepticism is appropriate, Book V discussed physiology, ..., Books VIII-XV were occupied by critical discussion of other philosophers. I find that reconstruction implausible: there is no reason to think that over half of *dem.* was negatively critical, and that only a fifth of it described the demonstrative method. In fact, Galen regularly refers to long discussions in *dem. of issues he deals with only briefly in the surviving treatises (see e.g. meth. med.* X 37; *Hipp. Plat.* V 219, 226, 722-723; *simp. med. temp.* XI 471). Given a knowledge of the difficulty of the subject matter and an acquaintance with Galen's generally expansive style, it is easy to imagine how the topics I mention in the text could come to occupy 15 books. (Note that two books of Galen's commentary on Aristotle's *APst.* discussed definition: *diff. puls.* VIII 764-765).

[62] Galen recognizes that categorical (*inst. log.* xiii) and hypothetical (ibid. xiv-xv) syllogisms may be used in demonstrations (note the medical examples at xiii 9, 12; xv 1).

[63] Cf. *inst. log.* xix 1, 5, 6; *Hipp. Plat.* V 224 (many of the Stoic syllogisms are useless 'as Chrysippus himself testifies by his practice—for nowhere in his treatises does he require those syllogisms for the proof of a doctrine'); ibid. V 781.

[64] See Al-Farabi, Commentary on Aristotle's *de Interpretatione*, 193 [Zimmermann, o.c. n. 45, p. 186].

been long and technical; but they will not have been—nor have professed to be—a comprehensive treatment of the subject.

What next of the axioms or first principles (archai)? Galen lays down certain formal conditions which any axiom must satisfy. An axiom must be 'primary', prōtos (e.g. *meth. med.* X 33; *pecc. dign.* V 75); that is to say, it must not itself require proof but be 'non-demonstrable', anapodeiktos (e.g. *meth. med.* X 34).[65] It must therefore be 'evident', enargēs (e.g. *pecc. dign.* V 94),[66] or 'self-crediting', ex heautou pistos. For first principles 'have their credibility (pistis) not through demonstration but from themselves' (*meth. med.* X 22).[67] Hence axioms will be universally accepted, they will be 'agreed upon by all men' (ibid.);[68] for they are 'naturally credible to all of us' (*subst. nat. fac.* IV 760).

The condition of universal agreement was of particular importance to Galen. 'As I said in *On Demonstration*, I was swamped by the amount of disagreement[69] among the doctors—and, turning to judge it, I realized

---

[65] The term ἀναπόδεικτος was ambiguous. Aristotle uses it to mean 'not capable of being proved'. Sextus (*M* VIII 223) says that it may mean either 'unproved' or 'not requiring proof' (cf. Apuleius, *int.* ix 188.4-11), and he adds that the Stoics use the word in their logic in the second sense. Galen stipulates that first principles do not require proof (see *nat. fac.* II 184; *meth. med.* X 50; cf. *inst. log.* viii 1). Does he also mean that they do not admit proof? At *opt. sect.* I 109 he says that 'we should ridicule those doctors who try to judge things apparent (τὰ ἐναργῆ) not by their sense-organs but by a proof'; and that perhaps suggests that evident truths cannot be proved. But at *nat. fac.* II 145 he remarks that 'we are accustomed to employ not only this mode of proof [i.e. demonstrative argument], but we also add arguments (πίστεις) based on what evidently appears which are cogent and compelling'; and he proceeds to assert that we can both prove that parts of the body have a δύναμις καθεκτική and also in some cases directly perceive the ἐνέργεια of that δύναμις. Galen's argument is not wholly clear, and he is probably not committing himself to the view that certain evident truths are also demonstrable. At *nat. fac.* II 117, however, he states that he will prove certain things which the old doctors 'asserted without proof, as being evident (ἐναργῆ)'. When he repeats the statement at ibid. II 175 he makes it clear that the items which the old doctors took to be evident actually are evident: proof is required here only because 'shameless sophists' (i.e. Erasistratus and Asclepiades) determined to deny the evident facts. In *nat. fac.*, then, Galen holds that what is evident does not require proof but may be capable of proof—and if what is evident is nevertheless disputed and denied, then it will be appropriate to produce a proof for it. Plainly there are difficulties with such a view: as far as I know, no surviving text deals with them.

[66] Cf. e.g. *opt. doct.* I 50, 52; *const. med.* I 251; *pecc. dign.* V 94-95; *Hipp. Plat.* V 782; *meth. med.* X 50, 972.

[67] Cf. e.g. *opt. doct.* I 52; *Hipp. Plat.* V 241; *simp. med. temp.* XI 462; *inst. log.* xvi 6, 7; xvii 7.

[68] Cf. e.g. *elem. Hipp.* I 458; *pecc. dign.* V 98; *Thras.* V 811; *meth. med.* X 40, 50; and the passage from *dem.* quoted by Philoponus, *aet. mund.* 600.3-601.16: 'In considering whether it was correctly agreed by everyone that being ungenerated implies being indestructible, we have noticed both that it is an undemonstrable, primary and self-crediting axiom, and also that it is supported by another evident axiom which we said a little earlier ran like this: whatever in no way admits the formula of generation will not admit the formula of destruction either'.

[69] διαφωνία, a semi-technical term in Pyrrhonism: see Sextus, *PH* I 26, 165 (and passim).

that I had first to train in demonstrative methods' (*meth. med.* X 469). The methods ensure that science starts from universal agreement on first principles. Hence the disputes which had upset Galen, disputes which raged both between and within the sects,[70] will not arise in a properly constituted art.

Further, there are material conditions which axioms must satisfy. Some axioms are 'logical principles', and 'that the demonstration of every doctrine depends upon the logical principles has been exhibited by us in almost all our treatises' (*Hipp. Plat.* V 782).[71] But evidently logical axioms will not by themselves suffice for any scientific proof. A second class of principles consists of those appropriate to the science in question. Such principles will state the 'what it is' of something ('one must state precisely what disease is, what a symptom is, what an affection is ...': *meth. med.* X 27). Equivalently, they will state the 'nature' of the object; for 'the nature of the thing we are investigating will be a principle for discovery (we learned this in *Demonstrative Methods* [i.e. *dem.*])—what, then, is the nature of putrefaction?' (*meth. med.* X 753). Or again, the special axioms state the 'essence' (ousia) of the object: 'What is a scientific account?—Clearly one which proceeds from the essence of the thing, as has been demonstrated in the treatise *On Demonstration*' (*Hipp. Plat.* V 593).[72]

All that is conventional wisdom. Galen has adopted much of it from Aristotle, salting it with something from the Stoa.[73] But axioms of the two types so far mentioned will not by themselves generate any medically useful theorems; for they cannot produce anything but necessary truths about the properties of diseases and the like. What is needed is an injection of contingency: the science of medicine is essentially empirical, and its axioms must include matters of empirical fact.

---

[70] For internecine strife among the Methodists see *meth. med.* X 35, 38, 53, 125; *adv. Iul.* XVIIIA 269; among the Erasistrateans: *nat. fac.* II 93. The existence of διαφωνία is said to have turned many doctors away from methodical inquiry: *const. med.* I 243 (see also *temp.* I 583: *us. part.* III 17; *alim. fac.* VI 454; *syn. puls.* IX 443-444). See also *in Hipp. morb. acut.* XV 446-452, where Galen distinguishes serious διαφωνία which is found among the doctors from the purely eristic διαφωνία which is all he sees in Pyrrhonian disputes; and note that Galen wrote a work περὶ ἀνατομιχῆς διαφωνίας (e.g. *nat. fac.* II 182). Medicine is better placed than philosophy; for the διαφωνία of the philosophers often cannot be resolved by appeal to τὰ ἐναργῆ—in philosophy nothing is evident (*Hipp. Plat.* V 766; *in Hipp. morb. acut.* XV 434-435).

[71] As examples of logical axioms Galen cites: 'things equal to the same thing are equal to one another; if equals are subtracted from equals the remainders are equal; ... nothing occurs without a cause; everything comes from something existing; nothing comes from what is completely non-existent; of everything it is necessary either to affirm or to deny' (*meth. med.* X 36-37). The force of 'logical' in the phrase 'logical axiom' is roughly that of 'a priori'.

[72] Cf. *Hipp. Plat.* V 219 (ὁ τῆς οὐσίας λόγος); *meth med.* X 40, 84, 161, 174.

Galen recognizes the need. Our eyes and ears and other sense organs supply us, he holds, with further axiomatic material; for among the first principles of an empirical science will be propositions known by empirical observation. There is no end to the list of such principles from Galen's writings. One illustration must suffice. In *Hipp. Plat.* Galen promises 'to show how you may discover scientific assumptions from which you may construct a genuine demonstration' about the seat of the regent part (V 226). His discussion is rambling; but it is clear that careful observation is the way to discover the appropriate axioms, and that among the axioms are such propositions as 'unforced inhalation is produced by a different set of organs and muscles and nerves from those which produce forced inhalation' (ibid. V 234), and that 'if you strip the brain of its bones and then wound or crush any one of its cavities you will render the animal not only immediately voiceless and breathless but also wholly devoid of perception and incapable of performing any movement based on impulse' (ibid. V 238).[74] Propositions of that sort are not abundant in Aristotle's *Analytics*: Galen saw that the axiomatisation of a practical, empirical science required him to admit a class of practical, empirical first principles.

7. *Definitions*

Axioms of the second of Galen's three types are statements of essence. It is an elementary Aristotelian truth that statements of essence are definitions, and we should therefore expect Galen to regard definition as among the principles of any science. But in fact Galen's attitude to definitions is curious, and it deserves a brief digression.[75]

Frequently, Galen seems to regard definitions with an uncompromising hostility. Doctors who dispute over meanings, he says, 'depart from

---

[73] For Aristotle axioms are primary and non-demonstrable (e.g. *APst.* 71b27-28). Aristotle does not explicitly require them to be self-evident or agreed upon, but he holds that they must be 'more convincing' than anything that is inferred from them (and Galen ascribes to 'Aristotle and his followers' the thesis that axioms must be 'self-crediting': *in Hipp. morb. acut.* XV 550). For self-evidence see Speusippus, fr. 30 Lang = fr. 35 Isnardi Parente = fr. 73 Tarán (Proclus, *in Eucl.* 179); for agreement see Sextus, *PH* II 135, 143, *M* VIII 314 (a Stoic requirement). On Aristotelian axiomatics see J. Barnes, Aristotle's *Posterior Analytics* (Oxford, 1975), pp. 98-100; on Stoic axiomatics see J. Brunschwig, 'Proof Defined' and J. Barnes, 'Proof Destroyed', both in Doubt and Dogmatism (above, n. 42).

[74] In truth, it is not clear whether these complicated sentences themselves express axioms or rather give the material from which appropriate axioms may be extracted.

[75] The topic of definition belongs properly to a discussion of the method of division; but any account of the principles of demonstration must at least touch upon the subject. See below, p. 95.

the matter of medicine and take up an inquiry suitable for logicians[76] or grammarians or rhetoricians—it is a logician's task to consider the correctness of names' (*die. decr.* IX 789). Such a task is contemptible: 'as we always say, following the divine Plato,[77] one should despise names but not despise knowledge of the facts. For the latter is important for men's safety and a slip there ends in destruction; but whether we use names properly or improperly, our patients neither benefit nor suffer from the fact' (*meth. med.* X 772; cf. *anat. admin.* II 581; *sympt. diff.* VII 46; *diff. puls.* VIII 496). Hence 'we do not insist in the matter of nomenclature—neither in this treatise nor in any other of our medical treatises' (*meth. med.* X 459).

Time and again in *meth. med.* Galen insists that he does not insist in the matter of names—'you may call it Theo or Dio if you like'.[78] Indeed his insistence becomes as tiresome as the pedantry he rejects.[79] But Galen insists that the insistence is not trifling. Terminological jousting may take the place of genuine scientific enquiry, and then the patient suffers. The Methodists 'depart from the utility of the art and turn to logical investigation. For the utility consists in discovering aids by which the patient will be cured; but they abandon this and dispute about names, talking of indications and counterindications and commonalities and goals and materials of aids and the rest—they think that by the distinction of names they are defended from their false assertions' (*meth. med.* X 630).

One particular form which word-chopping frequently took was a manic devotion to definitions—'I think that some of them wouldn't even buy a cabbage without first defining it' (*diff. puls.* VIII 569). For this new phenomenon Galen invented a name: it is the disease of philoristia, definitionitis (ibid. VIII 698; cf. 764). Definitions are usually wasted labour. Why try to define the term 'pulse'?—It is clear to everyone what it means. 'When they stretch out their arms, offer their wrist and ask the doctor to feel their pulse, should we suppose that they are uttering the word "pulse" in the way they might say "scindapsos"[80] or rather that they produce the sound to signify some thing?' (ibid. VIII 696-697).

---

[76] διαλεκτικοῦ: for a similarly pejorative use of the adjective see e.g. *diff. puls.* VIII 571.

[77] Cf. *subf. emp.* 46.25; *diff. feb.* VII 354. Galen is not quoting Plato verbatim: for Platonic parallels see e.g. *Charm.* 163A, *Crat.* 440C, *Soph.* 218C, *Plt.* 261E. Elsewhere Galen ascribes the same view to Hippocrates: *nom. med.* 22.13-24.33 MS.

[78] Cf. *meth. med.* X 70, 81; *diff. puls.* VIII 496. See also *nom. med.* 10.9-12 MS: Galen says to those who persist in worrying about words 'This fever is Zeno', or 'Apollonius'.

[79] See e.g. *meth. med.* X 43-45, 50, 54-59, 139, 155, 975; cf. e.g. *opt. med.* I 62; *Hipp. Plat.* V 725; *morb. temp.* VII 427; esp. *diff. puls.* VIII 493-497.

[80] σκινδαφός is a stock nonsense-word: cf. e.g. *diff. feb.* VII 348; *nom. med.* 8.20, 32.28-31 MS; Sextus, *M* VIII 133.

Such disputes are sterile. And sufferers from definitionitis can do worse than that: the arguments they produce are verbal sophisms, tricks which depend on trivial linguistic manoeuvrings (*caus. procat.* vi 47).

'I wish I could learn and teach things without their names, in order that we might not be exercised, by way of surplus, by the fuss about language in addition to the demands which the art lays upon us because of the study appropriate to it' (*diff. puls.* VIII 493—the opening sentence of the work). But we cannot teach and learn without using words. Let us then avoid useless disputes about language. Galen will use ordinary Greek (e.g. *meth. med.* X 42);[81] his prose will not be rhetorical—he does not carry an ivory-handled sword or use mascara (*soph.* XIV 587); he will not object to an occasional barbarism or solecism (e.g. *meth. med.* X 43; *alim. fac.* VI 584-585); the only thing that matters is clarity—'we think that that man speaks most finely who is able to reveal most lucidly what he means' (*diff. puls.* VIII 567; cf. *meth med.* X 81; *nat. fac.* II 1; *inst. log.* iv 5).[82]

Galen's distaste for definitionitis was no doubt justified in practical terms: pedantry can be a sort of charlatanry, and it can also be a tedious waste of time.[83] Galen's fulminations are a busy man's response to other people's trivial games.

Yet Galen sometimes appears to play the game himself.[84] Thus in an interesting passage at *meth. med.* X 602-604 he argues against applying the term ephēmeros to a certain kind of fever: the name is inappropriate because the fever is not a day-long distemper—'the word ephēmeros does not belong to the essence of such fevers'.[85] Arbitrary stipulations may thus be inapposite and dispute about words is not always futile. Again, ordinary language may itself be misleading. Consider the 'anomaly of the names' of diseases (ibid. X 81): some diseases are named from the affected part, some from a symptom, some from an alleged cause, some

---

[81] Cf. *inst. log.* xvii 7: one of the two most important rules to observe 'when arguing for or proving anything' is 'to understand the signification of the words in accordance with the custom of the Greeks'. See also e.g. *sympt. diff.* VII 45-46; *diff. puls.* VIII 567; *nom. med.* 15.1-25 MS (which refers to *dem.*); and *caus. procat.* vi 55-56, where a sophist's quibbling paradox is alleged to rest upon an abuse of ordinary Greek. See also below, n. 129.

[82] On all this see esp. *nom. med.* (M. Meyerhof and J. Schacht, Galen: Ueber die medizinischen Namen, ABA 1931.3 (Berlin, 1931)). On Galen's attitude to language see esp. K. Deichgräber, Parabasenverse aus Thesmophoriazusen II des Aristophanes bei Galen, SBA 1956.2 (Berlin, 1956).

[83] Galen had himself been attacked by 'the sophists' for improper use of language: *diff. puls.* VIII 567, 589.

[84] The fact that the sophists dispute over names requires Galen to indulge in the same sport on occasion (esp. *diff. puls.* VIII 493-500, 566-590).

[85] On ἐφήμερος see H. Fränkel, 'ΕΦΗΜΕΡΟΣ als Kennwort für die menschliche Natur', in his Wege und Formen frühgriechischen Denkens (Munich, 1960²).

from a similarity, and so on. 'One who strives for the truth must attempt in every way to avoid the beliefs superadded to the names[86] and to attend to the essence of the things' (ibid. X 84). Pedantry has its point. (Modern readers will reflect on the old controversy over the nature of hysteria, where debate was fouled by a 'belief superadded to the name').

As for definitions, Galen can be found to say that 'in the case of every object of inquiry you should replace the name by the definition' (meth. med. X 39);[87] and in some cases at least the replacement is not a simple or insignificant operation.[88] Why does Galen criticise his colleagues for their love of definitions? They err, he alleges, first in asking for definitions where no definition is needed, secondly for supposing that everything whatever can be defined, and thirdly for misunderstanding the nature of definitions—for 'definitions are not of words but of things' (diff. puls. VIII 574; cf. 571). Definitions are necessary for scientific advance but not for buying cabbages—Galen's opponents insist on defining their greengroceries. Some terms are primitive and unanalysable, they cannot be defined—Galen's opponents waste time by attempting to analyse the unanalysable. Definitions are attempts to state the essence of a thing, not to state the meaning of a word—Galen's opponents treat arguments about definitions as an armchair occupation whereas in fact it is a serious scientific enterprise.

There is thus a philosophical point to Galen's reflexions upon definition. We may distinguish among a name ('phrenitis'), its purely verbal definition ('fever accompanied by delirium'), its denotation (diseases of that sort), and the essence of what it denotes (a scientific account—or a 'real' definition—of what phrenitis actually consists in). If we are investigating phrenitis, then it is of great importance, Galen holds, to grasp the denotation of the term 'phrenitis'—to be able to pick out cases of phrenitis; and it is of equally great importance to establish the essence of phrenitis—to discover what the disease consists in and to determine its 'real' definition. As for the verbal definition of 'phrenitis', that is of no scientific significance, and disputes about it are trifling. All this is at bottom Aristotelian, and it also has some affinity to a referential theory of

---

[86] τὸ προσδοξαζόμενον τοῖς ὀνόμασιν: the need to avoid 'superadded beliefs', προσδοξαζόμενα, is a cardinal point of Epicurean epistemology (see Epicurus, ad Hdt. 50; Lucretius IV 465, 816). The notion is also found in the Pyrrhonian tradition (see Sextus, PH I 30; III 236; M VI 20).

[87] The point had been explained in dem.; see also meth. med. X 149-151.

[88] For examples see e.g. pecc. dign. V 58-59 (on ἁμάρτημα); opt. doct. I 42 (κατάληψις); temp. I 552 (θερμόν, ψυχρόν, ξηρόν, ὑγρόν); Hipp. Plat. V 274-275 (καρδία); nat. fac. II 2-3 (κίνησις); Thras. V 867-876 (ἰατρική, γυμναστική—the whole of Thras. is in effect a discussion of terminology, as Galen himself from time to time admits; but the discussion is neither trifling nor simple).

the meaning of general scientific terms. According to a theory of that type it is a mistake to try to produce some complex phrase synonymous with the term in question: instead of looking for a verbal definition, we should recognize that grasping the sense of the term 'phrenitis', say, is a matter of understanding its reference, of seeing that 'phrenitical' is true of a man just in case he is in a condition of that sort. And having thus grasped the sense of the term, we may proceed at once to a scientific investigation of the nature of phrenitis. In the light of such thoughts, Galen's objections to definitionitis may seem to be something more than intelligent reminders of the fatuity of terminological disputations.

8. *Knowledge of First Principles*

How are the axioms to be discovered? How shall we tell, of a putative first principle, first whether it is a truth and secondly whether it is a primary truth? 'The old philosophers say that there are two kinds of phenomena, first, those which are discerned by one of the senses ..., then those that impress the thought with a primary and non-demonstrable impact' (*meth. med.* X 36).[89] Thus 'the principles of every demonstration are things evident to perception and to thought' (*temp.* I 590).[90] Some principles, then, we grasp directly by thought (these must include the logical axioms and presumably at least some statements of essence); others are given to us by sense-perception. It is worth noting that Galen has no time for induction: 'we have proved in our work *On Demonstration* that inductions are not to be used for scientific demonstrations' (*Thras.* V 812).[91] Induction is logically disreputable (for familiar reasons); it is also epistemologically superfluous. For perception gives us general truths and not merely truths about the individual objects which on any particular occasion we happen to observe. We grasp 'common forms' in perception—as do all percipient creatures; for even a donkey, when it looks at its donkey-driver, recognizes him in one way as Dio, in another as a man (*meth. med.* X 134). The common form, and with it generality, is directly given in perception. Induction is otiose.

We must admit that we possess certain natural criteria for determining the truth about things (*Hipp. Plat.* V 723; *opt. doct.* I 48). It is evident that

---

[89] The distinction is a commonplace of Hellenistic philosophy: see e.g. Sextus, *M* VII 25. It represents, within the sphere of τὰ ἐναργῆ, the distinction (going back at least to Plato, *Rep.* 507B) between αἰσθητά and νοητά; it was perhaps first codified by Theophrastus (see Sextus, *M* VII 218 = Theophrastus, fr. 27 Wimmer).

[90] Cf. *meth. med.* X 39, which refers to *dem.*; *alim. fac.* VI 454.

[91] Cf. *sem.* IV 581; *simp. med. temp.* XI 469-471; *in Hipp. off. med.* XVIIB 909 (referring to Galen's works *On Example* and *On Induction*—cf. *lib. prop.* XIX 43).

this is so (*opt. doct.* l.c.). 'I say that you all possess natural criteria, and in so saying I am reminding you, not teaching or demonstrating—nor stating it on my own authority' (*Hipp. Plat.* l.c.). What are these criteria? They are, of course, first, our sense organs by means of which, when they are in their natural condition, we apprehend things evident to perception; and secondly 'the mind or the intelligence or whatever anyone likes to call it, by which we distinguish the consistent and the inconsistent and other things which belong to them, including division and collection, similarity and dissimilarity' (*Hipp. Plat.* l.c.). These natural criteria are 'creditable without demonstration' (*Hipp. Plat.* V 778). We may indeed refuse to credit them, but we cannot judge or assess them, for they are themselves the ultimate standards for assessing everything (*opt. doct.* I 49). Thus 'I judge objects of perception by what appears evidently to perception, objects of thought by what is grasped evidently in thought' (ibid.); and starting from 'what appears of itself and evidently to perception or to thought' (ibid. I 50), we proceed down 'the straight path of demonstration' (ibid. I 51).

The criteria are natural, but their employment requires more than a merely passive waiting for things to strike us. The doctor must seek out perceptions. Indeed—and this is a point on which Galen insists—he will often have to perform dissections in order that the evident facts may reveal themselves to him (e.g. *Hipp. Plat.* V 233-239, 263-264).[92] Moreover, our natural criteria must themselves be in good order. Your eyes may be sharper than mine, and my intellect may be keener than yours (*opt. doct.* I 52). We must not simply accept our perceptual and intellectual apparatus as we find it: we must train it (e.g. *temp.* I 597) and hone it to a fine acuity. Sometimes—notably in connexion with the sense of touch—that training may take a lifetime (*dign. puls.* VIII 767-773).[93]

It is clear, then, that men may not recognise what is evident as being evident. 'We must begin from something primary that is agreed upon by all men, and thence proceed to the rest; but most men choose principles which are disputed and then proceed without proof to the rest in the same way' (*meth. med.* X 32). Men rashly assent to what is non-evident: 'we must first show that genuinely evident things can never conflict with one another, and then learn to distinguish what is evident from what is not' (*pecc. dign.* V 44-45).[94] 'There are many falsities which resemble truths

---

[92] See M. Vegetti, 'Modelli di Medicina in Galeno', in Nutton, o.c. n. 7, at p. 49.

[93] Note that the sense of touch provides 'the primary items and as it were elements of the art involved in pulses, and if they are unknown nothing else can be firmly known' (*dign. puls.* VIII 771; cf. 776). On this passage see Deichgräber, o.c. n. 46, pp. 6-16.

[94] Just as we must distinguish true principles from apparent principles, so we must distinguish genuine from apparent proofs (*pecc. dign.* V 78). But that, philosophically speaking, is a much less formidable task.

among the principles of demonstrations', and only trained minds can
distinguish them (*Hipp. Plat.* V 782; cf. 796).[95] Moreover, 'false opinions, when they pre-occupy men's souls, make them not only deaf but
also blind to what other men see evidently' (*comp. med. loc.* XIII 117—
Galen has the Methodists in mind). 'Evident perception and thought' is
not a phrase denoting quick or casual or unthinking apprehension; in
fact, Galen suggests that it is synonymous with the 'apprehensive presentation' of the Stoics and with the 'persuasive and examined and
unmovable presentation' of the New Academy (ibid. V 778).[96]

Galen's epistemology has some original touches (the emphasis on
training is the most striking) but in essence it is traditional. It is also, as
Galen well knew, controversial. Galen speaks earnestly of 'training' our
natural faculties, and he supposes that those with 'trained' faculties will
be able to discriminate genuine from apparent axioms. He does not
explain how or by what process our faculties are to be trained; he does
not explain how a trained mind can be recognized as such, by itself or
by others; he does not explain how or by what marks a genuine grasp of
a genuine axiom is distinguished from a spurious grasp of a spurious
axiom. More generally, he does not take seriously the battery of
arguments which the Greek sceptics, Pyrrhonian and Academic, had
fired against the Stoic idea of 'apprehensive presentation'.

Moreover, there seem to be internal conflicts within Galen's account.
He insists, for example, on the need for careful and practised observation; yet he also says that 'if anything fails to come into our apprehension at a single onset, it is thereby definitely disputed, it requires demonstration, and no art ought to begin from such a thing' (*meth. med.* X 38). The
axioms must be accepted at first impression—yet they are also the
product of trained reflexion. Or again, the axioms must be universally
agreed upon. But 'remember this throughout the whole argument, that
we shall interpret our words in accordance with Greek habits, as was said
in our work *On Demonstration*, but the discoveries and inquiries and
demonstrations of the essence of the objects will depend not on what is

---

[95] Some argue that the brain is the seat of the regent part because it is located near
to the sense-organs. They rely on the proposition that 'the first principle in the case of
everything that has a function depends on something near to it'. But that proposition 'is
evident neither to perception nor to thought ... in such a way as to be primary and self-
creditable'. Hence the argument is no demonstration, even though its conclusion is true.
See *Hipp. Plat.* V 241. Contrast *Hipp. Plat.* V 797-798: Plato, in his proof of the triparti-
tion of the soul, uses the principle that 'the same thing cannot do or suffer opposites in
the same respect at the same time' (see *Rep.* 436B). That, Galen says, is an axiom, it
is 'something evident to thought'; but yet it is not 'clear to everyone', as Plato himself
recognises.

[96] For the Stoic φαντασία καταληπτική see e.g. Sextus, *M* VII 248; for the Academic
notion, ibid. VII 166.

believed by most men but on scientific assumptions' (*meth. med.* X 42).[97] The first principles are to be agreed upon by all men—yet they are not to be the opinions of most men.

Criticisms of that sort can be multiplied. Some of them are given an answer in parts of Galen's surviving corpus; others, no doubt, were considered at length in *On Demonstration*. But to the fundamental questions of the Sceptic Galen made, I suspect, no serious reply.[98] He was familiar with the work of the Pyrrhonists and the Sceptical Academics; he was equally aware of the replies of the 'Dogmatic' philosophers. Perhaps he believed that the Dogmatists had adequately answered the sceptical challenge and that he had no need to repeat their retorts. But in any case he plainly thought that the extreme Pyrrhonists were not worth taking seriously;[99] and he probably subscribed to the sensible view—a view shared by Ptolemy[100]—that the problems of scepticism were of no concern to a scientist whose business it was not to defend the possibility of knowledge but to describe the foundations upon which his science was constructed.[101]

9. Galen's Use of Deduction — (i) Negative

So much for Galen's theorizing about logic and the demonstrative method. What of his practice? Did he chop logic at his bedside consultations? Do his medical treatises stink of logic? Or is it the case with Galen, as with so many methodological gurus, that he did not himself follow the course he prescribed for others? Those questions are pressing, but they are not readily answered. Of Galen's clinical practice we know very little,[102] and we cannot determine by direct means whether or not he

---

[97] The same distinction is made by Aristotle, *Top.* 110a16-19, 148b20-23.

[98] In *opt. doct.* Galen attacks the sceptical views of Favorinus; but his attack is directed towards an alleged incoherence in Favorinus' special brand of scepticism—it does not attack Pyrrhonism in general.

[99] See esp. *diff. puls.* VIII 780-786; and note the dismissive references to ἀγροικοπυρρώνειοι at ibid. VIII 711, *praecogn.* XIV 628 (cf. *temp.* I 589; *art. sang.* IV 727: the Erasistrateans seek asylum in Πυρρωνεία ἀγροικία as though in a shrine). Galen was not a Sceptic; but he certainly had a sceptical cast of mind—he was sceptical in the sense in which all wise men are sceptical. See Frede, o.c. n. 10, pp. 68-69.

[100] See G.E.R. Lloyd, 'Observational Error in Later Greek Science', in Science and Speculation (above n. 27), at pp. 159-164. For some remarks on the connexions between Galen and Ptolemy see P. Manuli, 'Claudio Tolemeo: Il Criterio e il Principio', *Rivista critica di storia della filosofia* 1980, 2-26, at pp. 2-12.

[101] Cf. *simp. med. temp.* XI 462: sceptics of the senses merely suffer from an excess of melancholy—'for if they overthrow what appears evidently through the senses, they will have nowhere to begin their proofs from'. (The point is Epicurean: Lucretius, IV 469-485).

[102] The various case histories which Galen describes are the closest we can come to knowledge of his bedside practice. But such histories cannot be regarded as faithful

employed the artifices of the demonstrative method in his treatments of particular patients. In the case of Galen' treatises an opposite difficulty raises itself: Galen's extant works are formidably extensive, and a serious answer to the question of method would require long labours and a large volume. Here I shall do no more than adduce a few illustrative passages.[103]

First, let us consider the deductive aspect of the demonstrative method, and ask to what extent formal techniques of deduction figure in or stand behind Galen's writings. We should not expect too much here. Galen never uses symbolic logic in his treatises, and he rarely sets arguments out in a formal fashion. (He does not for example, normally number the premises of an argument, or indicate which rules of inference he is invoking). That is not surprising: an argument may be rigorous without being formally expressed, a piece of reasoning may depend upon self-consciously logical reflexion without displaying any technical logic in its finished shape. Formal reasoning is the scaffolding with whose aid a ratiocinator erects his tower of argument; when the tower is completed, the scaffolding is removed. If no logic is visible, it does not follow that no logic was vital. In any case, Galen himself remarks that demonstra-

---

reports of Galen's actual bedside cogitations. Note, however, Galen's account of his treatment of Eudemus, *praecogn.* XIV 606-619. At the end, Eudemus congratulates Galen on his prognosis: 'you have reasoned out logically (διαλεκτικῶς) the discovery of what will happen' (ibid. XIV 618). Compare Galen's treatment of Menander the orator (*caus. procat.* ii 11-iii 22) who had the ability to follow and assess the arguments of his doctors (ibid. ii 16).

[103] There are two general issues which I should like to have investigated. In each case the lack of scholarly tools (notably an index verborum to Galen) hampers research. First, Galen's writings span half a century and cover a wide range of topics. Did Galen's use of logic vary from one subject to another—from therapy to anatomy, from general physiology to detailed hygienics? (On this see Vegetti, in Nutton, o.c. n. 7: he distinguishes two opposing tendencies in Galen's thought—a 'high' medicine, marked by proof and an interest in theory and connected with anatomy and with Alexandrian medicine, and a 'low' medicine, marked by division and an interest in clinical practice and connected with the theory of the humours and Hippocratic medicine. I am unconvinced by all of Vegetti's story; on the topic of proof, I think it can be shown, especially from *meth. med.*, that Galen regarded the possibility of demonstrative proof as of prime importance to clinical practice). Again, did Galen's use of logic develop or change in the course of his long career? (Indeed, did his ideas about logic itself undergo development?) Genetic studies (which have bedevilled Aristotelian scholarship for the last sixty years) might produce exciting results in the case of Galen.—Secondly, it would be good to have a thorough investigation of Galen's literary technique—of his vocabulary, his syntax, his style. (And genetic research would not be out of place here either). An author's logical inclinations are generally revealed in his language, both in particularities of wording (technical terminology, grammatico-logical structure, etc.) and in his general tone or style (clarity of sentence-structure, attention to the articulation of arguments, etc.). Many passages of Galen's writings strike me as splendid examples of logical prose—but vague impressions of that sort are no substitute for precise investigation.

tions are generally simple—or at any rate, short.[104] And the simpler the reasoning the less need to leave it exposed on the surface of the text.

There are, however, a few paragraphs in which Galen's deductive expertise is explicitly displayed.

My first two examples are negative—Galen uses the arcana of formal logic in criticism of his opponents. In *simp. med. temp.* Galen devotes some time to the views of 'those doctors who begin their demonstrations from too great a distance' (XI 463)—who try to prove the powers of drugs from their colours or their smells or the like. Such doctors, he adds, often compound their errors: 'being untaught in demonstrative method, they talk inconclusive and non-demonstrative nonsense' (ibid. XI 465). For example, they argue that 'roses are hot because they are red'. They take as their assumption:

(1) Every fire is red

Galen grants them that; but what use is it to them? It would be ridiculous to infer that:

(2) Everything red is fire

still more ridiculous to infer that:

(3) Everything red is hot

Yet they wish to move, with the help of a second premiss, namely:

(4) Every rose is red

to the conclusion that:

(5) Every rose is hot[105]

And to get to that conclusion they require proposition (3). Perhaps, then, we might suppose that they meant to assume not (1) but:

(6) Everything hot is red

In that case 'they might perhaps have converted the axiom'[106] and so inferred proposition (3). But had they done so, then they would have

---

[104] See *Hipp. Plat.* V 655: the 'true account' of the site of the regent part can be given in a demonstration of '39 syllables—two and a half hexameters'; a second proof is longer—the equivalent of five hexameters. Logical complexity is not the same as length; but a short argument is unlikely to contain many complex logical moves—see further, below p. 87 f. and 92.

[105] The question was disputed among the doctors (*temp.* I 685); cf. *inst. log.* ii 1, where "rosewater heats" and "we are naturally heated by rosewater" are cited as illustrative propositions.

[106] Reading ἀναστρέψαντα (διαστρέψαντα, Kühn).

committed an elementary logical error; 'for it is contrapositives, not mutually converse propositions, which are true together'.

Galen had explained the logical distinction between contraposition (antistrophē) and conversion (anastrophē) 'in the logical methods' (see *simp. med. temp.*XI 500).[107] The operations apply both to universal categorical propositions ('Every A is B') and to conditional propositions ('If p, then q'). Take such propositions:

Every A is B   If p, then q

To apply contraposition you reverse the order of the terms and at the same time negate them:

Every non-B is non-A   If not-q, then not-p

To apply conversion you merely reverse the order of terms:

Every B is A   If q, then p

Plainly, contraposed statements 'are true together' while converted statements are not. (In saying that they 'are true together', Galen means that 'statements contraposed to true statements are themselves true' (*simp. med. temp.* XI 466): if X is the contrapositive of Y, and is true, then X is true).

Galen's victims thus commit two logical errors.[108] First, they state as an assumption a proposition which is inappropriate in its content (proposition (1) does not contain the relevant terms, for it refers to fire and not to hot things in general). Secondly, they assume a proposition which is inappropriate in its form (proposition (6) has the right content but it has the same form as (1)—and that form is logically inappropriate to the argument). Their inference is only intelligible on two assumptions: first, that they confuse (1) with (6); secondly, that they think they can infer (3) from (6). The second assumption betrays their ignorance of formal logic:

---

[107] Cf. *inst. log.* vi 3-4: categorical propositions 'convert by the interchange of the wording of the terms, i.e. when the subject becomes predicate and the predicate subject; they contrapose when, along with this interchange, they are true together ... In hypothetical propositions conversion occurs when the wording of the terms is intersubstituted, contraposition with their opposition' (i.e. contraposition occurs when intersubstitution is accompanied by exchanging each proposition for its contradictory opposite). That is not wholly satisfactory—but its inadequacy does not affect Galen's point in *simp. med. temp.*

[108] Galen actually says that they make three errors. The second and third are those I describe. The first appears like this in Kühn: πρῶτον μὲν ὅτι μὴ δείξαντες ὅτι πᾶν πῦρ ἐρυθρὸν ἀντιστρέφειν αὐτῷ, ὅτι πᾶν ἐρυθρὸν πῦρ πειρῶνται λόγον ἕτερον, ὡς ἀληθῆ (XI 466). That is nonsense: it is not clear to what error Galen is alluding, and I do not know how to emend the text. (Jim Hankinson has suggested to me that Galen imagines that his opponents, as an alternative to inferring (2) from (1), might unwarrantably assume (2) without argument).

they do not realize that contraposition and conversion are different operations.

A few pages later, Galen discusses a similar argument. Olive oil, he claims, is not pungent; even if we allow that oil produces hoarseness in the throat, it cannot be inferred that oil is pungent. For although it is true that:

(1) Everything pungent produces hoarseness

it is false that:

(2) Everything that produces hoarseness is pungent

Now Galen's opponents assume that:

(3) Oil produces hoarseness

and hope to conclude that:

(4) Oil is pungent

But they can reach that conclusion only if they use not (1) but (2). Galen's opponents thus tacitly infer (2) from (1): 'so here again comes the error based on conversion' (*simp. med. temp.* XI 499).[109]

Now Galen adds something new: the inference to (4) is invalid 'whether we make the premiss categorical or hypothetical—for nothing follows in the second figure from two universal affirmatives, and the conditional is not true of necessity'. If we express (1) and (3) in categorical form, then the two propositions take the form 'Every A is B, Every C is B'—and from such a pair of propositions (as Aristotle proves at *Prior Analytics* 27a 18-20) nothing whatever follows about the relation between A and C.

Suppose, then, that we express (1) and (3) in hypothetical form: 'If anything is *A*, it is *B*'. Then 'the hypothetical proposition—which Chrysippus and his followers call a conditional statement—is something we cannot assume as true either on the basis of perception or on the basis of logical implication. For such statements cannot be grasped through perception (or by perception or however you like to put it) ...'. At this point the published text degenerates into absurdity.[110] The conditional which Galen is talking about must be the complex proposition:

If (1) and (3), then (4)

---

[109] τὴν ἀναστροφὴν τοῦ συνημμένου (Kühn): proposition (1) is not, strictly speaking, a conditional, and perhaps we should excise τοῦ συνημμένου.

[110] I suggest: ... τὰ τοιαῦτα τῶν ἀξιωμάτων [πᾶν τὸ δακνῶδες καὶ χερχνῶδές ἐστι καὶ εἰ τι δακνῶδες τοῦτο καὶ χερχνῶδές ἐστι] ⟨...⟩ οὔτ' εἰ πᾶν τὸ δακνῶδες κτλ. (XI 499). The excised clause is a gloss explaining the difference between categorical and hypothetical propositions. The lacuna will have contained words to the following effect: 'nor can the conditional in question be proved by logic. Now if you converted proposition (1), you could infer (4). But'.

For Galen wants to show that, in Stoic no less than in Peripatetic logic, the argument from (1) and (3) to (4) is invalid; and the Stoics held that an argument is valid just in case the corresponding conditional proposition is true. (Corresponding to any argument is a conditional proposition in which the antecedent is the conjunction of the argument's premisses and the consequent is the argument's conclusion. Thus 'A1, A2, ... An: therefore B' is valid just in case 'If A1 and A2 and ... An, then B' is true).[111] Galen states that such complex conditionals cannot be grasped on the basis of perception. No doubt he went on to say that the conditional in question cannot be shown to be true by logical means either.

When the text recovers intelligibility, Galen is discussing contraposition and conversion. He presumably pointed out that neither in categorical nor in hypotetical form can (2) be deduced from (1): if you suppose that it can be, you are confusing contraposition and conversion.

Galen's diagnosis may seem tiresomely pedantic. But it is exact, and Galen shows clearly how attention to elementary logic will enable a doctor to avoid errors in his practice—errors which are potentially disastrous for his patients.[112]

10. *Galen's Use of Deduction—(ii) Positive*

For positive instances of Galen's use of deductive technique let us turn first to *Hipp. Plat.*. In two pages of that treatise Galen constructs six illustrative demonstrations in order to show how easily those who are skilled in logic can produce medical proofs.[113] The first illustration is clear: 'where the beginning of the nerves is, there is the regent part; the beginning of the nerves is in the brain; therefore the regent part is there' (V 655). The general form of the argument is this:

---

[111] For this Stoic thesis see Sextus, *M* VIII 415-417; cf. *PH* II 113, 137.

[112] At *nat. fac.* II 75 Galen reports that, according to Erasistratus, 'it is absolutely true that if anything flows from the veins, then one of two things—either there will be a wholly empty space or the neighbouring matter will flow in and fill the place of what is being evacuated'. Since the former is impossible (nature abhors a vacuum), the latter must be the case. Asclepiades objected to Erasistratus' argument: there are not two possibilities but three—the veins might contract or collapse. Later on (ibid. II 106) Galen reverts to Erasistratus' argument. 'The disjunction which he assumes for his proof should in truth be a disjunction not of two but of three items. If we employ it as a disjunction of two items, one of the premisses of the proof will be false; if as of three, the argument will be invalid'. Here Galen uses the terminology of Stoic logic; and he surely has in mind the Stoic classification of bad arguments—for he in effect accuses Erasistratus of the error the Stoics called ἔλλειψις (see Sextus, *PH* II 146, 150; *M* VIII 429, 434). Asclepiades saw that Erasistratus' argument would not do even though he was 'ignorant of logical study'(*us. part.* III 467; cf. 472, 473, 475): Galen called upon his knowledge of logical theory to show why it would not do.

[113] For some discussion of the physiological subject matter see I. M. Lonie, 'Erasistratus, the Erasistrateans, and Aristotle', *Bull. Hist. Med.* 38 (1964) 426-443.

Take anything you like, if it is A it is B
But X is A
Therefore: X is B

That is elementary. Galen's second argument has precisely the same logical form (ib. V 655). The third argument is slightly more complicated. It appears to have three premisses: Those veins are thickest which grow from their source; the veins are instruments of the nutritive power in us; the largest vein grows from the liver.[114] 'From that it was concluded that the liver is the source of the veins, from which again it followed that this organ is the source of the power we have in common with the plants' (ibid. V 657). That argument is best represented as follows:

(1) What the thickest vein grows from is the source of the veins
(2) The thickest vein grows from the liver
Therefore: (3) The liver is the source of the veins
(4) The veins are instruments of the nutritive power
(5) Whatever is the source of the instrument of anything is the source of that thing
Therefore (6) The liver is the source of the nutritive power.

The inference to (3) has the form we are already familiar with. The inference to (6) is a little more complicated (particularly as Galen expects us to supply premiss (5) which he does not state); but it is easy to see that it is formally valid—and Galen may well have regarded it as merely a variant of the form already used.[115]

---

[114] It is not clear from the text exactly what—or indeed how many—the premisses are. The antecedent of ὧν in ἐξ ὧν ἐπεραίνετο is obscure; nor does reference to the earlier, discursive, treatment of the argument provide any help. My first premiss is intended to represent what Galen refers to when he says: τοῦτο μὲν ἓν λῆμμα δι' ἐναργῶν ἀπεδείχθη (p. 486.20 de Lacy). The text at p. 486.17-20 is uncertain, and it is not clear what the ἐναργῆ are. But I think that the λῆμμα must be as I represent it. (Note that the first premiss to the argument is itself a conclusion from a previous argument which rested upon evident principles). The second premiss is clear enough (δεύτερον δέ ...: p. 486.21). The third premiss I read into p. 486.25, αὖθις δέ. That requires an emendation at p. 486.24 (omit μέν after ἁπασῶν—de Lacy retains μέν, but translates as though he had omitted it). There may be other ways of analysing this argument, but I doubt if they would be formally different from the way I suggest.

[115] In standard modern dress, the inference to (3) has the form

$$(\forall x)\ (Fx \supset Gx),\ Fa \vdash Ga$$

The inference to (6) has the form:

$$(\forall x)(\forall y)(\forall z)(Fxy \wedge Gyz \supset Fxz),\ Fab,\ Gbc \vdash Fac$$

It is possible to 'generate' the second form from the first: take the first form; replace 'Fx' by a conjunction (and, correspondingly, 'Fa' by a pair of premisses); replace the monadic

The remaining arguments have the same conclusion as the third argument. The fourth adds nothing new; the sixth appears to rest on a frail analogy. Here is the fifth argument. 'If we suppose that the right ventricle of the heart is the source of the vena cava, that will be contrary to what is observed and discovered in the dissections of fish. For in none of them does the heart possess a right ventricle, since those animals do not have lungs—and I have shown in the treatise *On the Use of Parts* why the right ventricle of the heart is both produced and destroyed along with the lungs' (ibid. V 658-659).

Since the argument is designed to prove that the source of the veins is in the liver, we must assume that Galen is implicitly presupposing a disjunctive premiss:[116]

(1) The source of the veins in animals is either the liver or the right ventricle of the heart

The form of the argument is, in part, a reductio ad absurdum; for Galen begins by making a hypothesis, viz:

(2) The source of the veins in animals is the right ventricle of the heart

He then takes it as theorem[117] that:

(3) Animals have right ventricles to their hearts if and only if they have lungs

But we know by observation that:

(4) Fish have no lungs

No doubt we also learn by observation (see *Hipp. Plat.* V 541) that:

(5) Fish have veins

From (3) and (4) we can infer that fish have no right ventricles to their hearts. But from (2) and (5) it follows that fish do have right ventricles. That is impossible; hence, by reductio, we reject hypothesis (2). But the

---

predicates by dyadic predicates. Hence the second form is, in a sense, a 'variant' of the first. Note that the 'variant' introduces relations (in particular, the relations expressed by '... is a source of ...' and '... is an instrument of ...'). The remaining three proofs also use relational terms. It is tempting to suppose that Galen is conscious of the fact and is deliberately choosing proofs which use his 'third kind' of syllogism (above, p. 69). But there is no explicit recognition of this fact in Galen's text. Nor have I come across any passage in which Galen expressly adverts to an employment of relational syllogistic.

[116] For the disjunction see *Hipp. Plat.* V 522, where the discursive treatment of the argument begins.

[117] It is not entirely clear whether (3) is part of the proof. Galen may mean that we observe directly that fish have no right ventricles—(3) is part of the explanation of why this is so, not part of an argument to show that it is so.

negation of (2), together with (1), entails the desired conclusion: the liver is the source of the veins.

That argument involves more steps and more types of inference than the other arguments in the passage, but it is not excessively complicated.[118] Galen does not handle it well. Granted, he is here summarizing a train of reasoning which he had earlier expounded at much greater length; but the sole purpose of the summary is to illustrate demonstrative technique. Galen does not explicitly state premiss (1); he omits premiss (5); he does not explain how the conclusion is to be inferred from the

---

[118] It is instructive (in more than one respect) to try to present Galen's argument in standard modern dress. Abbreviations: 'A (ξ)' for 'ξ is a (kind of) animal'; 'V (ξ, ζ)' for 'ξ is a vein of ζ'; 'L(ξ,ζ)' for 'ξ is a liver of ζ'; 'S(ξ,ζ)' for 'ξ is source of ζ'; 'H(ξ,ζ)' for 'ξ is the right ventricle of the heart of ζ'; 'G(ξ,ζ) for 'ξ is a lung of ζ'; 'f' for 'fish':

1	(1)	$[(\forall x)(\forall y)(Ax \wedge Vyx) \supset (\exists z)(Lzx \wedge Szy))]$	
		$v\ [(\forall x)(\forall y)(Ax \wedge Vyx) \supset (\exists w)(Hwx \wedge Swy))]$	Ass
2	(2)	$(\forall x)(Ax \supset)(\exists w)Hwx \equiv (\exists u)Gux)$	Ass
3	(3)	Af	Ass
4	(4)	$—(\exists u)Guf$	Ass
5	(5)	$(\exists y)Vyf$	Ass
6	(6)	$(\forall x)(\forall y)((Ax \wedge Vyx) \supset (\exists w)(Hwx \wedge Swy))$	Ass
6	(7)	$(Af \wedge Vbf) \supset (\exists w)(Hwf \wedge Swb)$	by 6
8	(8)	Vbf	Ass
3,6,8	(9)	$(\exists w)(Hwf \wedge Swb)$	by 3,6,7
3,6,8	(10)	$(\exists w)Hwf$	by 9
2	(11)	$Af \supset ((\exists w)Hwf \equiv (\exists u)Guf)$	by 2
2,3	(12)	$(\exists w)\ Hwf \equiv (\exists u)Guf$	by 3,11
2,3,6,8	(13)	$(\exists u)Guf$	by 10,12
2,3,4,6,8	(14)	$(\exists u)Guf \wedge —(\exists u)Guf$	by 4,13
2,3,4,5,6	(15)	$(\exists u)Guf \wedge —(\exists u)Guf$	from 5,8,14 by EE
2,3,4,5	(16)	$—[(\forall x)(\forall y)((Ax \wedge Vyx) \supset (\exists w)(Hwx \wedge Swy))]$	reductio
1,2,3,4,5	(17)	$(\forall x)(\forall y)((Ax \wedge Vyx) \supset (\exists z)(Lzx \wedge Szy))$	by 1,16

Here (1) is Galen's (1), (2) is his (3), (4) is his (4), (5) is his (5). I add (3), the trivial supposition that fish are animals. Line (6) represents Galen's (2), the ὑπόθεσις. The conclusion, (17), represents Galen's theorem that the source of the veins is the liver.

I do not suggest that this formal argument represents Galen's train of thought. Rather, my suggestion is this: had Galen attempted to set out his argument rigorously, using the formal logic which he expounded in *inst. log.* (and, presumably, in *dem.*), then he would have arrived at something roughly analogous, in length and complexity, to my formal argument. I say in the text that Galen's arguments are not excessively complicated. But surely (1) - (17) is pretty complicated? In a sense it is; but the complexity arises wholly from the conceptual complexity of the constituent propositions of the argument, and not from any esoteric principles of inference nor from the length of the argument. The conceptual density, if I may so put it, is brought out by my 'translation' of Galen's premisses: they are, from the point of view of their logical syntax, highly complex in structure. (Compare them to the standard illustrative sentences of ancient logic: 'It is day'; 'All men are mortal').

premisses. In this passage if anywhere we should expect precision and lucidity from Galen: we do not find it.[119]

In the six exemplary demonstrations in *Hipp. Plat.* Galen does not expressly advert to the logical form of his deductions. He presents deductions but he does not comment on them from a logical point of view. I cite, finally, a passage in which such an adversion is made. 'I want, while I am on this argument, to bring to mind a certain logical theorem which was exhibited in the essays *On Demonstration* and which is useful in the present context' (*simp. med. temp.* XI 613). The context is a discussion of the 'attractive' powers of drugs. Galen has presented the general theorem, proved elsewhere, that 'most attractions occur when there is a relatedness of qualities' (ibid. XI 611), i.e. that if A attracts B then A and B have something in common. He infers the specific theorem that 'purgative drugs are related to the humours that they attract' (ibid. XI 612). Hence 'we may expect that knēkos is phlegm-like ... and similarly for the Cnidian kokkos'. For knēkos and kokkos are purgative drugs which 'attract' phlegm.

It is at this point that Galen introduces the logical theorem. 'The theorem', he says, 'is this. Of demonstrations, some conclude that one thing belongs of necessity to another, others that it may possibly belong. But of the latter, some translate[120] into belonging of necessity when they follow necessary principles—as in the case just demonstrated by us. For the phlegmatic humour contained in kokkos and knēkos cannot be shown evidently, but belongs possibly and probably and contingently ...' (ibid. XI 613).

At first blush, Galen's theorem appears remarkable. You may have a proof, he says, which establishes that it is possible that so-and-so should be the case; and yet that conclusion may 'translate', under certain circumstances, into the conclusion of a proof that it is necessary for so-and-so to be the case. The possible can be translated into the necessary.

On closer inspection Galen's theorem turns out to be less remarkable. His statement of the theorem is not lucid, but he must surely have the following possibility in mind. There may be two distinct proofs, each concluding to the same proposition. Given the first proof, all we can say of the proposition is that it is possible or probable. Yet by considering the second proof we may go further and say that the proposition is necessary;

---

[119] The criticism is not new: Al-Farabi accused Galen of poor logic in these arguments—see F. W. Zimmermann, 'Al-Farabi und die philosophische Kritik an Galen', in A. Dietrich (ed.), Akten des VII. Kongresses für Arabistik und Islamwissenschaft, Abh. Akad. Wiss. Göttingen, phil.-hist. Kl. 3.98 (Göttingen, 1976), at pp. 410-412.

[120] μεταπίπτουσι : μεταπίπτειν is a technical term in Stoic logic (see M. Frede, Die stoische Logik (Göttingen, 1974), pp. 44-48). But I have found no Stoic parallel to the Galen passage, and Galen is probably using the verb μεταπίπτειν in a non-technical sense.

for in the second proof it follows from necessary principles.[121] It is indeed true that there may be pairs of proofs of that sort: Galen's 'logical theorem' does not perform the metaphysical conjuring trick of transforming the possible into the necessary—it makes the less exciting, but true, observation that what is proved possible by one argument may be proved necessary by another.

How does the theorem apply to the case of knēkos and kokkos? Galen's argument, fully articulated, runs thus:

(1) If A attracts B, then A is B-like
(2) If A purges B, then A attracts B
Therefore: (3) If A purges B, then A is B-like
Therefore: (4) If A purges phlegm, then A is phlegm-like
(5) Knēkos and kokkos purge phlegm
Therefore: (6) knēkos and kokkos are phlegm-like

Galen takes it as established that propositions (1) and (2) hold of necessity.

Now (6) can readily be shown to be true, by various considerations; but those empirical considerations will not show that it is necessarily true. Since, however, it can also be shown to follow from necessary principles—that is the point of argument (1) - (6)—we may conclude that it does in fact hold of necessity.

In what sense does (6) 'follow from necessary principles'? It is natural to suppose that Galen is relying on the following modal thesis:

If p is necessary, and q follows from p, then q is necessary.

Now that is a theorem of standard modal logic. But Galen's argument cannot in fact be justified by the theorem; for proposition (6) does not follow from the two necessary principles, (1) and (2), alone: it follows from the conjunction of (1) and (2) with (5)—and even if we allow that (1) and (2) are necessary, surely (5) is not necessary, so that the conjunction of (1), (2) and (5) is not necessary.[122]

---

[121] Put more rigorously, Galen's 'theorem' is this: For certain propositions, C, there may exist two proofs ⌜A₁, A₂, ..., Aₙ ⊢ C⌝ and ⌜B₁, B₂, ..., Bₘ ⊢ C⌝. Since the Aᵢs are not necessary truths, the first proof shows only that C holds as a matter of fact. Since the Bᵢs are necessary principles, the second proof shows that C holds of necessity.

[122] The point can be put more rigorously. Let 'Lp' abbreviate 'necessarily p'. Then the 'theorem' may be expressed as:

Given that ⌜A₁, A₂, ..., Aₙ: therefore B⌝ is valid.
then if L (A₁ and A₂ and ... and Aₙ), then LB.

Galen's argument is:

(1), (2), (5): therefore (4).

He assumes that L(1) and L(2). But in order to avail himself of the theorem he would require L ((1) and (2) and L (5)). Since it is false that L (5), it is false that L ((1) and (2) and (5)).

Perhaps Galen has made a logical error. Perhaps, on the other hand, the thesis he is implicitly appealing to is not the standard modal theorem I have just stated. Let us rewrite the last stage of Galen's argument in semi-Aristotelian form, thus:

(4*) Every phlegm-purger is phlegm-like
(5*) Knēkos is a phlegm-purger
Therefore: (6*) Knēkos is phlegm-like

Now we may select a modal thesis which is specific to categorical syllogistic; in particular, let us select this:

Given a valid syllogism 'Every A is B, X is A; therefore X is B', then if every A is necessarily B, then X is necessarily B

Since (4*) is supposed to follow from necessary premises, we can infer that every phlegm-purger is necessarily phlegm-like. Hence, with the help of the syllogistic thesis, we can infer the desired conclusion: knēkos is necessarily phlegm-like.

The thesis is not, strictly speaking, a part of Aristotle's syllogistic; but it is immediately derivable from a celebrated element in the modal syllogistic of the *Prior Analytics*—an element which some of Aristotle's successors saw reason to reject.[123] I suggest that Galen took Aristotle's part against his successors, and that the 'theorem' to which Galen appeals is in fact a controversial element in Aristotle's modal syllogistic. That suggestion goes beyond the wording of Galen's text. But even if it is wrong, the passage from *simp. med. temp.* shows how, in the middle of a detailed pharmacological treatise, Galen remained conscious of 'the logical methods'.

11. *First Principles*

So much for the deductive aspect of proofs. I turn now to the axioms. And here there is a multitude of passages to choose from; for in his medical writings, and especially in *meth. med.*, Galen keeps constantly in mind his own injunction to begin from the appropriate axioms. A minor

---

[123] The controversial element is the modal syllogism Barbara LXL; i.e.

LAaB, BaC; therefore LAaC

See Aristotle, *APr*. 20a 15-23; for Theophrastus' rejection of it see e.g. Alexander, *in APr.* 124.8-30; for later Peripatetics who accepted it see [Ammonius] *in APr.* 38.38-39.2. (The syllogism is valid just in case the necessity operator is taken to govern the predicate, A, only; i.e. if 'LAaB' is read as '(LA)aB', rather then as 'L(AaB)'. In fact that narrow reading turns Barbara LXL into a special case of Barbara XXX). If Galen is relying on Barbara LXL, then the modal operators in his premises must all be construed with narrow scope—and that will make the premises seem less plausible.

illustration of the negative effects of that injunction can be seen in the long account of the seat of the regent part (*Hipp. Plat.* V 227-284): a recurrent theme in Galen's criticism of the Stoic view is that they fail to adopt proper first principles—the propositions they argue from are not 'scientific assumptions', and that alone is enough to destroy their case.

As a positive illustration, consider Galen's discussion of fevers which involve putrefaction. He refers to *On Demonstration*, reminding us that we must begin the search for a cure by asking after the essence of putrefaction. Putrefaction is 'the alteration into a corrupt state of the whole substance of the putrefying body by the agency of external heat'. That, then, gives us an axiom for a proof; and Galen quickly infers that we must 'evacuate the part already corrupted, by any means, and reduce the remaining parts to precise symmetry by moderate exercises and cool breezes' (*meth. med.* X 753-754).

Galen's determination to drive his argument back to first principles is evident in many of the particular therapies in *meth. med.*. Here is one fairly typical example (X 414-415). A man has been wounded in the abdomen, and his intestines have extruded. The entrails have swollen. We suppose that the wound 'is small, so that the extruded and swollen entrails cannot be remitted'. 'Here, then, is not one of two things necessary, either to evacuate the swelling or to enlarge the wound?' (ibid. X 414). The former is better, if it can be done. (Galen does not say why it is better: perhaps the reasons are obvious; in any event, the point is of no methodical importance).

How, then, can the swelling be evacuated? There is an evident answer: 'if we can remove the cause by which the entrails are being swollen'. Here Galen relies upon an evident truth of thought: if *A* is causing *B*, then if *A* is removed, *B* will be removed (cf. *meth. med.* X 80). The next step, therefore, is to ask what the cause of the swelling is. 'Cooling from the surrounding air'. That, presumably, is something we know from perception; or rather, physics tells us that the cause must be found in one of the four primary elements (or in some combination of them), and observation indicates that in this case the cause is an excess of cold—and cold from the environment.

'So that the cure lies in its being heated'. One of the fundamental axioms of Galen's practice—another truth evident to thought—is that cures are provided by opposites:[124] if *A* is too cold, it is cured by the

---

[124] For this crucial principle see e.g. *meth. med.* X 100, 103-104, 116, 120, 178, 650, 739; cf. *const. med.* I 260-261; *nat. fac.* II 121; *san. tuend.* VI 361, 378-379. At *sect. ingred.* I 71 (and *introd.* XIV 678) the principle is ascribed to the Rationalists, at *san. tuend.* VI 34 to Hippocrates (cf. ibid. 369; *in Hipp. nat. hom.* XV 162—with e.g. Hippocrates, *nat. hom.* VI 52 L.).

application of heat; if too dry, by moisture; and so on. Thus a simple application of what we might call the axiom of therapy informs us that the protruding intestine should be warmed. 'Therefore one should soak a soft sponge in hot water and squeeze it out, thereby heating the entrails'—and it may help to add some warm and astringent wine, 'for that heats more than water and adds strength to the entrails'.

That procedure may not be successful. (Again, Galen does not explain why). If it is not, then we resort to the second of the two options: we enlarge the wound sufficiently to allow the remission of the entrails.

That short passage is typical of many in *meth. med.*. It exhibits the fundamental weakness of Galen's medicine—its reliance upon such imprecise and unquantified notions as those of heat and dryness.[125] It also exhibits the great strength of Galen's medicine—its rigour and clarity. For the passage is in effect an exercise in the analytical method. How is the desired result, A, to be achieved? Well, if A, then either B or C; if B, then D; if D, then E; .... If not B, then C; if C then X .... Within the analysis, there are brief arguments. The arguments do not expressly invoke any axioms but they implicitly rely upon certain first principles which Galen has already often mentioned. These short arguments are demonstrations.

At the risk of tedium, let me set out one of the component arguments in fully explicit form:

(1) Elemental opposites 'cure' (or remove) one another [Axiom]
(2) Heat and cold are elemental opposites [Axiom]
(3) Removal of a cause brings about removal of the effect [Axiom]
(4) Coldness of the air is causing swelling of the entrails [Observation]
Therefore: (5) If the coldness is removed the swelling will subside [from (4), (5)]
But: (6) Heat removes cold [from (1) and (2)]
Therefore: (7) Heat will reduce the swelling [from (5) and (6)]

The argument is valid. It rests upon first principles of medical science. It is not a remarkable argument, for it can be paralleled a hundred times from *meth. med.* alone. But it is, I think, a good argument.

---

[125] The notions are unquantified because Galen has no thermometer or other measuring device. He was conscious of this deficiency: e.g. *meth. med.* X 183, 650-651; *temp.* I 608-609; *cur. rat.* XI 285 (but contrast *ars med.* I 383). The notions are imprecise because it is not clear what the criteria for being e.g. hot are (wine at the same temperature as water is nevertheless 'hotter' than water—for the explanation see *temp.* I 658-659). Galen is aware that his terms 'hot', 'cold', etc. are multiply ambiguous (see esp. *temp.* I 538-552, 647-650, and passim—cf. e.g. *elem. Hipp.* I 464, 476); and he insists that he is referring to genuine hotness, etc.—to τὸ κατὰ δύναμιν θερμόν and not to τὸ κατὰ φαντασίαν θερμόν (e.g. *ars med.* I 381; *nat. fac.* II 129). But the imprecision remains. On these complex issues see G. Harig, Bestimmung der Intensität im medizinischen System Galens (Berlin, 1974).

12. First Principles and Physics

Quite apart from such particular arguments, there is another and far more significant way in which Galen's insistence on the demonstrative method and his eagerness to ascend to first principles affected his whole approach to medicine. A principal difference, in Galen's eyes and in ours, between Galenian medicine and the medicine of his rivals lies in the fact that Galenian physicians were required to be versed not only in human and animal physiology but also in natural science as a whole. In concrete terms, that meant that a Galenian had to be thoroughly acquainted with the classical theory of the 'primary elements' or of the four elemental qualities.[126]

You must know 'the nature of man'; but 'by physiology ... you cannot properly cure diseases until you have considered the nature of the body as a whole' (*meth. med.* X 17). For 'it is impossible to discover diseases without knowing the elements from which a body is primarily constituted' (ib. X 86). 'It was shown earlier ... that a doctor can do nothing about any of the uniform parts without what is called natural science ... and now our argument makes it plain that he cannot discover any complete therapy for the organic parts either without an acquaintance with that science' (ibid. X 186).

Galen's rivals do not study natural science. The Methodists and the Empiricists do no general physics at all, and the Rationalists will not consider anything more abstract than the organic parts (e.g. *meth. med.* X 184).[127] Since they do not study physics, they cannot effect proper cures.

---

[126] For the four basic qualities see esp. *meth. med.* X 186: 'if it is not conceded in the method that the four qualities are causes of generation and destruction, then it is possible neither to begin the method nor to progress in it nor to complete it; and to exhibit them acting upon and being acted upon by one another belongs to the study of the elements'; cf. ibid. X 16, 24, 49, 97, 100, 103, 174, 463.

[127] The Rationalists 'order us to depart from the highest reaches of natural science (φυσιολογία) and not to try to learn of the nature of man in the way in which the philosophers do, by ascending to the first elements'; they hold that nerves, arteries etc. are the στοιχεῖα of the φυσιολογία of man (*meth. med.* X 107). A Rationalist will say: "I stay within the boundaries of the art: you cross those boundaries and try to lead us to the foreign principles of natural science" (ibid. X 106; cf. *elem. Hipp.* I 459; *in Hipp. nat. hom.* XV 8; and see *nat. fac.* II 126: the Erasistrateans hold that the four basic qualities are 'beyond the scope of doctors and appropriate to physicists'). Whereas the Empiricists profess no proofs, the Rationalists have a theory of proof. They in effect defend the autonomy of medicine; and they could have appealed to Aristotle's authority in refusing to go beyond the 'proper principles' of their science (see *APst.* 88a18-b29). Galen is here Platonic (see *Rep.* 511C), and his criticisms of the Rationalists are strongly reminiscent of Plato's criticisms of those geometers who treat as principles propositions which should themselves be derived from higher principles (*Rep.* 510C). But Galen's point is not purely theoretical. He is not simply championing a Platonic view of the unity of science. Rather, he believes he can show that medicine cannot achieve its goal—that doctors cannot produce cures—unless it ascends to the first principles of general physics. He thinks he can disprove the Rationalists' unargued dogma that the boundaries of medicine are set by the organic parts.

The Rationalists do indeed 'attempt to ascend to the essence of the disease, recognizing that it is otherwise impossible to grasp the appropriate cure'; but they do not attain to those essences, and they are reduced to such prescriptions as 'Strengthen the weakness'—which Galen briskly dismisses as an 'empty phrase' (ibid. X 103). They cannot use drugs correctly; for 'every use of drugs is referred to the hot and cold and dry and moist as to a standard', and they lack the science to apply that standard (ibid. X 400). Nor can they cure wounded ligaments; for 'they do not know the nature of each part, which, as we have shown, depends upon the mixture of the elements' (ibid. X 410).[128]

Galen, by contrast, frequently bases his specific therapies on general science. He will regularly say such things as: 'this kind of disease it is most advantageous for doctors to have investigated—and anyone who is going to undertake the investigation correctly must first have considered the question of the elements' (*meth. med.* X 462). Since Galen has considered 'the question of the elements', he can cure fevers. He can cure your baldness because he has studied, 'in the scientific writings, the origin of hair' (ibid. X 1015). And because he knows 'what is said in the anatomy of that part and in the scientific writings on its functioning and use', he will cure you of priapism in three days (ibid. X 968-971).

Passages of that sort are legion in *meth. med.*; and Galen makes it plain that the ascent to the first principles of natural science is founded upon the requirements of the demonstrative method. In a word, logic shows the need for physics, and physics is indispensable not merely for general medical theory but also and especially for particular therapies.

The best way to grasp Galen's thesis is to follow through the argument of the first two hundred pages of *meth. med.* There is a strong and single thread of reasoning running through those pages, and it provides the basis for all the therapies that follow. But the argument is not clearly stated: Galen interrupts himself constantly, and the long polemical digressions do not aid the reader in following the argument—even if they add piquancy to the narrative. What follows is a summary: some of the elements in it will already be familiar; I shall generally let Galen speak for himself and not intrude with underlinings.

After a polemical exordium, the main argument of *meth. med.* begins at X 39. Galen promises that 'the whole of the ensuing account will make use of the methods which I established in the essay *On Demostration*. It will be 'a most timely fruit of my exertions', and it will also be a useful propaedeutic for 'amateurs of the greatest art, that which is concerned with the human soul'.

---

[128] Cf. *meth. med.* X 170, 184.

Since we wish to find cures for diseases, 'we must first know how many diseases there are in all' (X 40). That knowledge will come by 'division', and to provide a division we must first discover the essence (ousia) of disease, we must learn 'what a disease is'. From *dem.* we have seen that 'we cannot discover the essence of anything unless its concept (ennoia) is first agreed upon'.[129] And since that concept will be the foundation of our first principles, it must be agreed upon by everyone.

We grasp the common conception of disease by discovering 'to what real thing people generally apply the verb "to be diseased"'. Now it is plain that people 'think that they are diseased in a part of their body when they see its functioning impaired' (X 41). Thus the common concept of a disease is this: a man is diseased with respect to a part of his body if and only if the natural functioning of that part is impaired. This concept is derived from 'common Greek usage' (X 42; cf. *adv. Lyc.* XVIIIA 202-203; *caus. procat.* xii 157-159).[130] Hence 'we take as a principle agreed upon by all that the goal of the therapeutic method is to provide health for diseased bodies, i.e. to restore the natural functioning of their parts if it is impaired'.

Galen stresses that although the concept of disease rests upon common agreement, the essence does not; and we have now to advance from concept to essence. After a digression (X 42-49), the next stage of the argument opens with the statement that 'nothing happens without a cause' (X 50). That is 'a non-demonstrable axiom, agreed upon by everyone, because it is evident to thought'. It is needed here because we must discover the cause of disease. Galen's assumption is the Aristotelian one that the essence of a thing is 'what it is', i.e. its (formal) cause. And whereas the concept of a thing is determinable by considering common usage, essence requires special insight and knowledge. The concept of disease is the concept of 'whatever it is that accounts for an impairing of a natural function'; to specify the essence of disease requires us to determine what in fact so impairs the natural functioning of a part of the body.

The discussion which follows is anfractuous. At the beginning of Book II Galen sums up its results. There have turned out to be four things in

---

[129] Cf. *meth. med.* X 141; *const. med.* I 256; *Hipp. Plat.* V 593; *Thras.* V 807; *cur. rat.* XI 255; *adv. Iul.* XVIIIA 265-268; *in Hipp. praed.* XVI 517-518 ('it has been shown in *On Demonstration* that the best principle for everything that is going to be said is the concept of the thing under investigation. Since, therefore, all men give the name of phrenitis to that condition in which they see the mind damaged ...'); cf. also *ars med.* I 306 (the ἔννοια of a thing only gives its 'accidental' characteristics).

[130] The concept depends on ordinary usage—but it may require skill to extract it. 'Just as all men understand the word "man" and know to what it applies even though there is nothing definite and distinct in it for them (as there is for logicians), so it is with the word "fever": we find that men understand the word but are not capable of defining its meaning or explaining it cogently' (*nom. med.* 17.33-37 MS).

impaired bodies: first, the impaired activity; secondly, the disposition which causes that impairment; thirdly, the causes of the disposition; fourthly, the necessary consequences of the disposition (X 78; cf. *const. med.* I 273). Now since 'it is agreed by everyone that what is cured is the disposition which impedes the functioning' (X 80), 'we shall call a disease that disposition which impedes the functioning' (X 81).[131] And here we have the essence of disease: a disease of the body is a disposition which impairs the natural functioning of a bodily part.[132] (It does not matter that the label 'disease' is applied to this rather than to anything else— 'you may call it Dio or Theo if you like'. It does matter that this is the essence of disease and hence that this is what therapy aims to remove).

Galen's argument now rambles. He asserts that we need next to know two things, 'first, how a disease differs from an affection (pathos); secondly, that it is impossible to discover diseases without knowing the elements from which the body is primarily constituted' (X 86). It is only the second point which is genuinely significant[133]—but the second point has unparalleled importance in Galen's eyes, and upon it the special characteristic of his therapeutic practice depends.

Why do we now need to study 'the elements from which the body is primarily constituted'? Why must we learn physics? Knowing that a disease is an impairing disposition is still, in a sense, purely formal knowledge: we need to know what dispositions are impairing.[134] Now 'if you do not know how to distinguish the properties and the causes of the functioning from among the things that pertain to the parts of the body, how will you discover the disposition by which the functioning is primarily impaired?' (*meth. med.* X 92). In order to know what impairs a given function, you must know the cause of that function; for—by the 'axiom of therapy'—if X causes the functioning, then the contrary of X will cause its impairment.

---

[131] Cf. *const. med.* I 260: 'the therapeutic method begins from the disposition of healthy and diseased bodies'.

[132] At *meth. med.* X 80-81 Galen does not actually use the word οὐσία; but see the reprise of these pages at X 115-116.

[133] At *const. med.* I 273 Galen acknowledges the triviality of the first point: 'it will make no difference whether you call it a disease or an affection'.

[134] See *nat. fac.* II 9: 'as long as we are ignorant of the essence of the active cause, we call it a capacity' (δύναμις); *subst. nat. fac.* IV 760 (διὰ τὸ μὴ γινώσκειν ἥτις ἐστιν ἡ αἰτία τῶν ἔργων, ὄνομα θεμένων ἀπὸ τοῦ δύνασθαι ...). Talk of 'capacities' (or of 'dispositions') is a mark of—temporary—ignorance. Galen often says things like 'Urine is attracted to the kidneys by an attractive force'. That is the sort of pseudo-science at which Molière scoffed. Galen is perfectly aware that such formulae are vacuous—or rather, that they are purely formal truths. Unlike Molière, he saw clearly that they have an important place in the development of scientific understanding.

It is here that physics appears. We must discover 'what disposition is the efficient cause of the functioning' (*meth. med.* X 116). 'Now that, we said, was the right mixture of hot and cold, moist and dry—and for that reason the primary disease in the homoeomerous parts was shown to come about by their distemper (dyskrasia)' (ibid.). In particular, there are eight distempers, four simple and four compound,[135] and they underlie all diseases which affect the non-organic parts. The components of eukrasia and dyskrasia are the four basic qualities, the four elements of Galen's physical chemistry. 'Thus anyone who wants to grasp with knowledge the proofs of these things must begin from the account of the elements' (ibid. X 122).

That accounts only for diseases of the homoeomerous parts: what of organic malfunctioning? 'Since we have shown that all the functions come about by the agency of the homoeomerous bodies, and all the other parts of each organ provide it with some utility, the genus of diseases will be two-fold: one kind in homoeomerous bodies, another in whole organs. In homoeomerous bodies, the distempers; of whole organs, one disease is due to conformation, one to the number of the parts, one to the quantity of each, and a fourth to position; and there is a disease common to the homoeomerous and the organic parts—loss of continuity' (*meth. med.* X 125-126).

Disease is essentially an impairing disposition: there turn out to be thirteen generic types of impairing disposition (the eight distempers, the four diseases of the organic parts, and loss of continuity), and hence thirteen primary kinds of disease. Galen's list lacks symmetry and elegance: the eight distempers, taken by themselves, provide a pleasantly neat theory; the addition of the four organic diseases seems ad hoc; and 'loss of continuity' is appended without any attempt to integrate it into a unified theory. But Galen is not interested in elegant symmetry: his concern is for truth.[136] The discussion remains elegant so long as it is a priori. With the four elements, empirical considerations enter, and Galen's argument for the connexion between elemental distemper and bodily malfunctioning is wholly empirical: the connexion is observed,[137] not posited.

---

[135] Cf. *meth. med.* X 103-105: the four primary qualities, hot cold dry moist (HCDM) each account for a 'simple' διάθεσις; by pairwise combination they jointly produce a further four 'compound' διαθέσεις. Thus the eight δυσκρασίαι are characterisable as: H, C, D, M, HD, HM, DC, CM. See e.g. *temp.* I 559, 572-573.

[136] Cf. *temp.* I 524-534: some theorists associate each of the four pairings of the basic qualities with one of the four seasons; Galen rejects the association—it rests upon a theoretical passion for neatness, not upon observation.

[137] 'The connexion is observed': but (a) the connexions which Galen claims to have observed are often imaginary, and (b) the confines within which his 'observations' are made are determined to a large extent by the theoretical notions which he employs.

In order to cure disease you must know what diseases are; in order to know what diseases are you must know what causes them; in order to know what causes them, you must know what causes the functioning of the healthy body; in order to know what causes the functioning of the healthy body you must know general physics, i.e. the theory of the four elements. There are two things to observe about that argument. First, only its last stage is a posteriori: it is a contingent fact that general physics is needed at all. The body could have been so constructed that all its functionings were, so to speak, internally explicable. In fact, things are not like that; and because of that fact the doctor needs general physics.[138] Secondly, the argument presupposes throughout a commitment to the demonstrative method, and in particular to a search for first principles. A Rationalist doctor claims to know about the uses and functions of the body; but he wants to stop there—he sees no need for further investigation. Why may he not stop there? Because propositions about the uses and functions of the body are not first principles: they are explicable in terms of higher propositions—and the Rationalist, by stopping at functions, is effectively cutting himself off from any knowledge. If propositions about functions were principles, the Rationalist would be right; because they are not—and it is a contingent fact that they are not—he is wrong and lacks medical knowledge. It is because they do not know logic that Galen's opponents show no interest in physics (cf. meth. med. X 111-112).

Galen's next task is to introduce therapy into the therapeutic method. This is done by way of the notion of an endeixis or 'indication'. Galen explains that an indication is 'the as it were reflexion of the consequence' (meth. med. X 126). That is unilluminating. But light is soon shed. An 'indication' is expressed by way of a conditional sentence, and a therapeutic indication will be given by way of a sentence of the form 'If X is diseased in such-and-such a way, then X will be cured by such-and-such a therapy'. The characteristic feature of an indicative conditional is that 'the consequent is reflected in the antecedent' (ibid),[139] and that 'the consequent is discovered by starting from the very nature of the thing

---

[138] The doctor needs Galen's physics, i.e. the traditional four-quality theory, because that is the true physics. It is a contingent fact that the four-quality theory is true and its rivals—most notably atomism—false. At this point too, contingency enters Galen's argument.

[139] An ἔνδειξις is οἷον ἔμφασις τῆς ἀκολουθίας. At PH II 110-112 Sextus distinguishes four theories of the truth-conditions of conditional sentences. The fourth theory is that of 'those who judge conditionals τῇ ἐμφάσει'; these theorists 'say that a conditional is true if its consequent is included potentially in its antecedent'. Galen is surely alluding to that theory, but its provenance is uncertain: see Frede, o.c. n. 120, pp. 90-93.

and without appeal to experience' (ibid. X 127; cf. 157; *const. med.* I 251; *inst. log.* xi 1).[140]

'I am persuaded that there is a method for discovering what we are inquiring into, the first principle of which is the goal which is set by each disease; for loss of continuity requires unification ...' (*meth. med.* X 160). The indicative conditional in this case is: 'If X is diseased by loss of continuity, then X is cured by unification'. The consequent is 'reflected in' the antecedent in the sense that it can be inferred from the antecedent without the application of any empirical knowledge. More precisely, the indication relies on a general principle governing the relation between disease and cure: 'there are two kinds of primary indication—a natural state indicates its preservation and hence requires what is similar to itself, an unnatural state indicates its removal and hence requires what is contrary—for everything is destroyed into its contrary and by its contrary' (ibid. X 178; cf. *ars med.* I 381; *san. tuend.* VI 361).

Set out with pedantic completeness, the argument for a primary therapeutic indication will run like this:

(1) Curing a disease is removing the impairing disposition
(2) A thing is removed just in case its contrary is produced
Therefore: (3) Curing a disease is producing its contrary
(4) Unification is contrary to loss of continuity
Therefore: (5) If X is diseased by loss of continuity, X is cured by unification.

Each premiss in the argument—i.e. (1), (2), (4)—is a first principle; and the indication in (5) is reached by logical deduction from first principles—first principles which owe nothing to experience.

Now all that may seem highly trivial—it does not take a learned physician to discover an indication like (5). Galen agrees. While maintaining

---

[140] Cf. the definition of an indicative sign at Sextus, *PH* II 101: it is something which ἐκ τῆς ἰδίας φύσεως καὶ κατασκευῆς σημαίνει τὸ οὗ ἐστι σημεῖον (cf. *M* VIII 154). Sextus uses the term ἔνδειξις only once (at *PH* I 240, where he is reporting a view of the Methodists), but it is clear that his σημεῖον ἐνδεικτικόν is identical with Galen's ἔνδειξις. Sextus' whole discussion of signs is based upon the distinction between ἐνδεικτικὰ and ὑπομνηστικὰ σημεῖα. Sextus ascribes the distinction to οἱ δογματικοί (*PH* II 100, where κατ' αὐτούς picks up κατὰ τοὺς δογματικούς, 97). Scholars have generally supposed that the Dogmatists here are Stoics, and the distinction is often attributed to Chrysippus and the Old Stoa (see esp. Brunschwig, o.c. n. 73, pp. 139-140). Some scholars are sceptical: the distinction is common in the medical writers (where it helps to differentiate the Rationalists from the Empiricists), and it has recently been urged that medical theorising provides the origin and fount of the distinction (see D. Sedley, 'On Signs', in Science and Speculation (above, n. 27), at p. 240-241 n. 8). Note that at *inst. log.* xi 1 Galen apparently ascribes the standard definition of ἔνδειξις to the Peripatetics—ἔνδειξιν μὲν γὰρ καλοῦσι (where the subject of καλοῦσι ought to be those who have discussed categorical syllogistic).

that such primary indications are the starting-points for any therapy, he also admits that 'this is not yet a part of the art of medicine—or at any rate not a part of any great account, nor a part proper to medicine: it is something common to laymen too' (*meth. med.* X 158-159).[141] The doctor is the man 'who can discover the means by which what is shown by the primary indication will come about' (ibid.; cf. *opt. sect.* I 173).[142] Primary indications are not yet parts of professional therapy: the art comes in when we ask how unification will be achieved. And here, with the entry of therapy proper, it might be thought that logic will bow out: logic provides the abstract form and foundations of therapy, the physician produces the rest from his clinical experience. Yet that is not Galen's view. Logic is not to be pensioned off. On the contrary, Galen explicitly states that, if we are to advance beyond primary indications to a more detailed and professional prescription, 'we need a long argument and many particular indications and a precise logical method' (*meth. med.* X 169).

The first particular example which Galen expounds is the cure of 'hollow' wounds (*meth. med.* X 173-186). 'We must of course start from the nature of the thing' (ibid. X 174): in particular therapy, as in general therapeutic theory, we must start from first principles—from natures and essences. Now since 'every unnatural hollowness indicates filling' (ibid. X 168), and a hollowness of flesh must be filled with flesh, 'we must know something about the generation of flesh' (ibid. X 174). The generation requires material, which is 'good blood', and a craftsman or technician, which is 'the correct mixture of ⟨the four primary qualities⟩ in the part underlying' the hollowed area (ibid.). Here, then, is the first step away from the unprofessional primary indication towards the art of medicine proper. Galen states that what he says is 'clear'. In fact, it is far from clear. No doubt 'precise logical method' informs us that to fill a hollow with flesh we must generate flesh, and that the generation of flesh (as of anything else) demands a material and a technician. But it is not clear why the material must be blood—or the 'technician' the underlying flesh. Galen is omitting stages in the argument. In a full account he would presumably introduce more physiological and physical theory. In any

---

[141] See *cur. rat.* XI 255-256 for the distinction between 'primary reasoning' which rests directly upon first conceptual principles and is open to all, and 'secondary' reasoning which leads ever further from the principles and which is the province of the τεχνῖται 'who sometimes come to show things which are quite incredible to the layman—not only the sizes but also the distances of the sun and the moon and the earth ...'.

[142] The doctor must also determine whether what is indicated can be produced, either by nature or by art: *const. med.* I 264-265: cf. the aphorism of Herophilus: 'Asked who could become a perfect doctor, he replied "A man who can distinguish the possible and the impossible"' (Stobaeus, *Anth.* IV 37).

event, clear or unclear, the proposition Galen has now moved to relies upon technical scientific knowledge. The step taken at X 174 surpasses the competence of the layman.

'Let us assume, then, that the site of the wound is healthy and the flow of blood flawless in quantity and quality' (ibid. X 175). Then flesh will grow. But, 'as we said in our reasonings on nature', all change of quality is accompanished by the production of two sorts of waste matter; and so the generation of flesh will be accompanied by excretions (ibid.). The wound will come to contain pus and filth, the former of which makes the wound moist, the latter dirty; hence we shall need two drugs, one a drying and the other a cleaning agent, and we shall need to apply them continuously 'since nature is never at any time inactive' (ibid. X 176).

Such drugs come in different strengths. The drying agent appropriate to hollow wounds is a mild one; 'for if it is stronger it will not only exhaust the excessive part of the inflowing moisture but will also touch the inflowing blood itself and prevent the formation of flesh by using up the material' (ibid. X 177). (We are referred to *simp. med. temp.* for the pharmacological details). Now the drug must be compounded with a view not only to the state of the wound but also to the state of the patient's body: 'the moister the wound is, the more you need a drug which is more drying; but the moister the nature of the body may happen to be, the more you need a drug that is less drying' (ibid. X 178). For the flesh that is being generated must have the same degree of moisture as the old flesh of the patient's body. Again, a non-technical primary indication—'Unnatural moisture in a wound demands a drying agent'—leads to a professional indication for which pharmacological understanding as well as logical expertise is required.

Galen ends the account of the therapy by insisting upon its logical aspect: 'so you clearly see now how many theorems a man needs if he is going to cure a wound according to the correct method' (ibid. X 180).

Compare Galen's therapy with those of the rival schools. The Methodists content themselves with a primary indication—'hollow wounds must be filled and fleshed out'— and then appeal vaguely to experience as the provider of detail (ibid. X 180-182). The Empiricists know that particular drugs have worked on particular types of patient. But if they try a drug and find it is ineffective, they do not know what to do: 'the Empiricist sees that the drug he has applied has not fleshed out this patient; but because he does not know whether that is because it dries too much or too little, he cannot move to another drug' (ibid. X 184). The Rationalist will not proceed by method beyond the diseases peculiar to organic parts; consequently he is in the same position as the Empiricists with regard to the curing of wounds, which are diseases of the homoeomerous parts (ibid. X 184-185). Only Galen's method, which advances beyond the primary indications of the Methodist, systematises the disorganized observations of the Empiricist, and takes the theorising of the Rationalist to its proper end in physical science, can provide a reliable and scientific mode of therapy. And the superiority of Galen's method is attributable to logical theory. It is because Galenians are logicians, trained in the techniques of the demonstrative method, that they follow the therapeutic procedure of *meth. med.*. It is because Galenians are logicians that their patients recover.

Galen's science is jejune, his conceptual equipment is imprecise, his therapies are usually vague and sometimes silly. That is to say, he was practising medicine at a time when basic science was too primitive to support the art. But his method is in all respects admirable. He grasps the importance of argument—and of rigour and formality in argument. His insistence on the ascent to first principles is wholly correct. The demonstrative method, conceived of as Galen conceived of it, is an indispensable tool for scientists—and, in particular, for medical scientists. And the demonstrative method is nothing else but applied logic.

'But come', a passing Sceptic may urge, 'is this vaunted method really anything more than glorified common sense? Is it a technical discipline, an esoteric art, to be discovered by professional industry? Surely not: Galen is telling us something we have always known'. The Sceptic is largely correct. Galen's logical methods are common sense—at least, they are common sense organized and regimented. But that neither belittles Galen's achievement nor derogates from the importance of his prescriptions. For glorified common sense is a glorious thing. And common sense itself, as a wise man remarked, is the rarest of God's gifts.

FRIDOLF KUDLIEN

'ENDEIXIS' AS A SCIENTIFIC TERM:
A) GALEN'S USAGE OF THE WORD (IN MEDICINE AND LOGIC)

With its rather broad spectrum of meanings, 'endeixis' seems so fascinating a word that it might well have deserved a place in Professor C. S. Lewis' brilliant "Studies in words". No exhaustive study on 'endeixis' is known to us. What J. Barnes has offered (in his contribution to this symposion) is said from the logician's point of view when he has to deal with 'endeixis'. The following contributions concerned with 'endeixis' cannot fill the gap just mentioned, nor can they claim any brilliance. They can merely try to emphasize what seem to us to be the main aspects of the word's history in ancient and medieval medicine and philosophy, so far as it serves there the function of a technical term (in both fields, it can also be used in a non-technical way; see below). It may be kept in mind that our contributions on 'endeixis' are written by philologists. A clinical physician and Galenist (such as Professor L. Garcia Ballester) would doubtless have to say more about the role and importance of 'endeixis/indication' in clinical medicine.

Let me start, nevertheless, my own contribution with a brief information on what 'indicatio(n)' (one of the possible Latin equivalents of the Greek 'endeixis', see R. J. Durling's contribution) means in modern medical language; this might be helpful for those who are not themselves doctors. In Eulenburg's well-known "Medizinische Real-Enzyklopädie" (I have used the 1896 ed.), 'indicatio' is translated and explained as 'Heilanzeige, -aufgabe'. Note that a) the word is exclusively linked here with a therapy ('Heilen'), and some thing ('Aufgabe')—so that, as a 'Heilaufgabe', 'indication' has come to denote certain tasks of the doctor (one might say that the term, thus understood, serves as a kind of appeal in the positive sense whereas 'counter-indication' would then mean that the doctor must refrain from doing this or that). Furthermore, several sub-groups of 'indication' are enumerated here: 'indicatio causalis'; 'indicatio prophylactica'. Again, one has to keep in mind that in all these cases, 'indication' does not mean a mere 'sign' but rather an action (for instance, 'indicatio symptomatica' is not to be understood as 'what the symptoms show'; actually, it points to the treatment of certain symptoms of the disease in question).

This is more or less how doctors in our own time still understand and use the term 'indication'. As for the early history of the term in medicine, the Eulenburg article is aware of the fact that 'indicatio' is a translation of the Greek 'endeixis' and that it was Galen, above all, who used the word in the modern sense. But the Eulenburg article also suggests that the concept, if not the term itself, is already to be found in the Corpus Hippocraticum (how far this is correct, is a question that R. J. Durling will deal with).

Now, before coming to Galen's usage of the term, it seems useful to clear up a confusion caused by L. Edelstein who has translated, or rather paraphrased, 'endeixis' as 'knowledge (Wissen)'.[1] This is certainly debatable as Dr. Lloyd has recently remarked.[2] But one should be fair: In so far as, according to Galen and other like-minded Greek physicians, "the disease in itself is indicative of its own treatment", the technical term 'endeixis' together with its derivative forms must certainly imply a "knowledge" of the disease as well as of its treatment.[3] I think this is what Edelstein has had in mind.

In the circumstances, it does not come as a surprise to us that the term 'endeixis' together with 'endeiktikos', 'endeiknynai', 'syn-endeiknysthai', 'antendeiknysthai' occurs extremely often in Galen's chief work on therapy, the *MM*. This does not mean, however, that even there the term would be exclusively linked with therapy: Take for instance X 336, 1f. "the nature of the artery indicates indeed that the harder parts of its membranes are opposed to growing together". Although the word 'indicates' is here certainly used in the technical sense (note the connection with 'nature' to which we shall come later on), this is an anatomical/physiological remark but not one pointing immediately to therapy.

In other Galenic treatises, too, the word, though used as a technical term, occurs occasionally without (direct) reference to therapy; in such cases, it seems to mean, at first look, nothing but 'sign'. One may for example pick up a passage from Galen's commentary on the Hippocratic *Epidemiae* (CMG V 10,2,2 p. 220,11): Heavy breathing 'indicates (endeiktikon esti)' that there is an accumulation of heat ('thermasia') in the depths of the body. But one must be careful: If one would translate

---

[1] L. Edelstein, art. "Methodiker", RE Suppl. VI, 1935, col. 367 1.28.
[2] G. E. R. Lloyd, The epistemological theory and practice of Soranus' Methodism, in: id., Science, folklore and ideology. Studies in the life sciences in ancient Greece, Cambridge 1983, p. 184.
[3] Cf. M. Frede, The method of the so-called Methodical school of medicine, in: J. Barnes/J. Brunschwig/M. Burnyeat/M. Schofield (edd.), Science and speculation. Studies in Hellenistic theory and practice, Cambridge 1982, p. 4 (the quoted words are his).

'endeiktikon esti' here as "is a sign of ...", something would be missing. Obviously, 'endeiktikon' is not quite the same as 'sēmeion' or 'symptōma'. By the latter, the physician would be helped to draw certain conclusions that were, however, limited in themselves because they would concern nothing but the identification of the disease in question. 'endeiktikos/endeixis', on the other hand, is for a Greek doctor who uses this word as a technical term, always beyond the realm of these limited conclusions: By pointing to something that is not so much a mere fact but rather "is the matter", the word, thus understood, forces (or entitles) the doctor to become active against the disease in question. Modern clinical epistemology as represented in Eulenburg's "Real-Enzyklopädie" would understand the passage quoted from Galen's commentary on the "Epidemiae" as referring to an 'indicatio symptomatica'.

To make it still more obvious that 'sēmeion' and 'endeixis/endeiktikos' are not identical in principle, Galen is sorting out, from the bulk of 'sēmeia', a particular group which he uses to call 'sēmeia endeiktika (indicative signs)'. For this, one may compare for instance a passage in his treatise "On the 'synectic' causes".[4] This is again, even more literally, what modern doctors happen to call an 'indicatio symptomatica'.

This principal distinction between a 'sēmeion' and an 'endeixis' can be used to illustrate those principally different approaches or methods in clinical medicine as they existed in Antiquity. To find out who followed this or that approach or method, one had only to use the term 'endeixis' as a yard-stick: Adherents of the Empiricist school of medicine refused to use the term and concept 'indication' at all; they were led entirely by the 'observation (tērēsis)' of 'sēmeia/symptōmata' which 'reminded' them ('sēmeion hypomnēstikon', commemorative sign) of what "is mostly and in the same way being observed".[5] The Methodist physicians did use the term 'endeixis', but in a very simple—one might even say, primitive—way: For them, 'indicative' meant that the manifest state of a disease makes it immediately obvious for the doctor what must be done; there is, as they have it, no need of observation (in the sense given to it by the Empiricists) or of inferences made from assumed hidden causes of diseases.[6] Galen offers a characteristic description of the Methodists' usage of 'endeixis' in his MM (X 158): A stone in the bladder, just

---

[4] This passage is quoted, as fr. 78, in: K. Deichgräber, Die griechische Empirikerschule. Sammlung der Fragmente und Darstellung der Lehre, Berlin/Zürich 1965 (repr.), p. 140 (see esp. line 29).

[5] See for this ibid., p. 99, 20 (from Galen's De sectis) and p. 141, 22-24 (from the ps. Galenic Definitiones medicae).

[6] For the foregoing, see Frede's paragraph on 'indication', l.c. pp. 4-8.

"because it is against nature", is 'indicating' immediately that it is to be removed; an exarticulated joint, just because it is "out of its natural place", indicates immediately that it must be put back into its proper place. This, says Galen, is not 'technikon'; any layman could and would handle the matter in the same way, in such cases. The right approach, and the correct understanding and usage of 'endeixis' is alone that practised by the Dogmatist school of medicine (of which Galen would count himself a member): 'logos', reason, is needed for it. Therefore, Galen is explicitly talking of the 'endeixis logikē', in opposition to the "merely empirical (apo tēs empeirias monēs)" approach (so e.g. in *MM*, X 244,10). This alone would enable the physician to achieve what is absolutely vital for him if he wants to treat patients in a 'technikos', that is to say, scientific way: He must take into account the 'nature of the matter' ('physis tou pragmatos', or 'ousia'). From this, the proper 'endeixis' would offer itself. As for references, one may only look, in the *MM*, at X 104,12f. (where the then almost regularly used formula 'tēn endeixin labein ek tēs tou pragmatos physeōs' occurs for the first time) or at X 101,12f. ('endeixis ... apo tēs ousias', as opposed to 'apo tōn phainomenōn'). Again and again, Galen is fighting in his writings against the merely 'empirical' approach while usually contrasting this, in these passages, to the 'indication from the nature of the matter'. See for instance his commentary on the *Epidemiae* where 'di' empeirias' is opposed to 'ek tēs tou pragmatos physeōs endeiktikōs' (CMG V 10,2,2 p. 14,19f.). Here, as elsewhere, one might paraphrase the latter words as 'it follows logically from the nature of the facts' or 'it is in the nature of the matter that ...'. As for the importance of 'phenomena', 'symptoms', 'signs' in this connection, one may remember what has already been said on the 'indicative signs': When seeking for the true 'endeixis', the Dogmatist would not observe all possible signs/symptoms as such (as the Empiricist does) but select only those that are 'indicative of the cause (sc. of the disease)'[7] (here, 'cause', aitia, appears to be identical with 'nature', physis/ousia).

It is in exactly this sense that the term 'endeixis', together with its derivative forms, is being used mainly, if not exclusively, in Galen's principal work on the method of therapy, the *MM*: True 'endeixis' is always something 'logical', here. Every disease has got its own specific or 'natural (oikeiai) endeixeis' (X 918,5f.). These may point to different medical purposes, so that there is not only an 'endeixis therapeutikē' (the modern 'indicatio curativa') but also an 'endeixis prophylaktikē' (the modern 'indicatio prophylactica') as for instance X 248,9f. makes clear.

---

[7] Cf. Deichgräber, l.c. p. 99, 18 and 21f. (from Galen's *De sectis*).

Furthermore, there are 'endeixeis' that are 'basic' ones because they are presented by the whole system as such, so to speak (Galen calls them 'prōtai endeixeis', see e.g. X 155-157); their counterparts are those 'endeixeis' to be taken from details (for 'kata meros endeixeis' see e.g. X 169,1). This would mean that a particular organ ('morion') of the body may offer an 'endeixis', too (X 918,8f.). However, also certain things or factors that lie outside the body (though being in close contact with, and relation to it) may count, in this respect: When Galen remarks in his commentary on the Hippocratic *Epidemiae* (CMG V 10,2,2 p.92,19-21) that "as for the differences in therapy, there is an 'endeixis' from the habits (of the patient)", this is being worked out further in the *MM* (see X 918,6-8). Here, there is a brief enumeration of what Galen calls the 'synendeiknymena' (lit. 'that which indicates in addition'): Apart from the 'strength (dynameis)', the 'nature/condition (physis)' and the 'age (hēlikia)' of the patient, the 'season (hōra)', the 'surroundings (chōra)' and the 'habits (ethos)' would belong to these 'synendeiknymena'.

In a context of this kind, the 'counter-indication (antendeiknysthai)' comes in quite naturally. In the *MM*, one may look for instance at X 626,9 where Galen points out, in a discussion about venesection, that "some factors would in addition indicate phlebotomy" whereas some other would "counter-indicate it".

In our foregoing discussion, several allusions have been made to 'logic/logical', in connection with 'endeixis'. In a treatise particularly concerned with the inter-relations between medicine and philosophy, "That the best physician is also a philosopher", Galen makes this connection between 'endeixis' and 'logical' explicit: "One must also use the logical method to recognize what all the diseases are, with regard to species and kinds, and how, for every disease, one must take an 'endeixis' of the therapeutical measures ('iamata')" (*Scr. min.* II p. 6, 10-14).

Now, what does 'endeixis' precisely mean, in connection with what Galen calls the 'logical method'—what, in other words, is 'logical' about the 'indication' as understood and used in the medical epistemology of the Dogmatists? Or does 'logikos' here mean nothing but a general, unspecific reference to 'reason'? A key-passage to answer such questions is to be found in the *MM* (X 126f.). Here, Galen offers a definition: "First, we must explain this word 'endeixis' itself. We call 'endeixis' the 'emphasis' of the 'akolouthia'." Therewith, we encounter indeed two technical terms taken from philosophical epistemology. 'Emphasis' which has here the general meaning 'appearing in (something)' or 'reflection' (as in a mirror; for references, see LSJ s.v.), seems to have played a role in early Stoic doctrines of cognition: Chrysippus is credited, by Diocles Magnes, with having defined those 'phantasiai (presentations/impressions)' which occur 'as if being of existing things', as 'phantasiōn emphaseis' (Stoicorum Veterum Fragmenta II p. 24, 20f.); later on, 'emphasis' may also have served as a term in Stoic logic.[8] And 'akolouthia' which has here the sense of 'consequence', has likewise been a technical term in Epicurean as well as in later Stoic epistemology.[9]

When taken by itself, the definition of 'endeixis' presented in the *MM* is certainly somewhat "unilluminating" (as J. Barnes has justly remarked). However, in the context of this definition, Galen goes into more detail, taking great care to point out that it is not the 'facts' or 'the matter (pragma)' but the 'nature of the matter' from which one must start, to find out what would be 'consequent (akolouthon)'. He goes even so far as to claim here that, in the circumstances, the true method of therapy proceeds in principle 'without experience (empeiria)'. Our first reaction to this startling remark may be that of a slight shock. But it just shows how extremely important the "theory of the underlying, hidden nature of things" has been for Dogmatist medical epistemology.[10] Furthermore, this harsh neglect of 'empeiria' gains at least a certain justification from the fact that, in Galen's eyes, 'empeiria' was hopelessly compromised by its being used as a leading concept in the Empiricist school of medicine, where it meant (as we have had occasion to note) nothing but the mere 'observation (tērēsis)' and 'remembrance (mnēmē)' of phenomena and facts—whereas 'endeixis' alone, as Galen states in X 126f., guarantees the true 'finding (heuresis)'.

In exactly the same sense, Galen has used the term 'endeixis' in his philosophical treatise on logic, the *Institutio logica*. As Professor Mau has argued in his commentary,[11] 'endeixis' plays here the role of a logical proof. But it is a peculiar kind of proof: It's got nothing to do with an 'apodeixis' since this latter technical term (admittedly better known in Greek logic and epistemology than 'endeixis'—Galen has written a special treatise on it that is lost) means a proof that follows from 'true premisses' and is a 'logos' ('lōgos perainōn ex alēthōn lēmmatōn' as Galen puts it in the "Institutio logica"). 'endeixis', on the other hand,

---

[8] For this, cf. the discussion in M. Frede, Die stoische Logik, Göttingen 1974, pp. 90-93.

[9] See M. F. Burnyeat, The origins of non-deductive inference, in: Science and speculation, l.c. p. 206 with n. 33; D. Sedley, On signs, ibid. p. 263.

[10] See M. Frede, On Galen's epistemology, in: V. Nutton (ed.), Galen: Problems and prospects. A collection of papers submitted at the 1979 Cambridge conference, London 1981, p. 80 with n. 13 (offering further Galenic references).

[11] J. Mau, Galen "Einführung in die Logik". Kritisch-exegetischer Kommentar mit deutscher Übersetzung, Berlin 1960, p. 29.

is here defined by Galen as a 'heuresis tou zētoumenou ek tēs tou pragmatos physeōs kat' akolouthian enargē tou phainomenou'. This definition offers nearly all technical keywords which we have already encountered in the medical passages quoted above ('enargēs', evident— one may take it here to mean 'self-evident'—is also a technical term in philosophical epistemology elsewhere).[12] According to this definition of 'endeixis' as presented in the "Institutio logica", Mau understands the term as such as meaning a "Beweis unmittelbar aufgrund des Sachverhalts". I wonder whether this is not slightly imprecise: Strictly speaking, 'Sachverhalt' would rather correspond to the Greek 'pragma'. However, as Galen keeps repeating, 'endeixis' is not merely based on what "is the matter" but on what he refers to as the "nature of the matter" (for which, by the way, one may compare from earlier Greek philosophy a phrase such as 'tēn physin tōn pragmatōn ... eidenai' in Plato's "Protagoras'" 337 d). Apart from this minor point, I tend to agree with Mau's criticism of Professor Stakelum who argues that Galen's usage of 'endeixis' in the *Institutio logica* comes in fact very near to the Aristotelian 'hypothetical proof' (but this is rather a question for specialists in the field to decide).

If it is clear that Galen uses 'endeixis' as a technical term in the same way both in medicine and logic—has he then taken this term from philosophy, to apply it to medical epistemology? Or was it the other way around? And this provokes a further question: When, if not with Galen, did 'endeixis' as a technical, medico-philosophical term originate, and where—in medicine, or in logic?

With Plato, we meet the word 'endeixis' together with its derivative forms quite often—but never, as far as I am aware, in the technical sense we are concerned with here. As for Aristotle, Professor Mau (l.c.) reminds us of the fact that 'endeixis' as a technical term does not even occur in Aristotle's chief work on logic, the "Organon" (the word is to be found very rarely in other Aristotelian treatises, but again not in the technical sense). So far as medicine is concerned, it was the Methodists who—if Sextus Empiricus, our main source for this, can be trusted—first used the word in the technical sense (but, as we have seen, in a way different from how the Dogmatists used it). Now, if the Methodists did not coin the term: Where did they take it from? Professor Frede's answer to this is that it came "into use in later Hellenistic epistemology",[13] although Frede cannot tell us precisely where and when. Apparently, one is to tread very cautiously here: If a philosopher such as Philodemus, in the certainly relevant treatise "On signs", uses the word

---

[12] See Sedley, l.c. p. 266 n. 65.

'endeiknysthai', one would expect that it possesses its technical sense, here; but the opposite seems to be true[14] (in an equally non-technical way, the physician Aretaeus, for instance, uses 'endeiknysthai' in the sense of 'appear'; see CMG II p. 13, 19). Does it help that the distinction between 'indicative' and 'commemorative' signs (which we have met in Galen's description of the Empiricist standpoint, see above p. 105) is commonly thought of having originated in Stoic philosophy? Unfortunately not: Experts such as Burnyeat[15] and Sedley[16] are now emphasizing the unlikelihood of its preexistence in Stoicism. While pointing out that this distinction seemes "more familiar in medical theory", Sedley seems to think of the possibility that physicians originally formulated this distinction. Burnyeat, on the other hand, does not believe in "medical priority", in this respect; he thinks that what Sextus reports about the distinction between 'indicative' and 'commemorative' signs is "the philosophical version of a distinction which in the medical literature leads an independent and quite complicated life of its own". In other word: There seems no way of getting an answer to the questions raised above. One should then content oneself to note with J. Mau (l.c.)—who, incidentally, seems inclined to believe (although he does not say so in so many words) that it was Galen who introduced 'endeixis' into the technical vocabulary of logic, taking it from medical epistemology—that 'endeixis' in its technical sense, if it is not be found in Aristotle himself, occurs quite regularly in late commentaries on Aristotle's logical treatises, particularly in Alexander. I may also add that the term can be found in Olympiodorus' commentaries on Plato's *Phaedon* (see the Index in Norvin's edition).

Let me conclude this brief and sketchy survey by making two remarks of a more general character: To argue that something is "in the nature of the matter" or "follows logically from the nature of the facts" (or that the nature of the facts "points to" something) may turn out to be a rather ambivalent or even dangerous type of argument, scientifically speaking. First, it required a speculation on 'hidden' things or factors/causes if one claimed to recognize the 'nature' of a disease (this was what the Empiricists as well as the Methodists had to say against the Dogmatists' use or 'endeixis'). Secondly, there were several more specific dangers involved if the 'logical method' were to be used by doctors who would

---

[13] Frede, Method of Methodical school, l.c. p. 4f.
[14] For this see Sedley, l.c. p. 242 n. 8 (criticizing the De Lacy for having taken this in the technical sense of 'indication').
[15] l.c. p. 212.
[16] l.c. p. 241 (bottom).

prove to be 'dilettantes'; of this, Galen was well aware.[17] The nature of such dangers can be illustrated if we turn our direction to a different field of activity: Politicians, above all, seem to be particularly prone to use this type of argument if they want to convince people of something; the appeal, then, would be not so much to our intellectual or 'logical' capacities but rather to our emotions (the phrase 'this is logical, though' is often used in the same way and with the same intention). However, a physician such as Galen was in a somewhat privileged position, in this respect, for if he used the term 'endeixis' as meaning a 'scientific proof offered by the nature of the disease', he could rely on something that was at least not entirely unsolid: his (comparatively) thorough knowledge of anatomy and physiology (in fact, 'physis tou pragmatos' came to mean, in this connection, the anatomical structure, too: see in the *MM* X 455 and 522). Although there was admittedly a great deal of speculation in these two areas, too, the Dogmatists' use of 'endeixis', at least if practised by a physician of Galen's intellectual rank, was thus not without justification.

My other remark would concern the non-medical and non-philosophical meanings of the word 'endeixis', and the question how far these meanings may be related to the term in its technical sense 'indication'. It is clearly not of great interest for us to learn that the word could be used in the sense of 'tax-declaration'. Much more remarkable, however, is the fact that it could also be used as a technical term in the sphere of the law-court. Here, 'endeixis' meant that somebody 'denounced' another person before the legal authorities.[18] The implication was that, herewith, a criminal should not only be made known as such, but that the one who 'indicated' this also expected or even demanded from the authorities that an appropriate action—an action whose nature was thought to be 'indicated' beyond doubt on ground of the nature of the 'denounced' crime—was being taken. This appears to offer a good parallel to the term's usage in medicine and logic: By the word 'endeixis/indication' itself, an appeal is made, so to speak, to the physician to play the role of a 'judge', so that he would then take an appropriate action against the 'culprit', i.e. the disease. One may also remember in this connection that in modern German (with English, it is different) one and the same word 'anzeigen' is used to 'denounce' somebody, and to make it clear as well that for instance a certain therapy is 'indicated' (= should be applied in a certain case).

---

[17] See for this Frede, Galen's epistemology, l.c. p. 81.
[18] See for this Thalheim's art. "endeixis", RE V 2, 1905, col. 2551f.

RICHARD J. DURLING

'ENDEIXIS' AS A SCIENTIFIC TERM:
B) 'ENDEIXIS' IN AUTHORS OTHER THAN GALEN AND ITS
MEDIEVAL LATIN EQUIVALENTS

I wish to put two questions: 1) What is the prehistory of the term 'endeixis' in medicine?, 2) How was the Greek term translated into Latin in the Middle Ages?

Michael Frede has recently written: "The notion of indication is not of Methodist origin. It comes into use in later Hellenistic epistemology ...." [1] He does not specify his sources nor does he investigate the earlier history of the term in medical authors.

The term 'endeixis' and related forms occur three times in the Hippocratic Corpus, never in a technical sense or in the sense or senses familiar to us from Galen. The terms occur only in later writings at that, namely in the *Precepts* and *Letters*. [2] (I owe this information to the Hippokrates-Wörterbuch in Hamburg).

There is a hint of the concept but not the term in Hippocrates' *De locis in Homine* 34 (6.326.10-12 L.). Hippocrates is laying down rules to follow when one does not know the nature of an illness. He says: "When one has to do with an illness one does not know, one must give a purgative that is not strong; if the condition improves, the way is 'indicated' (dedeiktai hodos), one must treat by attenuation. If it does not improve, but deteriorates, the opposite." Littré has seen the significance of this passage in his Index (t. X) where under 'Indication' he cites the locus.

'Endeixis' does not occur in the writings of Apollonius of Citium, Dioscorides, Aretaeus (for whom see above and below note 4, however) or Soranus: it does occur in one prose writer before Galen, namely in Rufus of Ephesus' *Quaestiones medicinales* 34 (Kai ta men toiauta echei tina kai para tōn symptomatōn endeixin tou ginōskesthai). [3] The term has clearly won acceptance before Galen but its widespread use seems to have originated with him.

It is idle to speculate whether in fact the medical use of this important term goes back to early Hellenistic writers such as Herophilus and Erasistratus. [4] Fragments are an unreliable and unsatisfactory guide.

---

[1] M. Frede, in: Science and speculation ... Ed. by Jonathan Barnes et al., Cambridge 1982, pp. 4-5.
[2] 9.252.18; 352.7; 400.18 Littré.
[3] Ed. H. Gärtner (Teubner ed.) 1975, p. 6.20-21.
[4] Aretaeus once uses 'endeiknyntai' (p. 13, 19 Hude).

Second, the standard Latin translation of 'endeixis' in the Middle Ages was 'indicatio' and dates back at least to the learned judge of Pisa, Burgundio (ca. 1110-1193). Burgundio uses it 17 times in his as yet unpublished version of *De interioribus* (i.e. *De locis affectis*). When this was translated—or when the translation first circulated—we do not know. In what is possibly an earlier version, that of *De complexionibus* (i.e. *De temperamentis*) he had twice translated 'endeixis' by 'demonstratio' (as if 'apodeixis' were in question). Niccolò da Reggio in his rendering of Galen's *Subfiguratio empirica* followed Burgundio in the use of 'indicatio'.[5]

What classical antecedents did this use of 'indicatio' have? The "Oxford Latin Dictionary" recognizes for 'indicatio' only two meanings: 1) The setting of a price on a thing, valuation, and 2) A statement, declaration. The clue is to be found under the verb indico,—are 3 (of things): To be an indication of, reveal, disclose, show. Note that one of the examples given is from Celsus I. 8. 2: stomachum ... infirmum indicant pallor, macies. Celsus' source surely had 'endeiknyntai'.

I owe to Dr. Bylebyl the information that Gerard of Cremona in his version of the *Methodus medendi* (from the Arabic) used the term 'significatio' for the Greek term 'endeixis'.

It would be interesting to study what were the Latin equivalents for 'endeixis' adopted by the Renaissance translators: I suspect they also used 'indicatio'.

---

[5] See Karl Deichgräber, Die griechische Empirikerschule ... 2nd ed. Berlin/Zürich 1965, p. 44.5 ("Medicativam artem ab experientia et non ab indicatione dicimus sumpsisse consistentiam ...").

IAN CASSELLS

A BRIEF NOTE ON ARABIC EQUIVALENTS TO GALEN'S
'Ἔνδειξις'

The glossary in M. C. Lyons *An Arabic translation of Themistius' commentary on Aristoteles 'De anima'* (London 1973) gives the equivalent of ἐνδεικνύναι as دلّ (dalla), 'to show'. In Arabic the word ἔνδειξις is translated by a variety of derivatives from this verb:

τοῦτο ἤρχει μόνον ἀνδρὶ περὶ φύσιν δεινῷ τὴν χρείαν τῆς γονῆς ἐνδείξασθαι.
(Galen, *De semine*, Kühn IV 544.17-18)

هذا وحده قد كان ممّا فيه كفاية لرجل ما هو حكيم فى العلم بأمور الطبيعة فى **الدلالة** على منفعة المنى. =
(do. ms Istanbul, Ayasofya 3590, f. 180a 4-5)

Dictionaries define دلالة (dalāla) as 'sign, token, indication', a rather general and untechnical term to represent the precise medical significance of ἔνδειξις. This excerpt from Rāzī, a reworking rather than a translation, uses دليل (dalīl), which is even more appropriate in a medical context as it carries the additional sense of 'symptom':

κωλυθήσεται δὲ τῆς ποιούσης αἰτίας αὐτὸ τελέως ἐκκοπείσης. ὥστ' ἐν μὲν τοῖς ἐφημέροις ἡ τῶν πρακτέων ἔνδειξις ἐκ τοῦ πυρετοῦ μάλισθ' ἡμῖν ἔσται ... ἐν δὲ τοῖς ἄλλοις ὅσοι τὴν ἀνάπτουσαν αὐτοὺς αἰτίαν ἔχουσιν ἔνδον, ὁ πρῶτος σκοπὸς τῆς ἐνδείξεως ἀπὸ τῆς αἰτίας ἐστιν.
(Galen, *Methodus medendi*, Kühn X 661.7-662.1 & 3-5)

وإذا كانت اسباب المرض قد بطلت فليس يؤخذ منها على ما به **دليل** حمى مثل حمى يوم من غضب، وإذا كان السبب قائما لابثا ويولد المرض فخذ **دليل** العلاج منه ومن المرض نفسه ايضا.

(Rāzī, *Kitāb al-Ḥāwī* ed. Hyderabad 1963, v.14, p.62.1-4)

Form X of the same verb has the altogether more specialized meaning of 'to infer, to conclude, to act in accordance with':

εἴπερ μὴ ἐκ τῆς τοῦ πράγματος αὐτοῦ φύσεως ἔνδειξιν ἔλαβον.
(Galen, *Methodus medendi*, Kühn X 104.12-13)

متى كانوا **يستدلون** بنفس طبيعة الشىء. =
(do. ms Florence, Laurentiana 250, f. 231a 15-16.

The foliation of this ms runs in retrograde to the text).

ὥστε ἕκαστος τούτων ἀπὸ τῶν τῆς διαθέσεως τοῦ φλεγμαίνοντος μέρους, οὐx ἀπὸ τῶν ἑπομένων αὐτῇ συμπτωμάτων, ἔνδειξιν τῶν βοηθημάτων λαμβάνει. (Galen *Methodus medendi*, Kühn X 101 ult —102.3)

فكما ان كل واحد من هؤلاء القوم انما يستدل على مداواة العضو الوارم ورما حارا بحال ذلك العضو الذى فيه الورم = الحار، لا بالاعراض التابعة له.

(do. ms Laurentiana 250, f. 232b 7-10)

ὥστ' οὐx ἀπὸ τῶν περὶ τὸ φλεγμαῖνον μέρος φαινομένων συμπτωμάτων ἡ ἔνδειξις αὐτοῖς γίγνεται τῶν βοηθημάτων, ἀλλ' ἀπὸ τῆς οὐσίας αὐτῆς. (Galen, *Methodus medendi*, Kühn X 101.11-13)

واذ كان مذهبهم فى تعليمهم هذا فليس احد منهم يستدل على مداواة الورم الحار بما يظهر فى العضو الوارم من = الاعراض، بل انما يستدلوا بنفس طبيعة الورم الحار.

(do. ms Laurentiana 250, f. 233a 13-15)

The most exact counterpart of all emerged in استدلال (istidlāl), the verbal noun of this form X meaning 'inference' or 'indication', and it seems to have become virtually the standard translation:

xαὶ τὴν ἔνδειξίν γε τῆς θεραπείας οὐx ἐx τῶν φαινομένων λαμβάνεις συμπτωμάτων. (Galen, *Methodus medendi*, Kühn X 101.3f)

ولا تقتصر فى الاستدلال على المداواة بالنظر فى الاشياء الظاهرة للعيان. =

(do. ms Laurentiana 250, f. 233b ult - 233a 1)

οἷον ἐν ταῖς περὶ τῆς εὑρέσεως τῶν ἀφανῶν ζητήσεσι, τῶν μὲν τὴν ἀνατομὴν xαὶ τὴν ἔνδειξιν xαὶ τὴν διαλεχτιxὴν θεωρίαν ἐπαινούντων. (Galen, *De sectis*, Kühn I 76 ult -77.3)

مثال ذلك: أن أصحاب القياس فى طلب استخراج الاشياء الخفية يمدحون التشريح، والاستدلال من الشىء على = ما يحتاج إليه فيه، وعلم المنطق.

(do. ed. Cairo 1977, p. 38.7-9)

xαὶ δύο εἰσιν αὗται πρῶται τῆς ἰατριxῆς αἱρέσεις, ἡ μὲν ἑτέρα διὰ πείρας ἰοῦσα πρὸς τὴν τῶν ἰαμάτων εὕρεσιν, ἡ δ' ἐνδείξεως. (Galen, *De sectis*, Kühn I 65. 8-10)

وهاتان الفرقتان اوّل فرق الطبّ: إحداهما تسلك فى معرفة الاشياء النافعة فى التماس الصحة طريق التجربة، = والاخرى تسلك فى معرفة ذلك طريق الاستدلال على الشىء الذى يحتاج إليه بالشىء الذى من أجله احتيج إليه.

(do. ed. Cairo 1977, p. 14.4-6)

That ἔνδειξις was understood by the Arabs as a term of great precision is demonstrated by the next quotation, which carefully distinguishes a general ἔνδειξις from a specific ἔνδειξις as indication of general or specific treatment:

يجب ان يكون أخذنا للعلاج العام من الاستدلال العام وللعلاج الخاص من الاستدلال الخاص.

(Abu l-Faraǧ ʿAbdallāh ibn aṭ-Ṭaiyib, *Tafsīr Kitāb Ǧālīnūs fī ḥīlat al-burʾ* (Commentary on Galen's *Methodus medendi*) ms Leiden, Univ. Bibl., Or. 278/1, Maqāla 8, f. 62a 13f)

These examples make it fairly certain that an استدلال in a text surviving only in Arabic represents a presumptive original ἔνδειξις, which in this passage (not, alas, in those fragments of the Greek which do survive) is also strongly suggested by the context:

جعلت استدلالي على الاشياء التى اداوى بها من هذه الامور الخفية التى استخرجتها بتلك الظاهرة للعيان.

(Galen, *On medical experience*, ed. R. Walzer, London 1944, p.82.4-5)

Walzer's translation runs: I reach my conclusion on the things which I shall use for treatment of the disease by inference from those invisible matters which I discovered with the help of those perceptible to the eye. (do. p.153.29-31)

While a more extended study than this would reveal how soon Greek terminology became adequately represented in the developing Arabic scientific vocabulary, there is every reason to suppose that the Arab translators were fully aware of the special significance of ἔνδειξις.

I am much indebted to Dr. U. Weisser of Erlangen [now Hamburg] for the majority of the above references.

PEARL KIBRE

(revised by R. J. Durling)

A LIST OF LATIN MANUSCRIPTS CONTAINING MEDIEVAL VERSIONS OF THE *METHODUS MEDENDI*

I. *Constantinus Africanus (d. 1087)*

Constantinus Africanus' *Megategni* is a paraphrase made from the Arabic. It is headed by a dedicatory letter to his pupil Johannes, Inc. *Quamvis karissime fili Johannes ingenium acutissimum in litteris habeas* (TK² 1163),* a prologue, Inc. *Quoniam intentio gloriosissimi Galieni hoc in libro* ... (TK² 1282), and text beginning *Secta autem medicorum triplex est, una dicitur* ... (TK² 1417). Expl. ...*cum levi fuste suaviter percutiatur.*

1. Basel D III 8, 14c, ff. 146ra-184ra (Durling Film C-94-2, NLM)
2. Berlin Lat. fol.(?) 897, 14c, ff.155-(157v). TK² 1282 is in error as it listed Berne for Berlin.
3. Boulogne-sur-Mer 197, 13c, ff.88ra-144ra. (TK² 1163)
4. Cambrai 907 (806), 14c, ff.1-37 (TK² 1282)
5. Cambridge CUg 98(50), 14-15c, ff.7a-80b. (TK² 1163)
6. Cambridge CUpet 33, 13-14c, ff. 1ra-23rb. Pref. Inc. *O fili Iohannes* (TK² 970)
7. Cambridge CUsj 78 (D.3), 13-14c, ff.32r-61r. (TK² 1163)
8. Chartres 284(340), 13c, ff.164vb- ? . Ms. too badly mutilated to utilize. (Durling Film C-148-2, NLM)
9. Dresden Db 92-93, 15c, ff.46vb—The text contains the note: "Translatio libri Megategni sepe Galienum laudat et allegat in hoc opere ..."
10. Edinburgh EU 166(III), late 13c, ff.48v-75v. (TK² 1163) A university MS., probably of Parisian origin (C. P. Finlayson). Pecia numbers.
11. Erfurt EA f.249, 13-14c, ff.1-25v.
12. Eton 172, 13c, ff.83vb-110ra. Diels p. 92; N. R. Ker, Medieval Manuscripts in British Libraries, II (Oxford, 1977), p. 352; (Durling Film C-128-2, NLM)
13. Krakow Polsk. Akad. 1700, 14c, ff. 66ra-121rb (Durling Film C-148-1, NLM)

---

* TK² = Lynn Thorndike and Pearl Kibre, A Catalogue of Incipits of Mediaeval Scientific Writings in Latin, rev. and augm. ed. Cambridge, Mass./London, 1963.

14. Leipzig 1184, 14c, ff. 68ra-105ra.
15. London BLr 12.C.XV, 13c, ff. 118^r-(145^v).
16. London UL Aa(Gaza, Strongroom) No. 55, in R. Watson, Descriptive List of Fragments of Medieval Manuscripts in the University of London Library (London, 1976), p. 29.
17. Lüneburg Ratsbücherei D 2o 5, 3, 4, 15c, ff. 113ra-170rb. See Martin Wierschin, HSS der Ratsbücherei Lüneburg, Miscellanea u. Historica (Wiesbaden, 1969), pp. 10-15.
18. (Whereabouts unknown). A fragment is edited by L. R. Lind in the B. E. Perry Festschrift (University of Illinois Press, 1969), pp. 103-113.
19. Oxford BL canon. misc. 504, 14c, ff. 131ra-140vb. Expl. in *eis que oportuna* ... (Durling Film C-82-1, NLM).
20. Oxford Ob 231, 14c, ff. 107^v-135.
21. Oxford Ome 218, 14c, ff. 99^r-129^r.
22. Oxford Ome 219, 14c, ff. 161.
23. Paris PU 125, 13c, ff. 179-207.
24. Rome Ran 1456, 15c, ff. 114^v-119^r. "Excerpta ex libris Megatorum [sic]" Inc. *Precepit Ypocras ut medicus considerare⟨t⟩ sapienter naturam corporumque* ... Expl. *Corpus cum aliis alimentis. Finis excerptorum Constantini.*
25. Salzburg, Erzbischöfliches Priesterseminar 2164, 13-14c, ff.— (Kristeller, P.O. Iter Italicum III (1983, p. 37)) Not yet seen (24 Jan. 1984).
26. Vatican Vat lat. 2378, 13-14c, ff. 121ra-142vb. (Durling Film C-39-2, NLM).
27. Vatican Vat. pal. lat. 1094, 14c, ff. 253ra-288ra. (Durling Film C-49-1, NLM).

II. *Gerard of Cremona (d. 1187)*

Gerard translated the *Methodus Medendi* from the Arabic. The version is commonly referred to as De ingenio sanitatis, from the opening words: Inc. *Librum de ingenio sanitatis a te et a multis karissime Nero* ... Not included in the posthumous list of Gerard's versions, drawn up by his pupils.

1. Basel D I 12, 14c, ff. 130ra-155vb. Cirusia Ghalieni [sic], i.e. books 3-6 only. Diels p. 135 (s.v. De chirurgia). (Durling Film C-96-2, NLM).
2. Cambridge CUpet 33, 13-14c, ff. 241vb-258vb.
3. Cesena Dext. Plut. 25 cod. 2, 13c, ff. 1ra-47va. Books 1 (incomplete)-6. Inc. ... ⟨*vitu*⟩ *perare. Nam si eligendus esset discipulus*

[= ch. 2 of bk. 1, cf. 1490 printed ed. f. 383rb, 19th line from bottom] Expl. ... *quia substantia eius siccissima est.* (Durling Film C-77-1, NLM).

4. Cesena Sinis. Plut. 5 cod. 4, 14c, ff. 219ra-256rb. Expl. ... *quandoque difficile* (Durling Film C-40-3, NLM).
5. Chartres 284(340), 13c, ff. 80v-129v, 164v-187.
6. Chartres 293, 14c, ff.59-79.
7. Cues 296, 13-14c, ff. 27-71v. Ascribed to G. of C. in colophon.
8. Cues 297, 13-14c, ff. 45v-109v.
9. Eton 132, 13c, ff. 110ra-160ra. Cf. Ker, II 352-3.
10. Edinburgh EU 166(XI), late 13c, ff. 213ra-241vb. (Durling Film C-90-2, NLM).
11. Florence FLg 58, 14c, ff. 1ra-[67vb]. (Durling Film C-85-3, NLM).
12. Gdańsk (Danzig) Mar. F. 41, 14c, ff. 29ra-83vb. Durling, *Traditio* 37 (1981) 380.
13. Kassel 8o10, a.1332, ff. 53v-15r. (Durling, *Traditio* 37 (1981) 380).
14. London BM Harl. 3748, 14c, ff. 42vb112vb. Ascribed to G. of C. in titulus and colophon.
15. Madrid 1198, 14c, ff. 99ra147vb. Bks. 3-14 (latter incomplete) Inc. *Sicut operandi significationes Nero karissime* ... Expl. *quod locum vulnerant verum (?)* ... (Durling Film C-89-2, NLM).
16. Montpellier 18, 14c, ff. 224r273vb. Ascribed to G. of C. in titulus and colophon.
17. Munich Clm 11, 14-15c, ff. 16ra35va. Bks. VII-XIV. Inc. *Librum de sanitatis ingenio iam diu Neroni inceptum componere postposui* ...
18. Munich Clm 13206, 14c, ff. 11ra-65v.
19. Naples VIII D 34, 14c, ff. 57ra-72vb. Bks. 8-11. Inc. *In hac particula febrium curationem artificialiter ostendi:* Expl. *et via largior efficitur facile igitur currunt si* ... Diels p. 131 (s.v. *De febribus:* source not identified). (Durling Film C-151-4, NLM).
20. Oxford All Souls 68, 14-15c, ff. 113ra-192vb.
21. Oxford Balliol 231, 14c, ff. 330ra-390rv.
22. Oxford BL cm 366, 12-15c, ff. 143r-150v. Bk. 6 (fragment). Inc. ... *prodesse. Sed misceatur aliquando cum oleo confectum in modum stercoris columbini* ... [cf. 1490 printed ed. f. 402rb, 5th line from bottom]. Not in Diels.
23. Oxford BL e 19, 14c, ff. 68va86vb. *Cyrurgia Galieni* [i.e. bks. 3-6, 13-14]. Not in Diels.
24. Paris BN 6865 B, 13-14c, ff. 84ra-137vb.
25. Paris BN 6883, 14c, ff. 41r-77r. (Durling Film C-62-5, NLM).

26. Paris BN 9331, 13-14c, ff. 1ra-90vb.
27. Paris BN 11860, 13-14c, ff. 165ra-216va. Ascribed to G. of C. in colophon.
28. Paris BN 14389, 14c, ff. 257rb-279vb. Bks. I-XIII only.
29. Paris BN 15456, 13c, ff. 61ra-115vb. Ascribed in colophon to G. of C.
30. Paris BN na 1482, 14-15c, ff. 172ra-187vb, Bks. VII-IX, XIV partim.
31. Paris Mazarine (PM) 3598(1281), 14c, leaves unnumbered (ff. i^r-viii^r), ff. 1-233. Ascribed in colophon to G. of C.
32. Paris Université (PU) 125, 13c, ff. 99vb-(121va). Book VII, only.
33. Vatican Vat. lat. 2131, f. 60^r-v. Fragment of Bk. I.
34. Vatican Vat. lat. 2369, 14c, ff. 81ra-95rb. Bks. III-VI only. Colophon; Explicit *Cyrugia vulnerum Galieni* ... Diels p. 135 fails to identify the source. (Durling Film C-40-2, NLM).
35. Vatican Vat. lat. 2375, 14c, ff. 304ra-398vb.
36. Vatican Vat. lat. 2377, 13-14c, ff. 1ra-51vb. Bks. I-XIII. (Durling Film C-40-3 and C-76-1, NLM).
37. Vatican Vat. lat. 2378, 13-14c, ff. 1ra-42vb.
38. Vatican Vat. lat. 2379, 14c, ff. 1ra-62vb. Bks. I-XIII.
39. Vatican Vat. lat. 2386, 13-14c, ff. 145ra-156ra. Incomplete.
40. Vatican Vat. pal. lat. 1094, 14c, ff. 115rb-196vb. Bk. XIV is incomplete: expl. *poteris artificialiter curare.* (Durling Film C-49-1, NLM).
41. Vatican Vat. pal. lat. 1095, 14c, ff. 3vb-33rb. Bks VII-XIV only.
42. Vatican Vat. pal. lat. 1096, 14c, ff. 153ra-183va.
43. Vatican Vat. pal. lat. 1097, late 12c, ff. 22ra-114ra.
44. Vatican Vat. Reg. Suev. 1305, 14c, ff. 81ra-107ra.
45. Vatican Vat. Urb. 235, 14c, ff. 1ra-39rb. Bks. I-VI. Beautifully decorated, many marginal notes.
46. Vatican Vat. Urb. 236, 14c, ff. 1-23vb, 23ra-31vb: 'Cirurgia G.' [i.e. bks. III-VI, XIII-XIV].
47. Vienna, VI 2273, 14c, ff. 13ra-56vb. Ascribed to G. of C.
48. Wrocław IV. F. 25, 13c, ff. 168va-186rb. Bks. VII-XIV. (Durling Film C-103-1, NLM).
49. Wrocław IV.F.26, 13c, ff. 88vb-107vb. Bks. I-IV (incomplete). Expl. ...*quod fiunt ei vigilie: dolor ⟨spasmus et alienatio⟩.* ... Cf. 1490 printed ed. f. 397ra, lines 24-25.
50. Würzburg M.p.Med. F.2, late 13c. ff. 5ra-60ra. Expl. ... *Vulnus autem quod vocatur carnosum ex genere duri apostematis est.* (Durling Film C-145-2, NLM).

III. *Burgundio of Pisa (ca. 1110-1193)*

Burgundio translated only books VII-XIV of M.M. His version, entitled simply Therapeutica, was completed by Pietro d'Abano (bk.XIV, end). Inc. *Terrapeuticam methodum Eugeniane amicissime olim quidem inceperam* ... (TK^2 1563). Expl. *Hic ergo iam et hiis finiatur sermo.*

1. Basel D.I.5, late 14c, ff. 1ra-54vb (Liber XI has colophon ascribing the version to Burgundio of Pisa; Durling Film C-98-1, NLM).
2. Cesena Dextr. Plut. 23 cod. 1, 14c, ff. 1ra-46ra (Incomplete. Expl. *alterum vero flegmone* ...).
3a. Cesena Dextr. Plut 25 cod. 2, 13c, ff. 48ra-110vb.
3b. Cesena Sinis. Plut. 5 cod. 4, 14c, ff. 159ra-198rb (with Pietro's completion of bk. XIV; Durling Film C-76-1, NLM).
4. Cortona 109. 14c, ff. 40ra-79vb (Durling, *Traditio* 37 (1981) 380).
5. Dresden Db. 92-93, 15c, ff. 565va-608rb (Durling Film C-115-1, NLM). Omits the portion completed by Pietro d'Abano.
6. London BM Addit. 22,669, 14c, ff. 1ra-27vb. With Pietro's completion.
7. London Wellcome 285, 14c, ff. 1r-40. With Pietro's completion.
8. Madrid 1978 (L.60), 14c, ff. 2ra-45va.
9. Metz 178, 14c, ff. 53vb-70vb. "Incipit liber de ingenio de nova translatione ..." (TK^2 73).
10. Montpellier 18, 14c, ff. 203r-223vb. Book XI only. (TK^2 910).
11. Monza F.8/165, late 13c, ff. 405-419. Book XI only. (Durling, *Traditio* 37 (1981) 380).
12. New Haven, Yale Medical Library (Cushing MS), ff. 1r-35va.
13. Paris BN 6865 B, 13-14c, ff. 32ra-81vb; With Pietro's completion of book XIV.
14. Paris BN 9331, 13-14c, ff. 1ra-90vb. With Pietro's completion.
15. Vatican Vat. lat. 2375, 14c, ff. 511va-575rb. (Durling Film C-38-1, NLM).
16. Vatican Vat. lat. 2381, 14c, ff. 134rb-182vb. With Pietro's completion.
17. Vatican Vat. lat. 2385, 15c, ff. 187va-265va. With Pietro's completion.
18. Vatican Vat. Barb. 178, 1329 A.D., ff. 3ra-44ra. With Pietro's completion.
19. Vatican Vat. pal. lat. 1093, 14c, ff. 71ra-107vb. (Pietro's completion begins with the chapter: *Duplex autem est et hoc genus unum quidem* ...).

20. Vatican Vat. pal. lat. 1096, 14c, ff. 14vb-52vb. (Durling Film C-31-1, NLM).
21. Vatican Urb. 235, 14c, ff. 41ra-82rb. (Incomplete, Expl. ... *sine flegmone precedente*).
22. Vatican Urb. 247, 14c, ff. 205ra-242vb. Expl. as Urb. 235.
23. Venice VE San Marco fa 531 (Class. XIV cod. 6), a. 1305, ff. 68ra-106va. With Pietro's completion.
24. Vienna 2272, 14c, ff. 93ra-126vb.
25. Vienna 2294 (Res. 956), 14c, ff. 1r-82v. With Pietro's completion (Inc. *Duplex autem est* ...). In one additional MS. at least, this version from the Greek is attributed to Niccolò da Reggio.
26. Munich Clm 35, 14c, ff. 116ra-144v. "Translatus a Nicholao de Reggio de Greco in latinum" (TK2 col. 1563). Whether at any time Niccolò revised the original version by Burgundio, remains to be seen.

Acknowledgements

Professor Pearl Kibre wished to acknowledge the assistance of many librarians, and especially Mlle. Marthe Dulong for her assistance in transcribing MSS in Paris libraries, particularly the Bibliothèque Nationale. Also to Mrs. Dorothy Hanks, of the National Library of Medicine (History of Medicine Division) for introducing her to the medical manuscripts on microfilm at the NLM. Finally, she would like to express her appreciation and thanks to her research assistant, Irving Kelter.

Addendum

A further Latin MS, containing books 1-6 in Gerard's version and the remainder in Burgundio's is Salzburg Museum Carolino-Augusteum 4004, 14c, ff. 84r-161v. See Yates, Donald. Descriptive inventories of MSS microfilmed for the Hill Monastic Manuscript Library. Vol. I. Collegeville, Minn. 1981, p. 146.

URSULA WEISSER

ZUR REZEPTION DER *METHODUS MEDENDI* IM *CONTINENS* DES RHAZES

Der vorliegende Beitrag, der das Nachleben von Galens Schrift *De metho-do medendi* im arabisch-islamischen Mittelalter beleuchten soll, konzentriert sich im wesentlichen auf einen einzigen arabischen Text. Diese Einengung des Themas ist in erster Linie bedingt durch den gegenwärtigen Stand der Forschung zum Problem "Galen bei den Arabern". Freilich kann die Erforschung der arabischen Galen-Übersetzungen bereits eine längere Tradition vorweisen, die unter anderem durch eine Reihe von entsprechenden Textausgaben dokumentiert wird — Gotthard Strohmaier berichtete vor Jahren beim ersten Galen-Symposium darüber.[1] Auch steht es völlig außer Frage, daß die wissenschaftliche Medizin im Islam weitgehend von Galens Anschauungen beherrscht wurde. Art und Umfang der Nachwirkung einzelner galenischer Schriften in der arabischsprachigen Medizinliteratur indessen können wir noch kaum übersehen — wie denn der konkrete Nachweis antiker Vorlagen und Vorbilder der arabischen Ärzte überhaupt zu den dunkleren Kapiteln der arabistischen Medizingeschichtsforschung gehört. Es hat überdies den Anschein, daß bei Quellenstudien zu arabischen Texten besonders jene Teile des *Corpus Galenianum* nicht immer ausreichend berücksichtigt werden, die dem Nichtgräzisten schwer zugänglich, weil nur in der Ausgabe Kühns erreichbar sind. Dies gilt leider auch für eine so grundlegende Schrift wie die *Methodus medendi*; daher existieren für unsere fragestellung noch so gut wie keine Vorarbeiten. Bei dieser Sachlage erschien es am sinnvollsten, die Rezeption der *MM* durch die Ärzte des islamischen Kulturkreises an einem Einzelbeispiel näher zu untersuchen, und zwar an einem Werk des Rhazes, der zu ihren herausragendsten Vertretern gezählt werden darf. Inwieweit die im folgenden aufgezeigten Tendenzen als typisch gelten können, muß die zukünftige Forschung erweisen.

1. *Zur orientalischen Überlieferung der Methodus medendi*

Als Hintergrund für unsere Fallstudie über den *Continens* wollen wir zunächst kurz skizzieren, was bislang über die *MM* bei den Arabern be-

---

[1] Gotthard Strohmaier: Galen in Arabic: prospects and projects. In: Galen: Problems and Prospects. A Collection of Papers Submitted at the 1979 Cambridge Conference, ed. by Vivian Nutton. London 1981, S. 187-196.

kannt ist. Es kennzeichnet trefflich die Forschungssituation, daß die spärlichen Angaben, die in den beiden 1970 erschienenen Standardwerken zur Medizin im Islam von Fuat Sezgin und Manfred Ullmann zusammengetragen sind,[2] in der Zwischenzeit nur wenige Ergänzungen erfahren haben. Einzige Informationsquelle für den Weg der *MM* in den Orient ist die unschätzbare *Risāla* des großen Übersetzers Ḥunain ibn Isḥāq (gest. 260/873 oder 264/877) über die syrischen und arabischen Galen-Übersetzungen.[3] Ḥunain bespricht sie dort an 20. Stelle, als Schlußtext (Nr. 15) des alexandrinischen Lehrkanons.[4] Mit gewohnter Präzision umreißt er Ziel und Inhalt des Werkes: "Er (sc. Galen) verfolgt in ihm das Ziel darzulegen, wie eine jede Krankheit behandelt wird nach der dialektischen Methode; er beschränkt sich dabei auf die allgemeinen Symptome, auf die man achten muß, um aus ihnen abzuleiten, womit jede der Krankheiten behandelt werden muß, und er führt als einfache Beispiele dafür spezielle Fälle an."[5] Weiter berichtet Ḥunain, daß die Schrift in zwei Etappen für zwei verschiedene Adressaten abgefaßt wurde. Inhaltlich gliedert er sie nach Hauptthemen in vier große Abschnitte: a) Grundlagen der therapeutischen Wissenschaft nebst Widerlegung des Thessalos[6] und seiner Anhänger (Buch I-II), b) Krankheiten, die unter den Begriff "Lösung des Zusammenhalts" fallen (Buch III-VI), c) Krankheiten der Homoiomeren (Buch VII-XII) — der Inhalt dieses Teils wird anschließend noch weiter spezifiziert —, d) Krankheiten der zusammengesetzten Körperteile (Buch XIII-XIV).

---

[2] Fuat Sezgin: Geschichte des arabischen Schrifttums. Bd. III: Medizin — Pharmazie, Zoologie — Tierheilkunde bis ca. 430 H. Leiden 1970, S. 96-98; Manfred Ullmann: Die Medizin im Islam (Handbuch der Orientalistik, I. Abt., Erg.-Bd. VI 1). Leiden/Köln 1970, S. 45.

[3] Ḥunain ibn Isḥāq: Über die syrischen und arabischen Galen-Übersetzungen. Zum ersten Mal herausgegeben und übersetzt von Gotthelf Bergsträsser (Abhandlungen für die Kunde des Morgenlandes XVII 2). Leipzig 1925, S. 16-19 (arab.), S. 13-15 (Übers.). Die deutsche Übersetzung wird auch zitiert von Sezgin, loc. cit.; s. auch J. Schleifer: Zum Syrischen Medizinbuch. II. Der therapeutische Teil. *Rivista degli Studi orientali* 18 (1939/40), S. 347f. — Ibn Abī Uṣaibiʿa, der als einziger der mittelalterlichen arabischen Biographen ausführliche Angaben zur *MM* bringt (ʿUyūn al-anbāʾ fī ṭabaqāt al-aṭibbāʾ, ed. August Müller. Kairo, Königsberg 1882-1884, Bd. I, S. 93,21-94,6), schreibt nach dem Nachweis von Bergsträsser (in seiner Einleitung zur Edition, S. II-V) lediglich Ḥunains *Risāla* aus.

[4] S. Albert Z. Iskandar: An attempted reconstruction of the late Alexandrian medical curriculum. *Med. Hist.* 20 (1976), S. 239.

[5] Übersetzung leicht modifiziert nach Bergsträsser, loc. cit.

[6] Rez. A der *Risāla*, die Bergsträsser 1925 veröffentlichte, bietet hier den Namen "Erasistratos". Die richtige Lesart "Thessalos" findet sich in Rez. B, aus der der Herausgeber sieben Jahre später Nachträge lieferte, s. G. Bergsträsser: Neue Materialien zu Ḥunain ibn Isḥāq's Galen-Bibliographie (Abhandlungen für die Kunde des Morgenlandes XIX 2). Leipzig 1932, S. 16 (Zu S. 16,21 der ursprünglichen Ausgabe).

Über die Transmission des Textes erfahren wir von Ḥunain, daß insgesamt drei syrische Fassungen existiert haben.[7] Die erste Version aus der Feder des Archiaters Sergios von Rēšʿainā (gest. 536 n.Chr.) genügte den philologischen Ansprüchen des frühen 9.Jahrhunderts schon nicht mehr; Ḥunain fand insbesondere den ersten Teil (Buch I-VI), eine Jugendarbeit des Sergios, völlig unzulänglich. Er selbst versuchte zunächst auf Veranlassung und mit der Unterstützung von Salmawaih ibn Bunān (gest. 225/840), dem späteren Leibarzt des Kalifen al-Muʿtaṣim, den zweiten Teil jener älteren Übertragung, beginnend mit Buch VII,[8] anhand eines griechischen Manuskripts zu verbessern. Dieses mühselige Unterfangen gab er indessen bald zugunsten einer Neuübersetzung des zweiten Teiles auf. Unglücklicherweise wurde das Original dieser Neufassung, ehe es vervielfältigt werden konnte, bei einem Schiffsbrand vernichtet. Erst viele Jahre später schließlich machte sich Ḥunain auf Bitten von Buḫtīšūʿ ibn Ǧibrīl (gest. 256/870) noch einmal daran, eine vollständige syrische Version zu schaffen. Für den zweiten Teil der *MM* standen ihm drei griechische Textzeugen zur Verfügung, die es ihm erlaubten, nach seiner Gewohnheit als Übersetzungsvorlage einen kritisch erarbeiteten Mischtext zu verwenden. Von Buch I-VI konnte er dagegen nur eine einzige Handschrift von schlechter Qualität auftreiben; nach Beendigung seiner Übertragung erhielt er allerdings Gelegenheit, diesen Abschnitt an einem zweiten griechischen Kodex zu überprüfen. Die geringere Verbreitung des ersten Teils der *MM*, in dem Galen neben den Grundlagen der Therapie die Wundbehandlung bespricht, begründet Ḥunain im übrigen damit, daß er nicht zur obligatorischen Lektüre der Alexandriner zählte — was ein interessantes Licht auf die Lehrinhalte der spätantiken Schulmedizin wirft.

Auf jener zweiten syrischen Version Ḥunains basiert schließlich die Übersetzung ins Arabische, die wir seinem Neffen und Mitarbeiter Ḥubaiš ibn al-Ḥasan al-Aʿsam (gest. Ende des 3./9.Jhs.) verdanken;[9] Buch VII-XVI wurden überdies vom Meister selbst noch einmal durchgesehen. Dies scheint die einzige arabische Fassung geblieben zu sein. Nach

---

[7] Vgl. auch Rainer Degen: Galen im Syrischen: Eine Übersicht über die syrische Überlieferung der Werke Galens. In: Galen: Problems and Prospects (wie Anm. 1), S. 145f. (Nr. 55).

[8] Degen, loc. cit., gibt irrtümlich an, diese Verbesserung habe den zweiten Teil von Buch VII betroffen.

[9] Bergsträsser hat einen Teil des arabischen Textes unter terminologischen Gesichtspunkten untersucht (Ḥunain ibn Isḥaḳ und seine Schule. Sprach- und literargeschichtliche Untersuchungen zu den arabischen Hippokrates- und Galen-Übersetzungen. Leiden 1913, S. 69) und kommt zu dem Schluß, daß Ḥubaiš's Urheberschaft auch von den sprachlichen Merkmalen der Übersetzung her wahrscheinlich ist; s. auch die arabische Textprobe, ibid. S. 5f. (arab.) ≈ *MM* X 40,16-41,8.

Sezgin ist sie in sieben durchweg unvollständigen Textzeugen auf uns gekommen.[10] Im Gegensatz zu der Überlieferungssituation, die seinerzeit
Ḥunain antraf, enthalten sie mit nur einer Ausnahme sämtlich Fragmente des ersten Teils; nach derzeitiger Kenntnis sind Buch VII-IX im Arabischen verloren bzw. nur fragmentarisch in Zitaten erhalten.

Als kleinen Ersatz dafür bietet die arabische Überlieferung jedoch ein
anderwärts nirgends bezeugtes Addendum Galens zur *MM* — ein Nach-
trag, der, weil vom Autor erst postum angebracht, freilich von recht frag-
würdiger Echtheit erscheint. Ibn Abī Uṣaibiʿa überliefert ihn[11] auf die
Autorität des ägyptischen Arztes und Kommentators griechischer
Medizin[12] ʿAlī ibn Riḍwān (gest. 452/1061 oder 460/1067) hin. Einst-
mals, so wird berichtet, plagten diesen hartnäckige Kopfschmerzen infolge einer Überfüllung der Venen. Die Anwendung des Aderlasses brachte
ihm trotz mehrmaliger Wiederholung keinerlei Linderung. Da erschien
ihm im Traume der große Arzt Galen selbst und forderte ihn auf, ihm
die *MM* vorzulesen — so wie nach der damals gebräuchlichen Unter-
richtsmethode der Schüler seinem Lehrer den zu erarbeitenden Text laut
vorzutragen hatte. Als Ibn Riḍwān sieben Teile der Schrift rezitiert hatte — ein beachtliches Pensum für einen einzigen Traum —, unterbrach
ihn Galen mit dem Ausruf: "Da habe ich doch tatsächlich den Kopf-
schmerz, an dem du leidest, vergessen!" Natürlich beeilte er sich, dieses
Versäumnis wiedergutzumachen. Er empfahl seinem leidenden Kollegen
nämlich, sich am Hinterhauptshöcker schröpfen zu lassen, was in der
Tat die Beschwerden auf der Stelle beseitigte. Trotzdem werden wir gut
daran tun, unsere Studien auf die Nachwirkung jenes Textes zu beschränken, den Galen noch zu Lebzeiten veröffentlicht hatte.

Man darf davon ausgehen, daß die abschließende Zusammenstellung
und theoretische Begründung der universellen therapeutischen Prinzi-
pien Galens in der MM auch für die arabische Heilkunde grundlegend
wurde. Dafür bürgte bereits die Verankerung des Werkes im vorislami-
schen medizinischen Lehrplan, der die Medizin im Islam bekanntlich

---

[10] Die wohl dem Florentiner Katalog entnommene Angabe bei Sezgin loc. cit., S. 98,
am Ende des Codex Laurentianus 250 fehlten "einige Blätter", erwies sich bei einer
Überprüfung als stark untertrieben: Der arabische Text endet bereits eine Seite vor
Schluß des VI. Buches (*MM* X 545,10), umfaßt demnach noch nicht einmal die Hälfte
des Gesamtwerkes.

[11] Ibn Abī Uṣaibiʿa, loc. cit., I 10,19-24; französische Übersetzung von Max Meyerhof und Joseph Schacht: Une controverse médico-philosophique au Caire en 441 de l'hé-
gire (1050 ap. J.-C.) avec une aperçu sur les études grecques dans l'Islam. *Bulletin de l'Institut d'Egypte* 19 (1936/37), S. 36f.; s. auch Jacques Grand'Henry: Le livre de la méthode
du médecin de ʿAlī b. Riḍwān (998-1067). Texte édité, traduit et commenté. Part I: Introduction — Thérapeutique (Publications de l'Institut orientaliste de Louvain 20). Louvain 1979, S. 6f.

[12] Vgl. hierzu Iskandar, loc. cit., S. 240f.

formal und inhaltlich wesentlich mitbestimmte. Ein weiteres Indiz für die Wertschätzung der *MM* ist die Tatsache, daß sich mehrere arabische Ärzte veranlaßt fühlten, sie zu bearbeiten.[13] Die erste Epitome (*iḫtiṣār*) verfaßte nach dem Zeugnis von Ibn Abī Uṣaibiʿa[14] bereits Ḥunains jüngerer Zeitgenosse Ṯābit ibn Qurra al-Ḥarrānī (gest. 288/901). Auf uns gekommen sind drei spätere Beispiele, die alle noch der näheren Untersuchung harren: je eine Kurzfassung von Rhazes (mit vollem arabischem Namen Abū Bakr Muḥammad ibn Zakarīyāʾ ar-Rāzī, gest. 313/925) und von dem jüdischen Arzt Maimonides (Mūsā ibn Maimūn, gest. 601/1204)[15] sowie eine als "Kommentar" (*tafsīr*) bezeichnete Bearbeitung von Abū l-Faraǧ ibn aṭ-Ṭaiyib (gest. 435/1043).[16] Im übrigen ist noch für das 13. Jahrhundert die Existenz eines griechischen Codex der *MM* im islamischen Bereich bezeugt, und zwar im Besitz des Muwaffaq ad-Dīn Yaʿqūb ibn Siqlab (gest. 625/1237).[16a]

Der Nachweis der Nebenüberlieferung der *MM* im arabischen Schrifttum liegt, wie eingangs angedeutet, noch sehr im argen.[17] Ullmann hat aus den wenigen gedruckt vorliegenden Kompendien die Zitate und Verweise auf die *MM* zusammengestellt;[18] die Identifizierung dieser Fragmente freilich steht noch aus. Wenn wir vom *Continens* zunächst einmal absehen, finden wir die *MM* erwähnt im *Paradies der Weisheit* (*Firdaus al-ḥikma*) des ʿAlī ibn Sahl Rabban aṭ-Ṭabarī (gest. gegen 250/855),[19] im *Schatz der medizinischen Wissenschaft* (*aḏ-Ḏaḫīra fī ʿilm aṭ-ṭibb*),[20] dessen traditionelle Zuweisung an den schon genannten Ṯābit ibn Qurra in der For-

---

[13] S. die Zusammenstellung bei Sezgin, loc. cit., S. 98.

[14] Ibn Abī Uṣaibiʿa, loc. cit., I 219,29.

[15] Zur Epitome des Maimonides ist eine weitere, in hebräischer Schrift ausgeführte Handschrift der Pariser Bibliothèque Nationale (hébr. 1203) nachzutragen, s. S.M. Stern: Ten Autographs by Maimonides. In: S.D. Sassoon: Maimonides Commentarius in Mischnam. Copenhagen 1966, Bd. 3, S. 12. Sie gehört zu einer Serie von Kurzfassungen der sog. "Sechzehn Bücher" Galens; vgl. dazu auch Elinor Lieber: Galen in Hebrew: the transmission of Galen's works in the mediaeval Islamic world. In: Galen: Problems and Prospects (wie Anm. 1), S. 182.

[16] Möglicherweise im Rahmen seines Kompendiums der "Sechzehn Bücher" Galens; vgl. Max Meyerhof: Von Alexandrien nach Bagdad. Ein Beitrag zur Geschichte des philosophischen und medizinischen Unterrichts bei den Arabern. *Sitzungsberichte der Preußischen Akademie der Wissenschaften zu Berlin, phil.-hist. Kl.*, 1930, S. 425. Eine flüchtige Durchsicht des Leidener Codex (or. 178/1) ergab im übrigen, daß es sich eher um eine recht freie kürzende Bearbeitung als um einen Kommentar im eigentlichen Sinn handelt.

[16a] S. Ibn Abī Uṣaibiʿa, loc. cit., II 215, 18f.

[17] Im Syrischen ist eine Reihe von Zitaten aus der *MM* von J. Schleifer (loc. cit., S. 343f.) im sog. "Anonymen Syrischen Medizinbuch" identifiziert worden; s. auch Degen, loc. cit.

[18] Ullmann, loc. cit.

[19] Ed. Muḥammad Zubair aṣ-Ṣiddīqī, Berlin-Charlottenburg 1928, S. 292,8-13.

[20] Ed. G. Sobhy, Cairo 1928, S. 2,4-5; 7,15-20; 35,18-21; 45,19-46,6; 67,3-6; 76,7-15; 148,20f.; 173,10-16; 177,23f.

schung umstritten ist, im *Liber regius* (*al-Kitāb al-malakī* oder *Kāmil aṣ-ṣinā'a aṭ-ṭibbīya*) des Haly Abbas ('Alī ibn al-'Abbās al-Maǧūsī, gest. Ende des 4./10.Jhs.)[21] und im Drogenbuch (*K. al-Ǧāmi' li-mufradāt al-adwiya wa-l-aġḏiya*) des Ibn al-Baiṭār (gest. 646/1248).[22] Ferner sind der Sekundärliteratur Angaben über weitere Zitate in vier (zumindest im Original) noch unveröffentlichten Texten zu entnehmen. Es handelt sich um das *Viaticum* (*Zād al-musāfir*) des Ibn al-Ǧazzār (gest. 369/979),[23] das *Buch über die Kräfte der einfachen Heilmittel* (*K. Quwā l-adwiya al-mufrada*) des Ibn Abī l-Aš'aṯ (gest. 360/970),[24] das *Nützliche Buch über die Art des Unterrichts in der Heilkunde* (*an-Nāfi' fī kaifīyat ta'līm ṣinā'at aṭ-ṭibb*) des ebenfalls schon erwähnten 'Alī ibn Riḍwan[25] und die Schrift über die Prüfung der Ärzte (*K. Imtiḥān al-alibbā' li-kāffat al-aṭibbā'*) des Muwaffaq ad-Dīn as-Sulamī (gest. 604/1207).[26] An außermedizinischen Autoren sind hier zu nennen der Physiker Ibn al-Haiṯam (gest. 430/1039), von dem Ibn Abī Uṣaibi'a ein *MM*-Zitat über das fortwährende Streben nach Wissen (*MM* VII 1: X 457,11-14) überliefert,[26a] sowie der Philosoph Abū Naṣr al-Fārābī (gest. 339/950), der Galens Hinweis auf die niedere Herkunft des von ihm bekämpften Methodikers Thessalos in seiner Rhetorik-Schrift als Beispiel für die polemische Technik innerhalb der Rhetorik an-

---

[21] Steindruck Būlāq 1294/1877, Bd. II, S. 7,25-27; 21,14-30.

[22] Steindruck Būlāq 1291/1874, Bd. I 41 ult.-42,7; 152,1-4; Bd. III 22,18-19; 105,14f.; 121,27-ult.; Bd. IV 85,7-10; 85,18-21; 93,2f. (über den *Continens* des Rhazes, offenbar nicht unmittelbar aus der *MM*); ferner Verweise auf die *MM* in Bd. I 110 ult. und Bd. IV 67,30.

[23] Nach Gustave Dugat: Études sur le traité de médecine d'Abou Djàfar Ah'mad, intitulé: Zad el-Moçafir "La provision du voyageur". *Journal asiatique*, Vᵉ sér. 1 (1853), 323. Ibn al-Ǧazzār zieht die *MM* heran zu Fragen des Nasenblutens und der Blutstillung bei Verletzungen.

[24] Nach Albert Dietrich: Medicinalia Arabica. Studien über arabische medizinische Handschriften in türkischen und syrischen Bibliotheken (Abhandlungen der Akademie der Wissenschaften in Göttingen, phil.-hist. Kl., 3. F., Nr. 66). Göttingen 1966, S. 145. In der Einleitung seines Werkes (abgedruckt ibid. S. 144f.) weist Ibn Abī l-Aš'aṯ im übrigen darauf hin, daß die *MM* lediglich allgemeine therapeutische Regeln enthält (s. die beiden letzten Zeilen des arabischen Exzerpts).

[25] In Buch VI, Kap. 1, s. die Übersetzung der Stelle bei Malcolm C. Lyons: The Kitāb al-Nāfi' of 'Alī ibn Riḍwān. *Islamic Quarterly* 6 (1961), S. 67; vgl. auch Iskandar, loc. cit., S. 243. Der Hinweis bezieht sich auf die Polemik Galens gegen Scharlatane und Modeärzte in *MM* I 1.

[26] Ein Zitat aus *MM* VI, s. Dietrich, loc. cit., S. 198. Bei den Parallelen zu *MM* VI 4 (X 412,13-423,12), die Otto Spies und Hans-Jürgen Thies (Die Propädeutik der arabischen Chirurgie nach Ibn al-Quff. *Sudhoffs Archiv* 55 [1971], bes. S. 383-387) in der Chirurgie des Ibn al-Quff (Kitāb al-'Umda fī l-ǧirāḥa. Haidarabad 1356, Kap. XVII 1, Bd. II, S. 98-107) nachweisen, handelt es sich wohl nicht um direkte, sondern um durch Paulos von Aigina vermittelte Entlehnungen. Zu *MM*-Zitaten in den *Aphorismen* des Maimonides, vgl. u. S. 146.

[26a] S. Ibn Abī Uṣaibi'a, loc. cit., II 91,30-92,3; vgl. Strohmaier, loc. cit. (wie Anm. 1), S. 189.

führt.[26b] Der Titel des galenischen Werkes lautet an allen diesen Stellen *Ḥīlat al-burʾ*, eine Lehnübersetzung des griechischen Titels Θεραπευτική μέθοδος, die auf Ḥubaiš bzw. Ḥunain zurückgehen dürfte. Belege für den Alternativtitel *aṣ-Ṣināʿa al-kabīra* (*Megatechne*), der bei Ullmann verzeichnet ist, sind uns in unserem Material nicht begegnet.

2. Die Methodus medendi im Continens des Rhazes

Die relativ geringe Zahl von Verweisen auf die *MM* in der bislang erschlossenen arabischen Medizinliteratur erklärt sich ohne Zweifel primär aus den weniger strengen Zitiergewohnheiten der mittelalterlichen Gelehrten, insbesondere bei systematischen Darstellungen von allgemein akzeptiertem Lehrgut. Im islamischen Mittelalter dürfte jedes medizinische Handbuch in irgendeiner Form von der *MM* abhängig gewesen sein. Will man sich ein genaues Bild vom Ausmaß ihrer Verwendung durch arabische Autoren verschaffen, so bleibt nichts anderes übrig, als deren Schriften systematisch auf nicht gekennzeichnete sachliche Entlehnungen hin durchzusehen. Da dieses Verfahren außerordentlich viel Zeit erfordert — mehr Zeit jedenfalls, als für die Vorbereitung dieses Referats zur Verfügung stand —, haben wir für unsere Untersuchung einen Text ausgewählt, in dem die Herkunft der Quellenstücke in aller Regel vermerkt ist: den *Continens* (arabisch *al-Ḥāwī fī ṭ-ṭibb*).[27] Bekanntlich haben wir im *Continens* kein zur Publikation bestimmtes und dementsprechend durchgestaltetes Werk vor uns, sondern die gesammelten medizinischen Notizen des Rhazes, die von Schülern aus dem Nachlaß veröffentlicht wurden,[28] d.h. eine riesige, nur oberflächlich geordnete Kollektion von Exzerpten aus den Schriften älterer griechischer, syrischer und arabischer Autoren, teilweise mit Anmerkungen und Kommentaren des Rhazes versehen und durch Erfahrungen und Beobachtungen aus seiner eigenen Praxis bereichert. Der Inhalt dieses Zettelkastens in Buchform ist auf die Erfordernisse der medizinischen Praxis abgestellt: Er bezieht sich überwiegend auf pathologisch-ätiologische und therapeutische Fragen.

Der Überlieferungszustand des arabischen Textes ist, wie bei dessen gewaltigem Umfang und loser Gliederung kaum anders zu erwarten, ei-

---

[26b] S. Friedrich W. Zimmermann: Al-Fārābī und die philosophische Kritik an Galen von Alexander zu Averroes. Abhandlungen der Akademie der Wissenschaften zu Göttingen, phil.-hist. Kl., 3. F., Nr. 98, Göttingen 1976, S. 401-414, hier S. 104 mit Anm. 20; s. auch Strohmaier, loc. cit. (wie Anm. 1), S. 189.

[27] Vgl. zu diesem Werk Sezgin, loc. cit., S. 278-280; Ullmann, loc. cit., S. 130.

[28] S. Ibn Abī Uṣaibiʿa, loc. cit., I 314,14-17; vgl. dazu auch Albert Z. Iskandar: A Catalogue of Arabic Manuscripts on Medicine and Science in the Wellcome Historical Medical Library. London 1967, S. 1f. und 29f.

nigermaßen desolat. Alle bekannten Handschriften sind unvollständig; die Anordnung der einzelnen Teile differiert in den verschiedenen Textzeugen, und selbst über die genaue Anzahl der Bände herrscht keine Einigkeit. In 23 Bände wird das Werk unterteilt in der Haiderabader Druckausgabe,[29] die erstmals einen Gesamttext in der Ursprache allgemein zugänglich macht. Sie wird allerdings, wie schon wiederholt beklagt wurde,[30] den Anforderungen moderner Textkritik bei weitem nicht gerecht. So wurden nicht einmal alle verfügbaren arabischen Handschriften zur Textrekonstruktion herangezogen, geschweige denn die griechischen Vorlagen der Exzerpte. Da es uns nicht möglich war, zusätzliches Handschriftenmaterial zur Kontrolle des gedruckten Textes heranzuziehen, ist nicht auszuschließen, daß einige der nachfolgenden Aussagen aufgrund authentischerer Textfassungen später etwas modifiziert werden müssen.

Zum leichteren Verständnis des folgenden fügen wir an dieser Stelle eine grobe Übersicht über die Einteilung des *Continens* ein:

Band I-X   Spezielle Pathologie und Therapie a capite ad calcem
Band XI   Würmer, Gicht u. dgl.
Band XII-XIII   Wundbehandlung
Band XIV-XVI   Fieberlehre
Band XVII   Akute Krankheiten
Band XVIII   Krisenlehre
Band XIX   Uroskopie; Bisse, Vergiftungen
Band XX-XXII   Materia Medica, Pharmazie
Band XXIII   Diätetik; Dermatologie

2.1. *Zitate aus der Methodus medendi im Continens*

Wie gründlich Rhazes mit dem Text der *MM* vertraut war, erhellt bereits aus der Existenz einer Epitome aus seiner Feder.[31] Daß Galens Werk ihm als grundlegend galt, läßt sich aus einer Äußerung in seiner Schrift *Aphorismen* (al-Fuṣūl, auch *K. al-Muršid*, *Führer*, genannt) erschlie-

---

[29] Abū Bakr Muḥammad b. Zakariyya ar-Rāzī (d. 313 A.H. = 925 A.D.): Kitābu'l Hāwī fi't-tibb (Continens of Rhazes). (An Encyclopaedia of Medicine). Published by the Dāiratur l-Maʿārif-il-Osmānia. Hyderabad 1373/1955-1390/1970. Eine zweite, revidierte Auflage ist im Erscheinen begriffen; uns lagen bereits vor die Bde. 1-5, 1974-1979. — Klaus-Dietrich Fischer verdanke ich den Hinweis, daß der lateinische Continens, für den ebenfalls in der Literatur abweichende Band-Angaben zu finden sind, 25 Teile umfaßt.
[30] S. Albert Z. Iskandar: The medical bibliography of al-Rāzī. In: Essays on Islamic Philosophy and Science, ed. George F. Hourani. Albany, New York 1975, S. 41f. Vgl. auch Ullmann, loc. cit., S. 130; Dietrich, loc. cit., S. 46.
[31] Vgl. o. S. 127.

ßen.[32] Rhazes hebt dort in Aphorismus 268 hervor, die Behandlung der Fieber, insbesondere der akuten, sei so schwierig, daß sich daran sowohl die Wohltaten der Medizin als auch die wahren Qualitäten eines Arztes offenbarten. Als Anleitung für dieses Gebiet empfiehlt er dann an erster Stelle, noch vor einer Anzahl von Spezialschriften, die *MM*.[33]

Im *Continens* schreibt er neben dem Original auch verschiedene Bearbeitungen der *MM* aus. Sie können hier nur aufgezählt werden; ihre genaue Identifizierung muß einer späteren Untersuchung vorbehalten bleiben. An zwei Stellen zitiert Rhazes eine *Synopsis* (*Ǧawāmiʿ*), und zwar Passagen aus deren 4. und 8. Buch (II 208,7 ff. und XVII 41,1 ff.).[34] Wahrscheinlich bezieht er sich hier auf den entsprechenden Teil der *Summaria Alexandrinorum*.[35] Rund 28 mal beruft er sich auf Kurzfassungen, bei denen es sich, ungeachtet der unterschiedlichen Titelformen (*Muḫtaṣar*, *Iḫtiṣār[āt]*, einmal auch *Iḫtiyārāt*, *Auswahl*), vermutlich um ein und denselben Text handelt. Da nirgends ein Verfassername auftaucht, darf man diese Bearbeitung vielleicht mit jener Epitome in Verbindung bringen, die in Ḥunains *Risāla* Galen selbst zugeschrieben wird.[36] Es dürfte sich wohl um eine unechte Schrift handeln; im Griechischen ist meines Wissens nichts daraus erhalten.[37] Nach Ḥunain bestand sie aus zwei Teilen, was dem Befund im *Continens* zumindest nicht widerspricht: Nur zwei Zitate enthalten eine Stellenangabe (XI 50,13 f. und X 266,8-10), die sich im einen Fall auf das erste, im andern auf das zweite Buch jener Kurzfassung bezieht. Schließlich wird einmal (IV 52,5-8) noch ein Auszug mit dem Titel *Talḫīṣ* zitiert; sofern wir es hierbei nicht mit einer weiteren Titelvariante für die zuvor besprochene Epitome zu tun haben, könnte man hier an Rhazes' eigene Bearbeitung denken, die nach dem

---

[32] Bei diesem Werk handelt es sich um eine Art Einführung in die Medizin mit kritischer Bibliographie, s. Iskandar, loc. cit. (wie Anm. 30), S. 43; Ullmann, loc. cit., S. 134f.

[33] Rhazes' K. al-Muršid aw al-Fuṣūl (The Guide or Aphorisms) with texts selected from his medical writings. Edited with an introduction by A. Z. Iskandar (Revue de l'Institut des manuscrits arabes, vol. 7, no. 1). Cairo 1961, S. 90,9-14; übersetzt in: Abû-Bakr Mohammad b. Zakariyyâ ar-Râzî: Guide du médecin nomade. Aphorismes présentés et traduits de l'arabe par El-Arbi Moubachir (La Bibliothèque de l'Islam). Paris 1980, S. 122.

[34] Stellenangaben ohne Buchtitel beziehen sich im folgenden stets auf die arabische *Continens*-Ausgabe (wie Anm. 29).

[35] Vgl. dazu Sezgin, loc. cit., S. 150 (Nr. 15).

[36] Ḥunain, loc. cit., Nr. 70, S. 34 (arab.), S. 28 (Übers.); vgl. Ullmann, loc. cit., S. 59 (Nr. 96); Sezgin, loc. cit., S. 56 (Nr. 115).

[37] Allerdings zitiert auch der Oreibasios-Scholiast eine Synopsis Galens zu seiner *MM* (τῆς θεραπευτικῆς αὐτοῦ σύνοψις), deren Echtheit freilich ebenfalls fraglich ist, s. Oeuvres d'Oribase, ed. Cats Bussemaker et Charles Daremberg (Collection des médecins grecs et latins). Paris 1851-1876, Bd. IV, S. 528,12f. mit Anm. 3. Mit der von Ḥunain erwähnten dürfte sie nicht identisch sein, da sie nach dieser Stelle mehr als zwei Teile umfaßt haben muß.

Katalog in der unikalen Handschrift des Escorial eben diesen Titel trägt.
Doch wenden wir uns nunmehr den Fragmenten aus der *MM* selbst
zu. Zur Abgrenzung des Materials seien vorweg zwei Bemerkungen ge-
stattet. 1. Berücksichtigt werden nur mit entsprechendem Lemma eingeführte Texte. 2. Ein Exzerpt gilt als beendet, wenn Rhazes im nachfolgenden Satz eine neue Quelle einführt. Beide Einschränkungen
erscheinen notwendig, weil wegen der oberflächlichen Redaktion des
Textes und seines schlechten Überlieferungszustandes nicht auszuschließen ist, daß einerseits Zitate aus der *MM* ohne Herkunftsnachweis in einen fremden Kontext geraten sind und daß andererseits *MM*-Exzerpte
nach Einschüben anderer Provenienz ohne neuerliche Titelangabe still-
schweigend fortgeführt werden. Die Identifizierung solcher nicht ausdrücklich gekennzeichneter Entlehnungen muß Aufgabe weiter Untersuchungen bleiben.

Zwei Zusammenstellungen der *MM*-Zitate im *Continens* liegen bereits
vor. Ullmanns Liste ist mit 14 Angaben freilich bei weitem nicht vollständig;[38] Sezgin verzeichnet aus den ersten 19 Bänden der indischen
Ausgabe 98 Stellen.[39] Beim erneuten Durchsehen der in der Zwischenzeit abgeschlossenen Edition konnten zahlreiche Nachträge verzeichnet
werden. Allerdings erscheint es ratsam, auf die Angabe einer definitiven
Gesamtzahl zu verzichten, da sich zum einen längere Exzerpte oft als
Aneinanderreihung von weit verstreuten Stellen entpuppen und zum andern die Länge der Auszüge stark variiert, so daß eine absolute Zahl wenig darüber aussagt, wie intensiv Rhazes die *MM* benutzte. Statt dessen
versuchen wir eine grobe Abschätzung des Gesamtumfangs der zitierten
Texte. Rhazes beruft sich für knapp 300 Seiten des *Continens* (nach dem
Haiderabader Druck) auf unsere Galen-Schrift. Er reproduziert darauf
den Inhalt von rund 350 Seiten des griechischen Textes (nach Kühns
Ausgabe), wovon wiederum etwa 120 Seiten zusätzlich noch einmal als
Dubletten wiederkehren.[40] Rhazes hat also ein gutes Drittel der *MM* seiner medizinischen Materialsammlung einverleibt — ein Anteil, der sich
noch beträchtlich erhöht, faßt man nur die medizinisch relevanten Abschnitte des Originals ins Auge und klammert die weitschweifigen Einlei-
tungen, die zahlreichen Wiederholungen sowie die ausgedehnten Pole-
miken Galens gegen seine Berufskollegen aus. Wiederum ein Drittel der

---

[38] S. Ullmann, loc. cit., S. 45.

[39] S. Sezgin, loc. cit., S. 98; einige der Angaben beziehen sich indessen auf die oben
besprochenen Kurzfassungen.

[40] Für die *MM* ist diese Abschätzung eher etwas zu niedrig angesetzt, da einige der
Zitate im *Continens* noch nicht mit Sicherheit identifiziert werden konnten. — Die Veröf-
fentlichung eines detaillierten Nachweises der *MM*-Stellen im *Continens* wird von der
Verf. vorbereitet.

exerpierten Stellen wird zudem noch ein zweites Mal zitiert, einige wenige Angaben erscheinen sogar noch ein drittes Mal. Damit gehört die *MM* zu den am häufigsten zitierten Quellen des *Continens*.

2.2. *Zur Interpretation der Zitate*

Die eigentliche Auswertung und Interpretation dieses umfangreichen Materials ist bei weitem noch nicht abgeschlossen. Textvergleiche unter philologischen Aspekten, Fragen der Übersetzungstechnik, des Sprachgebrauchs u. dgl., mußten von vornherein zurückgestellt werden, weil der zur Verfügung stehende arabische Text hierfür nur eine allzu schwankende Grundlage abgeben könnte. Fürs erste haben wir die Galen-Exzerpte des Rhazes unter drei Fragestellungen durchgesehen:

1. Wie verfährt Rhazes mit seiner galenischen Vorlage?
2. Welche inhaltlichen Schwerpunkte lassen sich erkennen?
3. Wie äußert sich Rhazes selbst zu den exzerpierten Stellen?

2.2.1. *Zur Behandlung der Vorlage*

Neun von zwanzig Bänden des *Continens* beginnen mit meist umfangreichen Auszügen aus der *MM*,[41] in einem weiteren steht ein *MM*-Exzerpt wenigstens an zweiter Stelle. Darüber hinaus werden zahlreiche Einzelkapitel mit solchen Zitaten eingeleitet. Bei derartiger Häufung kann man die prominente Stellung der Materialien aus der *MM* wohl kaum auf bloßen Zufall zurückführen.[42] Rhazes selbst dürfte dafür verantwortlich sein, auch wenn er die abschließende Redaktion des *Continens* nicht selbst vorgenommen hat. Die Länge seiner Textauszüge bewegt sich zwischen einer halben Zeile (s. z.B. XXIII 1: 119,9 ≈ *MM* XII 3: X 824,2) und über 24 Seiten (XIII 82,17-107,3), allerdings mit Einschluß vereinzelter Anmerkungen des Kompilators. Gut die Hälfte der Zitate weist neben dem Buchtitel *Ḥīlat al-burʾ* eine Stellenangabe auf, gewöhnlich bestehend aus der Nummer des entsprechenden Buches der *MM*, in einigen Fällen ergänzt durch die Bemerkung ''gegen Ende''. Wenn diese Zahlen im vorliegenden Druck alles andere als verläßlich sind, so dürfte dies zumeist der Überlieferung anzulasten sein, da arabische Zahlwörter, zumal wenn unpunktiert geschrieben, bekanntlich reichlich Gelegenheit zu Verlesungen bieten. Bezeichnenderweise kann man die richtige Angabe bisweilen dem Apparat entnehmen. In einigen

---

[41] Die Bände XX-XXII, die die Materia medica behandeln, müssen hier ausgeklammert werden, da ihr Stoff alphabetisch angeordnet ist.

[42] Vgl. auch Ullmann, loc. cit., S. 130.

Fällen, zumal an so kritischen Stellen wie den Übergängen zwischen zwei Büchern, mag der Irrtum schon Rhazes beim Exzerpieren unterlaufen sein.

Größere Exzerpte geben nur selten einen einzigen fortlaufenden Sinnabschnitt der Quelle wieder. Das vorhin erwähnte längste Zitat beispielsweise umfaßt Passagen aus dem Ende von Buch IV (*MM* IV 7: X 296,12-300,15), aus Buch V Teile aus den Kapiteln 2 (X 310,14-316,10), 5-8 (X 327,16-345,5) und 11-15 (X 357,15-379,2) mit diversen Lücken und endet mit einer Paraphrase von *MM* VII 11 (X 512,15-513,4). Immerhin folgen die einzelnen Stücke hier in der ursprünglichen Anordnung aufeinander, wie es sich im übrigen in der Mehrzahl der Fälle verhält. Es kommen aber auch Exzerpte mit größeren Textsprüngen vor, so etwa, wenn sich an eine Reihe von Auszügen aus Buch VII 6 (X 471,1-496,5, mit Auslassungen) unmittelbar drei Zitate aus Buch XIV 15 und 16 (X 993,15-994,6; 997,12-1000,12; 1002,9-14) anschließen (VI 257,1-264,16). Während man hier jegliche Stellenangabe vermißt,[43] ist in wieder anderen Beispielen jeder Wechsel genau vermerkt, so u.a. zu Beginn des 8. Bandes (1,9-2,17), wo Rhazes Exzerpte aus *MM* IV 7 (X 297,10-14), VIII 5 (X575,5-10 und 577,13-17) und XII 1 (X 813,7-814,1 und 815,1-17) aneinanderreiht. Umgekehrt besagt der Einschub der Floskel ''es sagte Galen'', ''er sagte'' oder einfach ''Galen'' (mit oder ohne Wiederholung des Buchtitels) nicht notwendigerweise, daß Rhazes dort ein neues Exzerpt beginnt; derartige Lemmata können sogar mehrfach innerhalb eines fortlaufend ausgeschriebenen Passus auftreten. Im übrigen erleichtert die oft recht eigenwillige Textgliederung in der Druckausgabe nicht gerade die Abgrenzung der einzelnen Fragmente.

Untersucht man die Zitate aus der *MM* im Hinblick darauf, wie exakt Rhazes seiner Vorlage folgt,[44] so lassen sie sich grob in vier Kategorien einordnen:

a) Zitate im engeren Sinn, d.h. Textwiedergaben, die sich eng an den Originalwortlaut anlehnen und allenfalls kurze Lücken aufweisen.[45] Ob man einen Teil davon geradezu als wörtlich bezeichnen darf, ließe sich nur durch einen Vergleich mit Ḥubaiš's ursprünglicher Version der *MM* entscheiden.[46]

---

[43] Nur zu Beginn findet sich eine Stellenangabe (Buch IV). Man könnte daraus schließen, daß Rhazes die Exzerptenfolge ungeachtet der Auslassungen als ein zusammengehöriges Zitat auffaßte.

[44] Hier kann nur ein direkter Vergleich mit dem griechischen Original vorgenommen werden; ob Rhazes Abweichungen von diesem eventuell bereits in seiner Vorlage vorgefunden hat, ist dabei selbstverständlich nicht festzustellen.

[45] Hierunter rechnen wir auch Zitate, die zu Beginn stärkere Abweichungen aufweisen, sofern diese lediglich dazu dienen, den Kontext der aus ihrem Zusammenhang gelösten Textstelle klarzustellen.

[46] S. auch noch u. S. 137.

b) Paraphrasen, d.h. meist gekürzte sinngemäße Wiedergaben der Ausführungen Galens, wobei gelegentlich die Abfolge der Argumente geändert sein kann (vgl. z.B. XIII 106,18-107,13 ≈ *MM* VII 11: X 512,15-513,4).

c) Referate, die mehr oder weniger umfangreiche Passagen in wenigen Sätzen zusammenfassen. Beispielsweise verwendet Rhazes kaum sechs Zeilen auf die Geschichte von dem Fieberpatienten, den Galen unkollegialerweise hinter dem Rücken der behandelnden Ärzte durch Massagen, Bäder und leichte Diät in drei Tagen kuriert hatte,[47] während sie im Original rund vier Seiten in Anspruch nimmt (XIV 147,14-148,3 ≈ *MM* VIII 2: X 536,6-540,2).

d) Isolierte Aussagen, die aus ihrem ursprünglichen Zusammenhang, oft einer Aufzählung, herausgelöst und dem entsprechenden Themenkreis des *Continens* zugeordnet werden. Wenn Galen in *MM* XII 8 (X 867,10-868,7) ein Medikament aus Opium und Bibergeil gleichermaßen gegen Augen-, Ohren- und Zahnschmerzen empfiehlt, so verwendet Rhazes diese Belegstelle zweimal mit Bezug auf die Ohren, zweimal im Kapitel über die Zahnleiden sowie einmal in dem über die Augenkrankheiten — wobei er jeweils nur den gerade zur Diskussion stehenden Körperteil nennt.

Es ist auch ansonsten recht aufschlußreich zu verfolgen, was Rhazes von Galens Ausführungen übergeht. Wenn er beim Exzerpieren einzelne Sätze oder kurze Passagen wegläßt, so kann man dies vielfach damit erklären, daß er für seine Materialsammlung nur an den positiven Angaben Galens, den praktisch verwertbaren Aussagen zu einzelnen therapeutischen Problemen, interessiert ist.[48] In einer anderen Schrift mit dem sprechenden Titel *Bedenken gegen Galen* (Šukūk ʿalā Ǧālīnūs) beklagt er sich einmal expressis verbis über die Langatmigkeit Galens in der *MM*, die in Wahrheit nur dessen Unfähigkeit verbergen solle, für bestimmte Krankheiten genaue Ursachen anzugeben.[49] Rhazes' Bestrebungen, den

---

[47] Zur Interpretation dieser Stelle s. Jutta Kollesch: Galen und seine ärztlichen Kollegen. *Das Altertum* 11 (1965), S. 52f.

[48] Einer Anregung Vivian Nuttons folgend, haben wir die *MM*-Exzerpte im "Syrischen Medizinbuch" (vgl. o. Anm. 17) mit den Auszügen im *Continens* unter dem Gesichtspunkt verglichen, ob die Auswahl im ersten unter anderen Aspekten getroffen wurde, speziell, ob dessen Autor sich mehr auf die generellen Grundsätze der Therapie bei Galen bezieht als Rhazes. Wir konnten nicht bestätigen, daß im "Syrischen Medizinbuch" eher theoretisch ausgerichtete Passagen der *MM* ausgeschrieben sind. Tatsächlich sind nur zwei der dortigen Exzerpte nicht im *Continens* zu finden, *MM* XIII 15: X 913,2-914,3, über einen Fall von Leberentzündung, und das Kap. *MM* VII 10: X 510,3-14, eine resümierende Wiederholung der Grundsätze für die Anwendung konträrer Mittel zur Behebung der acht Dyskrasien.

[49] S. Iskandar, loc. cit. (wie Anm. 30), S. 44.

Text seiner Quelle zu straffen, fallen naturgemäß zuerst Galens Ausein-
andersetzungen mit den medizinischen Schulen seiner Zeit — insbesondere mit den Methodikern — zum Opfer. Sie hätten, rund 700 Jahre
später und nach dem Sieg des Galenismus, allenfalls noch historisches Interesse beanspruchen können. Ein eindrucksvolles Beispiel für Rhazes'
Fähigkeit, aus einem von Polemik nur so strotzenden Kapitel der *MM*
die maßgebliche Ansicht Galens herauszufiltern, ist seine Version von
MM IV 4 (X 256,1-264,15), wo Galen neun Seiten lang gegen die von
Thessalos eingeführte Kategorie des "chronischen Geschwürs" wettert,
die er selbst für unsinnig hält. Alles, was diese von Galen verworfene und
damit überholte Lehre und deren Widerlegung betrifft (X 256,3-257,18;
258,2-261,11; 261,16-18; 262,8-264,11), läßt Rhazes einfach vollständig
beiseite. Nur die dazwischen eingestreuten spärlichen Hinweise Galens
auf die Kriterien für die korrekte Abgrenzung und Einordnung des frag-
lichen Krankheitsbildes stellt er in seinem Exzerpt zusammen und liefert
so, ohne sich allzuweit vom Wortlaut der *MM* zu entfernen, mit nur 12
Zeilen Text (XIII 73,3-14) einen kompakten Abriß der galenischen Dok-
trin vom "bösartigen Geschwür".

Einen wichtigen Einblick in die literarische Werkstatt des Rhazes ge-
währen die Mehrfachzitate des *Continens* aus der *MM*. Zum Teil handelt
es sich um wirkliche Dubletten. So werden beispielsweise Galens Ausführungen über die schmerzhaften Darmgeschwüre, bei deren Behandlung
man gegebenenfalls der Schmerzstillung Vorrang einräumen soll (*MM*
XII 1: X 813,7-814,1), im Abschnitt über die Darmkrankheiten innerhalb von 70 Seiten zweimal zitiert (VIII 2,4-9 und 69,15-19), das zweite
Mal allerdings stärker paraphrasiert. Wir treffen sie im übrigen noch ein
drittes Mal — in verkürzter Form — in Rhazes' Zusammenstellung all-
gemeiner therapeutischer Grundsätze an (XXIII 1: 272,7-10). Damit
sind wir auch schon bei der zweiten, häufigeren Art von Mehrfachzitaten, bei der ein und dieselbe Stelle zu verschiedenen Problemkreisen herangezogen wird. Das Kapitel über das Fieber, das, bei gleichzeitiger
Schwäche des Magenmundes, von rohen Säften hervorgerufen wird
(*MM* XII 3: X 820,15-829,18), zitiert Rhazes zur Gänze sowohl in Buch
XIV (2,4-7,14) als Beleg für die Therapie von "Fiebern mit zusätzlichen
Symptomen" als auch in Buch XVI (76,14-81,14) unter der Überschrift
"Schleimfieber". Daß sich ein Zitat dieses Umfangs vollständig wiederholt, ist freilich die Ausnahme. In der Regel werden nur Teilstücke, oft
sogar bloß einzelne Sätze, aus einem Exzerpt in einem anderen Kontext
nochmals angeführt. Zur Frage der Blutstillung etwa zieht Rhazes an
einer Stelle (XIII 87,6-88,4) ca. zwei Seiten der *MM* aus (*MM* V 3: X
314,18-316,10); daraus taucht ein Absatz über Derivation und Revulsion
(ibid. 315,7-14) auch im Buch über die Entleerungsverfahren (VI 4,4-9)

auf, und ein weiteres Detail, die Behandlung uteriner Blutungen durch Schröpfen in der Region unterhalb der Brust (ibid. 315,16-316,1), kehrt im Kapitel über die gynäkologischen Erkrankungen (IX 2,4-5) wieder.

Soweit der Zustand des arabischen Textes eine schlüssige Aussage zuläßt, stimmen die Mehrfachzitate in keinem Fall im Wortlaut exakt überein. Dieser Befund führt uns von neuem auf das schon oben angeschnittene Problem der Zitierweise des Rhazes, das vor allem im Hinblick auf die Möglichkeit der Rekonstruktion ansonsten verlorener oder schlecht bezeugter älterer Schriften aus den Fragmenten im *Continens* von Belang ist. Geringfügige Differenzen zwischen den verschiedenen Wiedergaben einer Textstelle lassen sich ohne weiteres daraus erklären, daß Rhazes für die Zwecke seiner Materialsammlung keinen Wert auf absolute Texttreue legt. Dies bestätigt somit frühere Beobachtungen,[50] daß Rhazes im *Continens* lediglich sinngemäß zitiert. Problematischer sind jene Dubletten, wo die eine Fassung nahe am Original bleibt, während die andere es stark paraphrasiert. Kann auch dieses Phänomen noch einfach auf die Rechnung des freien Umgangs mit den Quellen gesetzt werden oder muß man nicht — wenigstens in einigen Fällen — doch eher von der Existenz verschiedener Vorlagen ausgehen? Bei einzelnen Beispielen hat es immerhin den Anschein, als gäben jeweils die Fassungen, die mit einer Stellenangabe versehen sind, den Originalwortlaut erheblich getreuer wieder als die ohne eine solche Kennzeichnung. Dieser Umstand ließe den Schluß zu, daß Rhazes im ersten Falle die *MM* selbst vor sich hatte, während er die stärker abweichenden Versionen nicht direkt, sondern über im Augenblick nicht näher charakterisierbare Mittelquellen zitierte, in denen er keine Buchangabe vorfand. Dies sind freilich noch rein spekulative Überlegungen,[51] die sorgfältiger Prüfung, möglichst auch anhand von Zitaten aus anderen Quellen des *Continens*, bedürfen.

2.2.2. *Inhaltliche Schwerpunkte*

Die Frage nach der Auswahl der *MM*-Exzerpte im *Continens* unter inhaltlichen Gesichtspunkten soll von zwei Seiten her, sowohl vom *Continens* wie auch von der *MM* ausgehend, beleuchtet werden. Zunächst wollen wir betrachten, wie intensiv Rhazes seine Quelle jeweils zu den einzelnen Hauptthemen seiner Sammlung heranzieht. Auf den ersten Blick schei-

---

[50] S. beispielsweise M. Ullmann: Die Schrift des Rufus "De infantium curatione" und das Problem der Autorenlemmata in den "Collectiones medicae" des Oreibasios. *Med. hist. J.* 10 (1975), S. 166f.; ders.: Die Taḏkira des ibn as-Suwaidī, eine wichtige Quelle zur Geschichte der griechisch-arabischen Medizin und Magie. *Der Islam* 54 (1977), S. 45.

[51] So wäre beispielsweise auch die Möglichkeit zu erwägen, daß die starken Differenzen sich durch Zitieren aus dem Gedächtnis erklären.

nen die Zitate recht ungleichmäßig über die 23 Bände des *Continens* verteilt zu sein. Dies beruht indessen nicht so sehr auf gezielter Auswahl,
vielmehr ist diese Verteilung durch den Inhalt der *MM* und die Gewich-
tung ihrer Themen von Galens Seite bereits vorgegeben.

Band XVIII über die Krisen enthält keinen Verweis auf die *MM*. In
Band VII über die Krankheiten verschiedener Brust- und Bauchorgane
finden sich lediglich zwei kurze Exzerpte über den Hydrops. Von den
drei Zitaten in Band XVII über akute Krankheiten sind zwei sogar noch
identisch. Der Mangel an Zitaten im gynäkologisch-geburtshilflichen
Teil des *Continens* (Band IX) spiegelt den Umstand wider, daß dieses
Thema in der *MM* nur am Rande berührt wird. Immerhin weiß Rhazes
aus den wenigen Andeutungen das Beste zu machen; so nutzt er selbst
eine Bemerkung über den Verlust der Zeugungskräfte, der den Samen
außerhalb der Fortpflanzungsorgane befällt (*MM* VII 6: X 474,11-13),
für diesen Kontext (IX 76,4-6), während sie Galen lediglich als Parallele
zu der Qualitätsminderung anführt, die seiner Ansicht nach die Milch
durch den Transport erfährt. Die Exzerpte in den drei (in vier Teilen gedruckten) Bänden pharmakologisch-pharmazeutischen Inhalts (XX-
XXII) erreichen insgesamt nur einen Umfang von knapp sechs Seiten;
dies entspricht der Tatsache, daß Galen in seinen bewußt allgemein ge-
haltenen Ausführungen nur ganz sporadisch einzelne Heilmittel erwähnt. Nach zunehmender Länge der Zitate geordnet, folgen nun Band
XIX mit drei sich teilweise überschneidenden Auszügen aus *MM* XIII
6 über Bisse giftiger Tiere, Band IV mit je einem längeren Exzerpt über
den Brustabszeß und die Tracheaverletzung sowie Band XI mit sieben
kurzen Stücken über so disparate Themen wie Würmer, Gicht, Elephan-
tiasis und Skirrhus. Auch zu den Krankheiten der Harn- und Ge-
schlechtsorgane (Band X) und den Kopf- und Hirnkrankheiten (Band I)
war der *MM* nur spärliches Material zu entnehmen. Etliche Dubletten
bringen die Auszüge in Band III über Leiden der Ohren, der Nase und
der Zähne auf einen Gesamtumfang von sechs Seiten. In Band VIII über
die Darmkrankheiten machen die *MM*-Stellen insgesamt ca. neun, in
Band II über die Augenleiden rund zehn Seiten aus. Der Doppelband
XXIII enthält einiges zur Diätetik, ferner Auszüge über allgemeine
therapeutische Maßnahmen wie Schmerzstillung und Entleerung sowie
drei Stellen zur Dermatologie aus der *MM*. Zum Thema ''Purgieren''
zieht Rhazes in Band VI rund 17 Seiten aus, und die umfangreichste
Auswahl zur Therapie eines einzelnen Körperteils (ca. 28 Seiten) finden
wir in Buch V über den Magen; diesem Organ widmet ja auch Galen
ein ganzes Buch (*MM* VII). Den zweiten Rang in der Gesamtstatistik
nehmen die *MM*-Auszüge in den drei Bänden über die Fiebertherapie
ein: Zu den rund 16 Seiten über das kontinuierliche Fieber (Band XV)

steuert ein einziges langes Zitat aus dem ersten Drittel von *MM* IX den Löwenanteil bei; Band XVI, der die von Schleim verursachten, die hektischen und die mit Bewußtseinsverlust einhergehenden Fieber behandelt, enthält u.a. zu den beiden letzten Fragen umfangreiche fortlaufende Exzerpte aus *MM* X und XII (insgesamt 23 Seiten); in Band XIV über die allgemeine Fieberbehandlung und die Faulfieber schließlich belaufen sich die Zitate auf etwa 31 Seiten. Mit weitem Abstand den größten Umfang erreichen jedoch die Entlehnungen zum Problem der "Lösung des Zusammenhaltes" im zweiten Teil von Band XII (der erste Teil, die "Schwellungen" behandelnd, bietet ca. 5 Seiten Exzerpte) und in Band XIII mit insgesamt rund 90 der *MM* entnommenen Seiten.

Das Resultat dieser Übersicht läßt sich folgendermaßen zusammenfassen: Am häufigsten zieht Rhazes die *MM* zu Fragen der Wundbehandlung heran; es folgen die Themen "Fiebertherapie" und "Magenkrankheiten". Hervorzuheben ist ferner, daß Rhazes auch für jene Gebiete, die Galen nur gelegentlich streift, Detailinformationen aus der *MM* zu gewinnen weiß.

Der Eindruck, daß Rhazes' Auswahl im großen und ganzen das Themenspektrum seiner Vorlage widerspiegelt, wird weiter bestätigt, wenn man umgekehrt die Frage stellt, wie groß der Anteil der einzelnen Bücher der *MM* an den Exzerpten im *Continens* ist. Aus dieser Sicht eröffnen sich aber auch einige neue Aspekte. Rhazes' vorrangiges Interesse an positiven medizinischen Informationen beispielsweise wird einmal mehr daran deutlich, daß die beiden ersten Bücher der *MM* lediglich durch drei winzige Zitate aus Buch II vertreten sind; zwei davon betreffen die Etymologie der Krankheitsnamen ἐπινυκτίς (arabisch: banāt allail, 'Töchter der Nacht', XXIII 2 2: 125,5-6 ≈ *MM* II 2: X 84,9-11) und χολέραι (arabisch: al-ḥaiḍa, V 193,15-16 ≈ *MM* 2: 82,9-11).[52] Aus Buch XI über die Faulfieber, die keine zusätzlichen Symptome aufweisen, entnimmt Rhazes nur ganze vier Stellen. Es folgen in einigem Abstand Buch III über die allgemeine Wundbehandlung (ca. 14 Seiten nebst drei kurzen Dubletten), Buch IV über die Wunden mit weiteren Komplikationen (ca. 15 Seiten), aus dem Rhazes u.a. an einer Stelle (XIII 70,18-75,5) fortlaufend ausgewählte Abschnitte aus Kap. 1-6 (*MM* X 235-291) wiedergibt, und, etwa gleichauf, Buch XIII über die Phlegmone. Mehr als das Doppelte exzerpiert Rhazes aus Buch IX über die kontinuierlichen Fieber in zwei langen, sich gegenseitig ergänzenden

---

[52] Die dritte Stelle, paraphrasiert in XI 317,6-10, behandelt das Hinken infolge einer Phlegmone als Beispiel dafür, daß nicht die Functio laesa, sondern die sie verursachende Diathese die Indikation für das ärztliche Eingreifen gibt (*MM* II 1: X 80,8-12). Im Arabischen steht anstelle von "Phlegmone" hier übrigens "harte Geschwulst" (waram ṣulb).

Zitaten aus Kap. 1-5 (*MM* X 600-627) in *Continens* XIV 187,4-189,1 und
XV 7,11-18,7 sowie einem nur dreizeiligen Zitat aus *MM* IX 16. Im
Gegensatz dazu sind die je 31 Seiten ausmachenden Zitate aus Buch VIII
über die Eintagsfieber und aus Buch XIV über die Schwellungen (mit
Ausschluß der Phlegmone) weit über den *Continens* verstreut. Im ersten
Falle kommen noch rund 14%, im zweiten Falle sogar rund 40%
Mehrfachzitate hinzu. Den Hauptteil der 34 Seiten umfassenden
Exzerpte aus Buch X über die hektischen Fieber macht ein langes Zitat
aus Kap. 5-11 (*MM* X 687-732 ≈ XVI 13,17-28,11) aus; hier gibt es nur
10% Dubletten. Aus Buch VI, dem zweiten Teil der speziellen Wundbehandlung, führt Rhazes mehr als die Hälfte (39 Seiten im *Continens*)
an, 30% davon sogar mehrfach; der größte Teil davon entfällt auf zwei
einander überschneidende Auszüge aus Kap. 2-4 (*MM* X 386-423,
ausführlicher in XIII 6,18-21,17 und knapper gefaßt in XII 182,13-
189,14) sowie ein weiteres langes Zitat aus Kap. 5 (*MM* X 424-442 ≈
XIII 129,12-136,18). Stärker verteilt über den *Continens* sind die Zitate
aus Buch XII über die von zusätzlichen Symptomen begleiteten
Faulfieber; von den ca. 41 Seiten, die Rhazes insgesamt übernimmt,
wiederholt er rund 60% anderwärts noch einmal. Mit 48 Seiten exzer-
piertem Text steht Buch VII über die Behandlung von Dyskrasien am
Beispiel des Magens an zweiter Stelle; alles in allem freilich liegen die
Auszüge des *Continens* aus diesem Teil der *MM* weit an der Spitze,
werden doch nicht weniger als 60% sogar noch ein drittes Mal
wiederholt. Für den hohen Anteil an Mehrfachzitaten sind hauptsächlich
drei umfängliche Auszüge aus Kap. 4-11 verantwortlich, die einander
stark überschneiden. Zwei davon laufen fast ganz parallel (V 2,7-20,19
≈ *MM* X 465-518 und, etwas später einsetzend, V 137,13-142,16), das
dritte, kürzere umfaßt nur einen Abschnitt aus Kap. 6 (*MM* 471-496 ≈
VI 257,1-262,10). Am vollständigsten jedoch hat Rhazes seiner Stoff-
sammlung Buch V der Galen-Schrift, über die Wunden der Gefäße und
des Kopf- und Brustraumes, einverleibt, nämlich zu drei Vierteln (58
von 78 Seiten). Hierzu tragen besonders zwei umfangreiche Zusammenstellungen von Passagen aus Kap. 2-15 (*MM* X 310-379 = XIII
85,19-106,16) bzw. Kap. 2-7 (*MM* X 310-337 = XII 200,11-213,12)
bei, die einander im einzelnen nur wenig überschneiden.

Fassen wir auch hier kurz zusammen: Die Zitate aus den vier Büchern
über die Wundbehandlung einerseits und aus den fünf Büchern über die
Fiebertherapie andererseits halten einander im Umfang fast die Waage.
Der leichte Vorsprung der Fieberbücher — hier liegt auch die Zahl der
Mehrfachzitate erheblich höher — widerspricht nur scheinbar unserem
ersten Resultat, wonach Rhazes die *MM* am häufigsten für chirurgische
Fragen heranzieht. Die Diskrepanz erklärt sich nämlich leicht aus der

unterschiedlichen Disposition der beiden Texte. Da Buch XII im Grunde mehr von den möglichen Begleitsymptomen des Fiebers als von diesem selbst handelt, wird es im *Continens* weniger in den Fieberbüchern als in verschiedensten anderen Zusammenhängen benutzt. An dritter Stelle folgen die Zitate über die Magenkrankheiten aus Buch VII; sie erreichen ungefähr den gleichen Umfang wie die Exzerpte aus den beiden letzten Büchern der *MM* zusammen, die — nach der Definition Ḥunains — die Krankheiten der zusammengesetzten Körperteile behandeln. Buch VII erreicht im übrigen die höchste Quote an Mehrfachzitaten.

2.2.3. *Zu den Kommentaren des Rhazes*

Abschließend wollen wir nun noch den Inhalt der rund 95 Anmerkungen des Rhazes zu seinen Exzerpten aus der *MM* betrachten, die in der Regel durch das Lemma lī 'von mir' eingeführt werden.[53] Die Fragestellung erscheint vor allem deshalb von Interesse, weil Rhazes, der allgemein als eine der selbständigsten Persönlichkeiten unter den Ärzten des islamischen Kulturkreises gilt, gern als Kronzeuge für die Kritik an den Lehren Galens im Mittelalter bemüht wird, bislang aber für den Bereich der Medizin noch wenig stichhaltiges Belegmaterial dazu beigebracht worden ist.[54] So warten wir beispielsweise noch immer auf die Veröffentlichung der bereits erwähnten Schrift *Bedenken gegen Galen*, die neben Kritik an den philosophischen Anschauungen Galens, wie sie bei den Gelehrten des Islam fast schon zum guten Ton gehörte,[55] auch kritische Äußerungen zu seinen medizinischen Vorstellungen enthalten soll.[56]

---

[53] Zum Inhalt solcher Anmerkungen im *Continens* s. die kommentierte Auswahl bei A.Z. Iskandar: Ar-Rāzī aṭ-ṭabīb al-iklīnikī. Nuṣūṣ min maḫṭūṭāt lam yasbuq našruhā. *Al-Mašriq* 56 (1962), S. 217-282; s. auch Max Meyerhof: Thirty-three clinical observations by Rhazes (circa 900 A.D.). *Isis* 23 (1935), S. 321-372.

[54] In der Zusammenstellung von Ahmed Mohammed Mokhtar (Rhazes contra Galenum. Die Galenkritik in den ersten zwanzig Büchern des "Continens" von Ibn (!) ar-Rāzī. Diss. Med. Bonn 1969) wird der Begriff "Kritik" außerordentlich weit gefaßt. Nur ein Teil der dort besprochenen Stellen enthält tatsächlich kritische Äußerungen zu Galen bzw. abweichende Ansichten des Rhazes. Ähnlich steht es mit den drei Fällen von angeblicher Galen-Kritik nach Georges Debsié (Pathologie und Therapie der Hämorrhoiden bei Avicenna. Diss. Med. Heidelberg 1970, S. 48f.): Bei Überprüfung am Text des *Canon* entpuppen sie sich durchweg als zustimmende Äußerungen Ibn Sīnās.

[55] Vgl. dazu J. Christoph Bürgel: Averroes "contra Galenum". Das Kapitel von der Atmung im Colliget des Averroes als ein Zeugnis mittelalterlich-islamischer Kritik an Galen, eingeleitet, arabisch herausgegeben und übersetzt (Nachrichten der Akademie der Wissenschaften in Göttingen. I. phil.-hist. Kl. 1967, Nr. 9). Göttingen 1967, bes. S. 276-290.

[56] Vgl. Shlomo Pines: Razi Critique de Galien. In: Actes du VIIᵉ Congrès international d'histoire des sciences, Jerusalem 1953 (Collection des travaux de l'Académie internationale d'histoire des sciences 8). Paris o.J., S. 480-487; s. auch Iskandar, loc. cit. (wie

Rhazes' Zusätze zu den Auszügen aus der *MM* im *Continens* sind recht unterschiedlicher Natur. Einige stellen schlicht technische Anmerkungen dar wie jener Querverweis auf Galens Besprechung der mit Ohnmacht verbundenen Fieber in *MM* XII 5 und 6 im Anschluß an das Zitat aus *MM* XII 2: X 820,5-10 (s. XVI 208,15-209,2). In einem anderen zitierten Text verweist Galen für die Diskussion der Therapie jener warmen Dyskrasie des Magens, die mit Fieber einhergeht, auf die entsprechende Stelle in den Fieberbüchern der *MM* (*MM* VII 9: X 508,14-16). Dies veranlaßt Rhazes zu dem Hinweis, er selbst reihe dieses komplexe Krankheitsbild im *Continens* unter die Magenkrankheiten ein (V 17,10-18,1). Mehrfach enthält der als Eigentum des Rhazes gekennzeichnete Passus lediglich die unmittelbare Fortsetzung des betreffenden Galen-Zitats (s. z.B. XIII 207,9-208,4 = *MM* V 4: X 324,4-13 oder V 18,6-10 ≈ *MM* VII 9: X 509,13-510,2): Der Einschub des Lemmas lī dürfte hier auf einen Irrtum der Redaktoren bzw. einen Überlieferungsfehler zurückgehen.[57] Es kommt auch vor, daß Rhazes in einem Zusatz eine näher bezeichnete Galen-Stelle mit eigenen Worten resümiert (XV 36,13-17 ≈ *MM* X 3: X 674,13-675,3).[58] Hier schließen sich sachlich jene Zusammenfassungen an, mit denen Rhazes am Ende eines Exzerpts aus der *MM* die wesentlichen Aussagen Galens noch einmal hervorhebt. So zählt er etwa zum Abschluß der Diskussion verschiedener Schmerzursachen in *MM* XII 7 (X 854,3-856,11) alle noch einmal der Reihe nach auf (XXIII 1: 229,12-14). Wenn Galen empfiehlt, bei einem durch eine Stichverletzung des Muskelkopfes ausgelösten Krampf als ultima ratio eine Defektheilung anzustreben, indem man den Muskel völlig durchtrennt (*MM* III 9: X 220,4-7), so hebt Rhazes den springenden Punkt noch einmal hervor mit den Worten:[59] ''Man darf den Muskel nur dann durchtrennen, wenn die [übrigen] Behandlungsmethoden nicht anschlagen und wenn der Fall dringlich ist'' (XII 152,5-6). Ähnlich

---

Anm. 30), S. 43f. Anders beurteilte dies Maimonides im Vorwort zur 25. Abhandlung seiner Aphorismen (vgl. Bürgel, loc. cit., S. 289f., dazu auch ibid, S. 285); danach betrifft Rhazes' Kritik lediglich die innere Logik der Argumentation Galens. Zu Rhazes' Galen-Kritik vgl. noch Gundolf Keil, Ahmed M. Mokhtar und Hans-Jürgen Thies: Galen-Kritik bei Rhazes. Zur Wertung der Autoritätskritik im islamischen Mittelalter, *Med. Monatsschr.* 25 (1971), S. 559-563, bes. S. 561f.

[57] Einmal wird Galen unmittelbar im Anschluß an das lī ausdrücklich als Urheber des Folgenden namhaft gemacht (XII 209,13-210,7 = *MM* V 6: X 331,3-16 und 332,13-17). Hier ist vielleicht ein Textverlust anzunehmen, dem die gesamte Anmerkung des Rhazes zum Opfer gefallen ist.

[58] Derartige Referate können auch zur Einführung eines Auszugs dienen, s. z.B. XXIII 1: 2,8-9, wo Rhazes zunächst feststellt, nach Galen fördere der Schlaf die Verdauung, ehe er den entsprechenden Beleg (*MM* VII 6: X 490,9ff.) anführt.

[59] Dagegen scheint Mokhtar (loc. cit., S. 64-66), der die Galenstelle im übrigen nicht zu verifizieren vermochte (s. ibid, S. 25), diese Anmerkung irrtümlich als Kritik an Galen zu verstehen.

verhält es sich bei Rhazes' Kommentar zu *MM* V 10 (X 351 ult.-354,12), wo Galen als Illustration zur Indikation aus der Natur des betroffenen Organs die Therapie von Wunden des Ohres anführt. Ohne nähere Begründung lehnt er zunächst die Anwendung des Galmei-Wundmittels am Ohr ab, weist aber am Ende des Abschnitts darauf hin, daß das Ohr wegen seines trockenen Temperamentes besonders stark trocknende Mittel erfordere. Von diesem Grundsatz ausgehend, kann Rhazes nun eine ausdrückliche Begründung für Galens erste Angabe nachliefern (III 4,8-9): Da die Galmei von leimiger Beschaffenheit ist, mangelt es ihr an der für die Anwendung am Ohr erforderlichen Trockenheit.

Unter den Zusätzen des Rhazes finden wir ferner gelegentlich sprachliche Glossen. Beispielsweise erläutert er aṣ-ṣifāq, einen gängigen arabischen Terminus für 'Bauchfell', mittels des transkribierten Fremdwortes περιτόναιον (X 222,10, zu *MM* XIV 13: X 988,5).[60] Oder er weist einmal darauf hin, daß Galen an der kommentierten Stelle das Wort 'Wunde' (qarḥa) ausnahmsweise in der speziellen Bedeutung von 'Gefäßruptur' (ḫarq al-ʿurūq) verwende (XIII 87,2, zu *MM* V 3: X 314,1). An einer Stelle korrigiert er sogar eine Ungenauigkeit der arabischen Version der *MM*: Galen gibt an, die unteren, fleischigen Teile des Magens heilten bei Verletzungen nur schwer (*MM* VI 4: X 419,17-420,1); im Arabischen steht hier für γαστήρ fälschlich baṭn 'Bauch', wie Rhazes klar erkennt und in seiner Glosse richtigstellt (XIII 21,6). Auf eine Korruptel der Vorlage Ḥunains scheint der folgende Fall hinzudeuten. *MM* V 9 (X 345,6-13) spricht Galen davon, daß bei Verletzungen der fleischigen Teile des Zwerchfells nicht nur Phlegmonen des Zwerchfells selbst, sondern auch solche der vom Bauchfell umspannten Organe auftreten und Komplikationen verursachen können. Im Arabischen nun werden beide Membranen mit dem Terminus al-ḥiǧāb bezeichnet, der gewöhnlich nur für das Zwerchfell gebraucht wird, so daß man die zweite Satzhälfte in der arabischen Version interpretieren müßte: "sondern auch [Phlegmonen] dessen, was jenseits des Zwerchfells liegt". Rhazes glossiert dies mit der Bemerkung "er meint die Brust" — die die Intention Galens nicht trifft —, fügt aber sogleich hinzu: "Hier liegt eine Unklarheit in der Erörterung vor, zu der schon Ḥunain Zweifel anmeldete" (XIII 97,19-20).

In die Nähe der Glossen zu stellen sind jene erläuternden Zusätze, die den Sinn aus dem Zusammenhang gerissener Zitate verdeutlichen oder aber im Zitat nur angedeutete Sachverhalte aus dem weiteren Kontext

---

[60] Im Zusammenhang mit der Anweisung Galens, bei der Hernienoperation ein Stück des Bauchfells zu entfernen. An seine sprachliche Glosse schließt Rhazes hier sachliche Erläuterungen an.

der Stelle ergänzen. Die isolierte — und in solcher Verkürzung mißver-
ständliche — Feststellung, Honig sei das beste Heilmittel für innere Verletzungen (*MM* IV 7: X 298,9), präzisiert Rhazes (XIII 84,7) durch die
Anmerkung "sofern eine Reinigung erforderlich ist". Oder wenn Galen
vorschreibt, völlig durchtrennte Nerven wie andere Wunden zu behandeln (*MM* VI 3: X 408,7-10), so hebt der Kommentar erläuternd hervor,
daß hier — anstelle der spezifischen Therapie, die bei anderen Nerven-
verletzungen angezeigt ist — die allgemeine Wundbehandlung indiziert
sei, deren Ziel im Auffüllen und Vernarben der Wunde bestehe (XII
15,14-15).

Bisweilen spezifiziert Rhazes allgemein gehaltene therapeutische Rat-
schläge Galens. Beispielsweise zählt er, wo sich seine Quelle mit der Nen-
nung von Arzneimittelgruppen begnügte, die in Frage kommenden Mittel einzeln auf (vgl. die Diaphoretika in XI 313,7-10, zu *MM* XX 1: X
80,10, oder die Mittel, mit deren Hilfe man nach Knochenbrüchen Kal-
lus verschiedener Härte erzielen kann, in XIII 237,1-2, zu *MM* VI 5: X
440,8). An anderer Stelle empfiehlt Galen, darauf zu achten, daß das
Kleinkind, das einem Patienten mit kalt-trockener Dyskrasie des Magens
als lebende Wärmflasche dienen soll, keine feuchte Haut habe (*MM* VII
7: X 502,17-503,1). Hier fügt Rhazes die konkrete Anweisung an, den
Körper des Kindes zuvor mit schweißhemmenden Mitteln zu behandeln
(V 15,20).

Bei einer Reihe von längeren Zusätzen bleibt noch im einzelnen zu
prüfen, inwieweit sie Ansichten Galens (eventuell aus anderen Werken)
referieren bzw. eine abweichende Meinung oder eigene Erfahrung des
Rhazes wiedergeben. Hier nur ein Beispiel: In seinem Kommentar zu
Galens Operationsvorschriften für eine verhärtete Lippe (*MM* XIV 16:
X 1002,6-13) warnt Rhazes vor dem Vorgehen gewisser nachlässiger
Operateure (sāhūn), die Haut und darunterliegendes Gewebe mit einem
einzigen Schnitt abtrennten, was eine Verkürzung der Lippe zur Folge
habe. In umso strahlenderem Licht läßt er dagegen die Vorzüge der von
Galen beschriebenen Technik erscheinen, die er noch einmal in allen
Einzelheiten wiederholt (VI 218,18-219,4). Ob Rhazes hier auf konkrete
Erlebnisse mit zeitgenössischen Kollegen anspielt oder ob er sich viel-
mehr auf eine literarische Quelle bezieht, muß vorläufig offenbleiben.

Auf die eigene Erfahrung beruft sich Rhazes im übrigen in unserem
ganzen Material nur an einer einzigen Stelle, und zwar im Zusammenhang mit Galens Bericht über den Fall jener vornehmen Römerin, die
an Herpes litt. Da sie sich weigerte, das von Galen verordnete galleab-
führende Mittel einzunehmen, nahm dieser schließlich Zuflucht zu einer
List: Nachdem er die Patientin zu einem Molketrunk überredet hatte,
mischte er diesem heimlich Purgierwinde bei (*MM* XIV 17: X 1007,

10-1008,8). Diese Geschichte gibt Rhazes Gelegenheit, seine eigene Beobachtung anzubringen, daß Molke Gelbgalle abführt und die Schärfe der Leber beseitigt (VI 127,4-5). Damit begibt er sich freilich in einen gewissen Gegensatz zu Galen, der die Heilung jener Frau ja weniger der Molke als der zugesetzten Skammonia zugeschrieben hatte.

Dies führt uns schließlich auf Modifikationen oder Teilkorrekturen, die Rhazes an Galens Lehren anbringt. Wenn dieser (*MM* VI 7: X 298,1-4) eine Reihe von Drogen mineralischer Herkunft bei inneren Verletzungen für kontraindiziert hält, so gilt dies nach der Ansicht von Rhazes nur für die orale Einnahme, während sie per anum verabreicht in vielen Fällen Anwendung fänden (XIII 84,1-2). An anderer Stelle ergänzt Rhazes die Angabe seiner Quelle (*MM* III 3: X 175,15-18), daß Schweißbildung entweder von der Schwäche der eingeborenen Wärme oder von übermäßiger Nahrungsaufnahme herrühre, durch die Beobachtung, daß umgekehrt auch bei Nahrungsmangel Schweiß auftrete. Auf den ersten Blick scheint er damit Galen zu widersprechen; indem er den nachgetragenen Fall darauf zurückführt, daß Nahrungsmangel die eingeborene Wärme schwäche (XIV 232,8-9), ordnet er ihn indessen doch wieder in die galenischen Kategorien ein.

Kritik an Galen, freilich recht milde Kritik, übt er allenfalls an zwei Stellen. Im Anschluß an seine Wiedergabe der Ausführungen Galens über die verschiedenen Grade der Austrocknung des Körpers sowie die im jeweiligen Falle angemessene Diät (*MM* VII 6, nach X 496,6) bemängelt Rhazes, daß für keinen dieser Zustände differentialdiagnostische Zeichen angegeben würden (V 13,10). Zum zweiten merkt Rhazes zu *MM* X 9 (X 701,3-12) an, es habe den Anschein, als sei Galen, der hier kalt-feuchte Heilmittel ohne styptische Eigenschaften als Mittel der Wahl bei hektischen Fiebern empfiehlt, der hierher gehörige Kampfer unbekannt (XVI 19,5) — womit er zweifellos recht hat. Einige Zeilen später, wo Galen die Eignung des Essigs für solche Fälle erwägt, kommt Rhazes noch einmal auf seinen Einwand zurück, mildert ihn aber beträchtlich ab (XVI 19,8-9): "Ich sehe, daß Galen den Kampfer nicht erwähnt, sei es, daß er ihn nicht kennt, sei es, weil er kräftig trocknet", d.h. eine unerwünschte Nebenwirkung hat — was das vermeintliche Versäumnis Galens im Lichte einer wohlüberlegten Ablehnung erscheinen ließe.

Aufs Ganze gesehen erweist sich Rhazes in den hier ausgewerteten Kommentaren und Ergänzungen zu den *MM*-Exzerpten im *Continens* weniger als Kritiker denn als sachkundiger Ausleger der Lehren Galens, über die er nirgends entscheidend hinausgeht. Wirklich überzeugende Beiträge zur arabischen Kritik an Galen als Arzt lassen sich aus unserem Material nicht gewinnen.

3. *Ausblick*

Wir konnten hier noch keine umfassende Übersicht über die Rezeption
der *MM* im arabisch-islamischen Mittelalter vorlegen, doch darf aus
unserer eingehenderen Untersuchung dreier spezieller Aspekte anhand
des *Continens* wenigstens soviel als allgemeines Ergebnis festgehalten werden: Der Einfluß der *MM* auf die Darstellung der internistischen wie der
chirurgischen Therapie in der Medizinliteratur des Islam muß außerordentlich hoch eingeschätzt werden. Zu einer differenzierteren Würdi-
gung ihrer Bedeutung bedarf es weiterer Detailstudien. Einen unmittelbaren Vergleich mit den Verhältnissen im *Continens* erlaubt
beispielsweise eine andere arabische Exzerptensammlung, in der im
übrigen nur Werke Galens ausgeschrieben wurden: Die *Aphorismen* (*K.
al-Fuṣūl*) des Maimonides, die, wie wir nachträglich anhand der engli-
schen Übersetzung der hebräischen Version (das arabische Original liegt
noch nicht im Druck vor) feststellten, rund 180 Zitate (mit Buchangabe)
enthält.[61] Ein weiterer Schritt wäre die Untersuchung von Schriften, deren Autoren den Inhalt der *MM* wirklich assimiliert und in ihre eigenen
Darstellungen integriert haben. Bei der Aufarbeitung der arabischen
Überlieferung des galenischen Werkes selbst schließlich müssen neben
der nur teilweise erhaltenen Version Ḥubaiš's vor allem die verschiedenen arabischen Bearbeitungen der *MM* berücksichtigt werden.

---

[61] The Medical Aphorisms of Moses Maimonides. Translated and Edited by Fred
Rosner and Suessman Muntner. Bd. 1-2. New York 1973. Es handelt sich um die folgenden Aphorismen: I 7, 60; III 13-15, 24, 30, 51, 67, 82, 83, 89-93, 105-108, 110, 113;
VII 6, 7; VIII 10, 11, 23, 36, 37, 40-43, 47, 48, 61-63, 74; IX 17-20, 39, 46-49, 56, 57,
68-70, 75-78, 86, 92, 114-120a, 124-126; X 1-4, 15-18, 32, 47, 51, 60-71; XII 8-11, 20,
21, 24, 33, 34, 37, 46, 47; XIII 9, 13, 41, 42; XIV 1, 6, 11; XV 15-25, 28, 33, 34, 36-43,
46-48, 54-57, 65; XVI 12; XIX 11, 13, 16, 33-37; XX 8, 9, 30; XXI 5, 6, 12, 16, 19,
26-28, 39, 40, 92-94; XXIII 33a, 42, 43, 52, 68, 97. Im Abschnitt XXV, in dem Maimonides Inkonsistenzen im Werk Galens aufzeigen will, erwähnt er die *MM* in Aph. 7, 43,
47, 53, 55.

FAYE MARIE GETZ

THE *METHOD OF HEALING* IN MIDDLE ENGLISH

The first translation of Galen into English that has as yet been identified is found in British Library, Sloane MS 6 from the fifteenth century. The translation was made about 1400 from the version of *Methodus medendi* known as *De ingenio sanitatis*, a twelfth-century translation from Arabic made by Gerard of Cremona. The English version covers all of Book III and three and a half chapters of Book IV.

That such a translation should exist at all will perhaps come as a surprise to some medical historians, who have long regarded the Middle English medical texts as a kind of backwater, a curiosity representative more of the degeneration of medical knowledge than of its dissemination. However, recent work on the subject of Middle English medical texts has shown that during the late fourteenth and fifteenth centuries, translation was the principal means of conveying medical knowledge in the vernacular, and that translators selected their copy texts from among the best authors the Latin textual tradition had to offer.[1] Apart from the Galen translation, famous Latin authors such as Bernard Gordon, Gilbertus Anglicus, Guy de Chauliac, a number of Salernitan writers, and a host of anonymous texts awaiting identification can be found in Middle English. What is more, Middle English medical literature survived into the Modern English printed tradition. One may cite Petrus Hispanus and Friar Thomas Multon as notable examples.[2] In short, Middle English medical literature is an important witness to the transmission and dissemination of medical knowledge and it deserves at least some of the attention that hitherto has been reserved for Arabic, Syriac, Hebrew, and Latin translations.

In order to allow the reader to compare the Galenic text in three of these languages: Middle English, Latin, and the original Greek, I have reproduced the Middle English chapter headings and incipits with their Latin and Greek counterparts. These chapter headings do not have an

---

[1] See Faye Marie Getz, 'Gilbertus Anglicus Anglicized'. *Med. Hist.* 26 (1982), 436-442 and my forthcoming edition of the Middle English Gilbertus Anglicus for the University of Wisconsin Press for a discussion of translation in Middle English medical literature. A recent edition of a Latin medical text and its Middle English counterpart is Linda E. Voigts and Michael R. McVaugh, A Latin Technical Phlebotomy and Its Middle English Translation (Philadelphia, 1984).

[2] For Multon, see my 'Charity, Translation, and the Language of Medical Learning in Medieval England', *Bull. Hist. Med.* 64 (1990), pp. 1-17.

exemplar in the Latin MS used for comparison and are in my text enclosed in square brackets. The Latin text used is in British Library, Harley MS 3748, from the fourteenth century (*De ingenio sanitatis* in this MS names Gerard as its translator; the text is found on ff. 42-112v). This MS has been corrected against the printed text of Gerard's translation found in Galen's *Opera*, edited by Diomedes Bonardus, vol. II. Venice: P. Pincius, 1490 (ff. 167-221). Folio numbers are given to Sloane MS 6 alongside the Middle English citations, to Harley MS 3748 alongside the Latin, and to the 1490 edition in square brackets underneath the Harley folio numbers. The Greek text offered for comparison is taken from C. G. Kühn's edition *Claudii Galeni Opera Omnia*, vol. X (Leipzig, 1825, repr. 1965). It should be remembered that the exact Latin exemplar for the Middle English text is as yet unknown and that the Middle English is many times removed by repeated translation from the Greek. Hence the equivalents in Latin and Greek are approximate.

The most distinctive feature of this particular translation is the use of linguistic 'doublets', that is, pairs of synonyms used to translate a single Latin word. The most common is 'essencion or being', which appears in sections I, III, and IX below, and which is used to translate Latin 'essencia'. This text shows a number of other such doublets, and they served as a major aid to the development of modern English medical vocabulary.[3]

I

Sloane MS 6 f. 183r — [In þis book ben vii chapitres contened. And in þe first he putteþ vnder what þing out of kynde a sekenes is conteyned].

Riȝt dere frende Nero, as it acordeþ þe significaciouns of wyrchyng for-to be considered of þe essencion or beyng of kynde and of þe sekenes, so it is nedeful þat þe science or þe connyng of þo þings with which curacioun or helyng schal be giffen.

Harl. MS 3748 f. 53rb — Sicut operandi significationes Nero karissime
[1490 ed. f. 174rb] — ab essencia nature morbi convenit considerari, sic et eorum sciencia cum quibus curatio dabitur ab eadem essencia perpendi necesse est.

---

[3] Middle English letters that may be strange to most readers are as follows: 'Þ' or 'þ' represent the 'th' sound. 'ȝ' in this text stands for modern 'gh'.

Kühn, p. 157

Εἴπερ οὖν, ὦ Ἱέρων, ἡ ἔνδειξις ἐκ τῆς τοῦ πράγματος φύσεως ὁρμωμένη τὸ δέον ἐξευρίσκει, τὴν ἀρχὴν τῆς τῶν ἰαμάτων εὑρέσεως ἐκ τῆς τῶν νοσημάτων αὐτῶν ἀνάγκη γίγνεσθαι

II

f. 184r

[Þe ii chapitre in which he determineþ of cure of wondes þat bene in fleschy membres repreuyng þe worchyng of Tesyle].
Wherfore I schal bigynne at som symple woundes as þus. A wonde beyn in þe ouerparty of fleschy membres is most symple.

f. 53vb
[f. 174va]

Undé incipiam a quibusdam simplicibus, verbi gracia, vulnus in superficie carnosorum membrorum existens simplicissimum est.

p. 162

Πρόδηλον δ' ὡς ἀπὸ τῶν ἁπλουστάτων ἄρξηται. τί δ' ἁπλούστερον ἕλκους ἐπιπολῆς ἐν σαρκώδει μορίῳ;

III

f. 186r

[Þe iii chapitre in which he treteþ of þe cure of holowe woundes and howe þei schalle bene cured].
Þerfor bigyn we of þat doctrine and science which we haue taken of Ypocras. Þerfor I sey þat þe wytte and þe bygynnyng of þis craft owe to be taken of þe essencion and beyng of nature of þingis.

f. 54va
[f. 175ra]

Incipiamus ergo ab ea sciencia et doctrina vulnerum quas ab Ypocrate suscepimus. Dico ergo quod ingenium et initium huius artis ab essencia nature rerum sumi debeant.

pp. 173-174

Εἴπωμεν οὖν ἡμεῖς ἤδη τὴν Ἱπποκράτειόν τε ἅμα καὶ ἀληθῆ μέθοδον ἑλκῶν κοίλων ἰάσεως, ἄρχεσθαι δὲ δήπουθεν αὐτὴν ἐκ τῆς οὐδίας χρὴ τοῦ πράγματος.

IV

f. 189r

[Þe iiii chapitre in which he determineþ þe cure of woundes in as miche as woundes].

Here forsoþe schal I begynne of þe cures of þam
þat al only bene woundes.

f. 55va
[f. 175vb]
p. 186

Hic autem incipiam de curis eorum que sola
vulnera sunt.

Ἐπὶ δὲ τὴν τοῦ ἕλκους θεραπείαν μόνου μετέρχεσθαι
χαιρός.

V

f. 191v

[Þe v chapitre in which he techeþ þe wytte to
cure solucion in þe which þer is lesyng of
skynne].

were forsoþe will He dispute of woundes which
bene nedeful for-to be souded and heled.

f. 56rb
[f. 176rb]
p. 197

Hic autem volumus disputare de vulneribus
que necesse est solidari et sanari.

Ἐπὶ δὲ τὸ τῆς οὐλῆς δεόμενον ἕλκος ἐπάνειμι,

VI

f. 192r

[Þe vi chapitre in which he techeþ to remove
superflue flesch of woundes].

Now forsoþe bihoueþ vs to turne agayne to þe
þings which we lefte of woundes to be cured,
and for-to schew how we mow drawe out þo
þings whiche bene superflue in woundes.

f. 56vb
[f. 176va]

Nunc autem oportet nos ad ea que de curandis
vulneribus dimissimus redire, id est, ostendere
qualiter ea que vulneribus sunt superflua
possumus evellere.

p. 200

ἀλλὰ γὰρ ἐπὶ τὸ λεῖπον ἔτι τῆς περὶ τῶν ἑλκῶν
ἀπιέναι χρὴ μεθόδου.

Λείπει δ᾽, ὡς οἶμαι, τὸ περὶ τῶν ὑπεραυξανομένων
σαρκῶν εἰπεῖν,

VII

f. 193r

[Þe vii chapitre in which he reprehendeþ or
reproueþ metoycens, þat is experimentours,
and confermeþ logiciens].

Wherfor I sey þat metoycens all þair studie
putte in þair experiments may nowise be turned
fro one medicyne to anoþer.

f. 57ra
[f. 176vb]

Quare dico methoicos omni studio in suis experimentis imposito nequaquam posse de una ad aliam verti medicinam.

p. 204

δῆλον δ', οἶμαι, κἀπὶ τούτων ἐστὶν ὡς ὁ μὲν ἐμπειρικός, εἰ καὶ ὅτι μάλιστα διωρισμένῃ χρήσαιτο τῇ πείρᾳ, τό γε μεταβαίνειν ἐπὶ τὸ προσῆκον εὐμηχάνως οὐκ ἔχει.

VIII

f.194v

[Þe viii chapitre in which Galiene determineþ of cure of woundes and of þe maner of þo þings which comeþ aboue in woundes].

Bot siþe þis resoun as me þink is wele diffinite, þus of me i-turne aȝeyn to þo þinge which I disputed first, saiyng euery sekenes which is wonte for-to come in woundes. And I schal bigyn at euyl complexioun.

f. 57va
[f. 177ra]

At cum hec ratio, ut video, a me bene sit diffinita, revertor ad ea que primitus disputavi, dicens unumquemque morbum qui in vulneribus solet evenire. Et incipiam a mala complexione.

p. 211

'Επεὶ δὲ καὶ περὶ τούτων αὐτάρκως διώρισται, πάλιν ἐπὶ τὴν ἀρχὴν ἀνέλθωμεν τοῦ λόγου, μιγνύντες ἁπάσας τὰς συμπιπτούσας ἕλκει διαθέσεις ἀπὸ πρώτης ἀρξάμενοι τῆς δυσκρασίας.

IX

f.195v

[Þe ix chapitre in which is schew how a wounde is to be cured when þere appereþ contrary significacions].

Of which þing as me semeþ I haue schewed as it bihoued openly þe medicynes of woundes, forwhi þat bihoueþ first to be considered is to be taken of þe essencion or beyng of þe sekenes.

f. 57vb
[f. 177rb]

Qua de re patenter, ut video, medicinas vulnerum prout oportuit ostendi nam quod primitus considerari oportet ab essencia morbi sumendum est.

pp.214-215

Τὸ μὲν οὖν καὶ τὰς κράσεις τῶν σωμάτων καὶ τὰς ὥρας τοῦ ἔτους καὶ τὰς φύσεις τῶν μορίων ἐπιβλέπειν χρῆναι τὸν μέλλοντα καλῶς ἕλκος ἰάσασθαι δεδεῖχθαί μοι νομίζω σαφῶς· καὶ ὡς μὲν πρῶτος σκοπὸς τῆς ἰάσεως ἐκ τῆς διαθέσεως λαμβάνεται μόνης,

X

f. 197ʳ

[Þe x chapitre in which he techeþ for-to knowe þe witte of curyng of þe self denotacions of woundes].

Here forsoþe wil I dispute of þe denocacions of woundes. I sey þerfor þat if any man sey þat wounds som bene bolnes oþer putred or roten or filthi oþer cancrous oþer erisipilar oþer with akyng and oþer with-out akyng and sich oþer
...

f. 58ʳᵇ
[f. 177ᵛᵃ]

Dico ergo quod si aliquis dixerit quod vulnera, alia sunt tumida alia putrida alia corrosiva alia erisipilata alia cancerosa alia cum dolore alia sine dolore et similia ...

pp. 221-222

Ἐν γὰρ τῷ παρόντι συγκεφαλαιώσασθαι βούλομαι τὸν ἐνεστῶτα λόγον ἐπὶ τὰς οἰκείας διαφορὰς τῶν ἑλκῶν ἐπανελθών· ἵν᾽ εἴ τις κἀντεῦθεν ἔνδειξίς ἰαμάτων ἐστί, μηδὲ ταύτην παραλίπωμεν. τὸ μὲν οὖν φλεγμαῖνον ἕλκος καὶ τὸ σηπόμενον ἀναβιβρωσκόμενόν τε καὶ γαγγραινούμενον ἐρυσιπελατῶδές τε καὶ καρκινῶδες ἀνώδυνόν τε καὶ ὀδυνῶδες, τά τ᾽ ἄλλα τοιαῦτα λέγουσιν ὡς διαφορὰς ἑλκῶν.

XI

f. 198ᵛ

[Here endeth þe þrid boke of Galiene Le ingenio sanitatis, þat is, of witte of hele.

f. 199

Here begynneþ þe ferþe boke contenyng vii chapitres. In þe first he setteþ bi-fore some comoun þings of accidentes and sekenes comyng to woundes].

Of all it be knowen þat seperacione of iuncture which is called dissolucion or lousyng of vneuenhed be a sekenes comyng to euery membre, neþeles it is noȝt noted with one worde.

f. 59ra
[f. 178ra]

Quamquam notum sit quod separatio iuncture que inparitatis dissolutio dicitur sit morbus unicuique membro eveniens non tamen uno vocabulo denotatur.

p. 232

Ἔν τι γένος ἦν νόσου καὶ ἡ τῆς συνεχείας λύσις, ἐν ἅπασι μὲν τοῦ ζῴου τοῖς μέρεσι γινομένη, προσαγορευομένη δ' οὐχ ὡσαύτως ἐν ἅπασιν.

XII

f. 200r

[Þe ii chapitre in which he techeþ to eschewe yuel complexion].

Also somtyme þise þre bene medled to-gidre and som-tyme tuo. Neþeles it bi-houeþ noȝt to be schewed þe cure of þise componed, siþen I disputed in my presence singulerly of þam.

f. 59va
[f. 178rb]

Quandoque hec tria commiscentur et aliquando duo horum tamen compositorum curam non oportet ostendi et sigillatim de eis presencialiter disputavi.

pp. 236-237

ἐνίοτε δὲ καὶ μίγνυσθαι συμβέβηκέ τινας τῶν εἰρημένων διαθέσεων, ἢ καὶ πάσας ἅμα. χρὴ δ' οὐ πασῶν δήπουθεν ἅμα λέγεσθαι τὴν μέθοδον τῆς ἰάσεως, ἀλλ' ἑκάστης ἰδία.

XIII

f. 201r

[Þe 3 chapitre in which he techeþ to hele woundez by her first causez].

Ouer þat I will diffinich som oþer þingz I sey. Þerfor no-þing for-to schew þe primityue significacion of curyng, siþe it is bitokned of þe essencion of þe sekenez and þe nature of þe seke membre and of þe gode complexion [201v] of þat þae enuyrowneþ us.

f. 59vb
[f. 178vb]

Preterea quedam alia volo diffinire. Dico ergo nichil primitivam significationem curationis ostendere cum [60ra] ab essencia morbi et natura membri infirmi et ab aeris complexione nos circumdantur et similibus denotetur.

pp. 242-243

Καὶ γὰρ αὖ καὶ τοῦτο καιρὸς διορίσασθαι ἤδη, τὸ μηδὲν τῶν προκαταρξάντων τῆς διαθέσεως αἰτίων

ἐνδείκνυσθαι τὴν θεραπείαν, ἀλλὰ μὲν ταύτης
ἔνδειξιν ἀπ' αὐτῆς ἄρχεσθαι τῆς διαθέσεως,
ἐξευρίσκεσθαι δὲ τὰς κατὰ μέρος ἐνεργείας ἀπό τε
τοῦ πρώτου σκοποῦ καὶ τῆς τοῦ πεπονθότος μορίου
φύσεως καὶ τῆς τοῦ περιέχοντος κράσεως,

XIV

f. 202ᵛ [Þe 4 chapitre in which he techeþ of þe cure of
þe worst woundes after techyng of oþer].
He is no gode leche þat perniciously laboreþ in
wordez bot also for he scheweþ þe crafte of
woundez to be cured.

f. 60ᵛᵃ Non est igitur bonus medicus qui in verbis per-
[f. 179ʳᵃ] niciose laborat sed qui viam et artificium curan-
dorum vulnerum ostendit.

p. 250 Οὐκ οὖν ἐν ὀνόμασι μιχρολογεῖσθαι καλόν, ἀλλ'
ἄμεινον εἰπεῖν τινα μέθοδον ἰάσεως ἑλκῶν,

XV [last line]

f. 203ᵛ Þerfor tyme scheweþ no tokne of curyng bot
noumbre of daies.

f. 60ᵛᵇ Tempus ergo nullum signum curandi
[f. 179ʳᵇ] demonstrat nisi numerum dierum.

p.253 ὁ χρόνος δὲ τί πλέον ἡμᾶς διδάξει τοῦ τῶν ἡμερῶν
ἀριθμοῦ

Although it is important to study the Middle English Galen as a discrete
text, its significance to the history of medicine cannot fully be appreciated
unless it is seen also in its manuscript context. Sloane MS 6 is a surgical
compendium, translated for the most part from Latin into English, and
containing a wide variety of information not only on surgery itself, but
also on phlebotomy, the nature of matter and the elements, and the
philosophical principles that underlie the working of the human body.
Within this compendium, the Galenic text supplies the theoretical basis
for learned surgery in general, and for wound treatment in particular.

The contents of the MS are as follows:

1. Johannitius, *Isagoge* (ff. 1-9), in English. Attribution supplied in
   a later hand ff. 1 and 9. Incipit: *Medicyne is divided in two partys,
   þat is theory and practys.*[4]

---

[4] The *Isagoge* found in this MS has been noted by Glending Olson, Literature as
Recreation in the Later Middle Ages (London, 1982), pp. 40 (note), 41.

2. Anon. 'Table of knowinge of symple medicynez' (ff. 10-18), in English. Avicenna cited on f. 14.

3. Anon. Treatise in English on the four elements, humours, complexions, and related topics (ff. 18-19ᵛ). Galen's *De complexionibus*, and Seneca are cited on f. 19. Incipit: *Element is a symple and leste particle*.

4. Anon. Table of Aristotelian causes in English (ff. 20ᵛ-21ᵛ).

5. Richardus (Anglicus?), 'Þe knowyng of medicynies after þer operacion'. Examples of medicines that can be known by the way in which they affect the body (ff. 22-32ᵛ), in English. Attribution on ff. 22 and 32ᵛ. Incipit: *Calefactives. Al medicine þat is hote*.

6. Bernard Gordon (no attribution). 'The mirrour of flebotomie' (ff. 33-40ᵛ), in English. Incipit: *Flebotomye is ane vniversale evacuacion*.

7. Anon. Treatise on cupping (ff. 41-42ᵛ), in English. Incipit: *Ventosyngz forsoþe bene done*.

8. Haly Abbas, *Liber regius* (excerpts). Sections concerning laxatives, astrology, and prognosis (ff. 43-50ᵛ), in English. Attribution on ff. 44ᵛ and 50ᵛ. Incipit: *No man oweþ to take a purgyng*.

9. Table of contents to 6, 7, and 8 above.

10. William of Parma (Saliceto). Surgery in English (ff. 53-140ᵛ). Attribution on f. 53. Incipit: *It is purposid to þe my gode frend*.

11. John of Arderne. Treatise on fistula in ano, haemorrhoids, and related topics (ff. 141-174ᵛ), in English. Attribution on f. 141ᵛ. Incipit: *I, John Arderne fro the first pestilence*.[5]

12. Illustrations in ink of various methods of healing, including spiritual healing, pharmacy, herbalism, astrology, bloodletting, and cupping. Many pictures of surgical instruments. Captions in English (ff. 175-177ᵛ).[6]

13. Anon. How to make medicinal syrups (ff. 178-179ᵛ), in English. Incipit: *About þe confeccion of surypes ben 7 canons*.

14. Anon. Tables for uroscopy (ff. 180-182), in Latin.

15. Galen, *De ingenio sanitatis*, books III and three and a half chapters of book IV (ff. 183ᵛ-203ᵛ) in English. Attribution on ff. 194ᵛ and 198ᵛ. Incipit: *Riʒt dere frende Nero*.

The relationship of the Galenic text to its Latin counterpart has been established above by comparing the Middle English with the Latin text.

---

[5] The Arderne translation has been edited by D'Arcy Power, John of Arderne: Treatises of Fistula in Ano, etc., Early English Text Society 139 (1910, repr. 1968). A new edition of Arderne in Latin and Middle English is being prepared by Peter Murray Jones.

[6] The illustrations found in this MS are discussed by Peter Murray Jones, Medieval Medical Miniatures (London, 1984), pp. 33, 91-94, 109, 110, 123-125, 130, 131, figs. 6, 41, 49, 56, and 60.

Can something similar be done with the compendium as a whole, that is, can a Latin compendium be found that is a counterpart for Sloane MS 6? The possibility cannot be ruled out, but what seems more likely is that the compiler of Sloane MS 6, instead of translating word-for-word a Latin compendium, took excerpts from other MSS (in the case of the *Isagoge*, perhaps a version of the Articella), translated them if necessary, and then assembled them in a form that suited his own specific needs.[7] This would of course explain why the MS as a whole is composed of a number of booklets that were copied by different scribes and compiled into a single MS in the fifteenth century.

The two processes discussed briefly above, translation and compilation, have been for the most part underexploited as sources of historical evidence. This is especially unfortunate since both processes point directly to the interests of people during a particular time period and give us direct evidence of some of the texts available to these people.

This is not to suggest that the Middle English *De ingenio sanitatis* is a significant witness to the Greek or even the Latin textual tradition. It is after all remote from anything Galen himself wrote and indeed is only a fragment of the complete text.[8] What the Middle English text does show, however, is that Galenic medicine was alive and flourishing in fifteenth-century England and was, by means of translation and compilation, reaching a new readership whose language was not that of university professors, but of the lay person.

Acknowledgements

I would like to thank the Keeper of Manuscripts of the British Library and the Librarian of the Wellcome Institute Library for the generous use of their facilities. I would also like to thank the Wellcome Institute Library, who funded me in this research. Prof. George Rigg of the Centre for Medieval Studies, University of Toronto, corrected the Middle English and Latin texts as always with great patience and learning. Finally, Dr. Vivian Nutton of the Wellcome Institute provided advice on Galen and Galenism that was indispensible to this study.

---

[7] This process has been examined in Latin texts by M. B. Parkes, 'The Influence of the Concepts of Ordinatio and Compilatio on the Development of the Book'. In: Medieval Learning and Literature, edited by J. J. G. Alexander and M. T. Gibson (Oxford, 1976), pp. 115-141. The provenance of Sloane MS 6 has yet to be studied.

[8] Thorndike and Kibre have noted in their Catalogue of Incipits of Mediaeval Scientific Writings in Latin, rev. and aug. ed. (London, 1963) a Bodleian Library MS (E musaeo MS 19) from the fourteenth century that is entitled 'Cirurgia Galieni' and that is a series of extracts from *De ingenio sanitatis* (col. 1495). The Sloane translation may have been derived from an abridged version of the Latin text that, like the 'Cirurgia Galieni', circulated separately.

JEROME J. BYLEBYL

TEACHING *METHODUS MEDENDI* IN THE RENAISSANCE

Assessing the influence of *Methodus medendi* on Renaissance medicine is in some respects like trying to find the hay in a haystack.[1] The medical literature of the period is immense, the dominant outlook was one of staunch Galenic orthodoxy, and this particular treatise lent itself to frequent discussion and citation. Galen devoted the greater part of the work to the treatment of wounds and fevers, and these were also among the topics most frequently discussed by the medical and surgical authors of the sixteenth century, the period with which I shall be chiefly concerned. In addition, *Methodus medendi* dealt in passing with a wide range of other issues, both practical and theoretical, which also attracted the notice of later readers. For example, it was the work quoted most frequently, and at greatest length, by Pierre Brissot in the tract of 1525 that helped launch the great bloodletting controversy of the sixteenth century.[2] Again, as Temkin has noted, book twelve of the *Methodus* contains Galen's only comments about the possible existence of a natural spirit in the veins, and this passage was commonly cited in the many discussions of this important physiological issue.[3]

But while references to *Methodus medendi* were common enough, there is also a sense in which the influence of the treatise is as elusive as the proverbial needle. It was not, after all, Galen's primary aim to set forth his views on derivation and revulsion or on the natural spirits, nor even

---

[1] Two recent articles that are directly relevant to the theme of *Methodus medendi* in the Renaissance are Donald G. Bates, "Sydenham and the medical meaning of 'method'", *Bull. Hist. Med.* 51 (1977) 324-338; and Jeffrey Boss, "The Methodus medendi as an index of change in the philosophy of medical science in the sixteenth and seventeenth centuries", *Hist. and Philosophy Life Sci.* 1 (1979) 13-42. Two other authors have discussed the broader concept of method and its relationship to Renaissance medicine: William P. D. Wightman, "Quid sit methodus? 'Method' in sixteenth century medical teaching and 'discovery'", *J. Hist. Med.* 19 (1964) 360-376; and Andrew Wear, "Galen in the Renaissance", in Galen: Problems and Prospects: A Collection of Papers Submitted at the 1979 Cambridge Conference, ed. Vivian Nutton (London: The Wellcome Institute for the History of Medicine, 1981), pp. 229-262, esp. pp. 238-245, "Medical Method".

[2] Pierre Brissot, *Apologetica disceptatio, qua docetur per quae loca sanguis mitti debeat* (Paris, 1525), passim.

[3] *Methodus medendi*, 12, 5 = X 839-840; Owsei Temkin, "On Galen's pneumatology", in his *Double Face of Janus* (Baltimore: The Johns Hopkins University Press, 1977, pp. 154-161. For Renaissance discussions, see, e.g., Francesco Valles, *Controversiarum medicarum et philosophicarum* (1564), Bk. 2, ch. 16, fol. 40r; André du Laurens, *Historia anatomica* (Paris, 1600), Bk. 6, Q. 22, p. 314.

to discuss the treatment of wounds and fevers. Rather, it was to propound a general method of treatment, applicable to all diseases in all circumstances. Thus the true measure of the treatise's influence would be whether and to what extent its principles were observed in the day to day practice of physicians. It is, however, notoriously difficult for medical historians to attain insights into the realities of medical practice at the grassroots level, and it would be particularly difficult in the present instance because the test of fidelity to the Galenic method would not be the treatment per se, but the inner intentions which led the physician to it. That is, did he act on the basis of rational insight into all of the circumstances that are relevant to the particular case under treatment—in other words, did he follow the curative indications—or did he simply do what is commonly done in similar cases?

If it is not possible to say how well Galen's method was practiced in the Renaissance, I hope to shed some light on how well it was taught, though even here the situation is complicated by the fact that Galen himself did not speak with a single voice in laying down his approach to therapeutics. In *Methodus medendi*, he is almost wilfully fastidious in his demands for a proper treatment: the physician must be able to make very precise diagnostic distinctions, involving insights into the underlying etiology and pathology of the disease; he must in addition be prepared to take account of complications in the disease; beyond this, he must make allowance for such quintessentially individual factors as the patient's natural temperament and present strength, and the condition of the air that surrounds him; and somehow he must balance all of these indications in devising a specific course of treatment for the particular case in question. But Galen did not always follow so rigorous a protocol in outlining therapeutic strategies. For example, in his lengthy work *De compositione medicamentorum secundum locos* we find two rather less complicated approaches. Sometimes remedies are recommended for a given kind of disease based only on rational insights into its essence and cause, and without reference to those indications that are unique to each case.[4] Or he might omit reasoning from indications altogether, and give only the names of diseases together with recipes to be used in curing them.[5] In the opening words and elsewhere in the treatise he refers the reader

---

[4] See e.g., *De compositione medicamentorum secundum locos*, 8, 6 = XIII 187-220, where Galen first reviews the various kinds of hepatic affections that can occur, and then evaluates hepatic remedies with regard to which kinds of affection they are good for, mentioning nothing besides the diagnostic category as the basis for selection.

[5] E.g., ibid., 9, 5 = XIII 288-306, where the discussion of dysentery amounts to little more than a collection of recipes gleaned from earlier writers. But see p. 305 for passing reference to individualization of treatment.

to *Methodus medendi* for the general principles from which these remedies are derived, but it is difficult to avoid the conclusion that listing diseases and remedies is, by Galen's own standards, a profoundly amethodical approach to therapeutics.[6]

It would therefore appear that Galen himself found it impossible to adhere consistently and rigorously to his own method of treatment, and so it should come as no surprise to learn that his Renaissance followers frequently fell short of it in their teaching, and were not always cognizant of the discrepancy. In fact, of the two major courses of the standard medical curriculum, each embodied one of the variant approaches to therapy that we also find in Galen. Thus the course on the theory of medicine often served as the forum for explaining the basic principles of methodical treatment as well as the physiological and etiological conceptions which it presupposes. But the course on the practice of medicine was focussed not on teaching the students how to apply this general method, but on how to diagnose and cure all of the major diseases. To be sure, the lectures on practice were fitted out with many of the trappings of methodical treatment, but there is a basic difference between inculcating a general method, and teaching the causes, signs, and cures of all diseases by enumeration. The latter approach tends to encapsulate therapeutic reasoning within the lectures or textbook, placing the burden on the teacher to explain what must be done for every disease; the former would ultimately place the burden on the student to learn how to rationally derive the cures that are appropriate to each case on an individual basis, which is, I take it, the true methodus medendi.

But because the traditional course on medical practice was in conflict with *Methodus medendi*, it can serve as a rather sensitive index of how well the latter was appreciated. Therefore, rather than focus on the idealized expositions of the *Methodus medendi*, I shall give primary attention to the criticisms that were voiced of the lectures and textbooks on practice, and to the various efforts that were made to bring them more into conformity with the Galenic method. As we shall see, external critics of the genre saw that its approach was fundamentally different from that of *Methodus medendi*, but there was almost no acknowledgement of these deficiencies within the genre itself.

A major exception were the public lectures on practice that Giovanni Battista da Monte delivered at the University of Padua for a few years in the early 1540s. Da Monte denounced the whole tradition of teaching

---

[6] E.g., ibid. 1, 1; 6, 1; 8, 6 = XII 378-379; 894-905; XIII 187-198. The treatise begins with the statement that therapy is indicated not only by the affection, but also by the temperament of the patient and the nature of the affected part. But the second of these three factors is largely ignored in what follows.

the practice of medicine by the enumeration of all the particulars, and made clear his intention to focus instead on teaching the general methodus medendi and its application. Considering the time, the place, and the individual, this was perhaps the last, best hope of making *Methodus medendi* the primary basis on which medicine was to be practiced, but as we shall see, the experiment apparently ended in failure after just a few years. In addition, though, Da Monte also cultivated bedside precepting as the best way to teach the application of the method to individual cases, and in this respect he seems to have had a more lasting impact on the development of clinical instruction.

Before I come directly to these matters, I should first note that although *Methodus medendi* was available to European physicians long before our period through the Latin versions of Constantine, Gerard and Burgundio, it became far more accessible through the new translation by Thomas Linacre and its many printed editions, the first in 1519.[7] This was one of a number of important Galenic treatises that Linacre translated, and based on a survey of sixteenth and seventeenth century critical reaction, Richard Durling has recently concluded, "Linacre's competence, then has never been in serious doubt. His successors could only make minor improvements, often in the light of Greek manuscripts unavailable to him. They respected his work too much to repeat it."[8] And in his chronological census of Renaissance editions of Galen, Durling reported that Linacre's translation enjoyed at least thirteen separate reprintings during the sixteenth century.[9] This made it ninth in the list of most frequently printed works of Galen, and it is very much longer than all but one of the works that precede it on the list.[10]

Because *Methodus medendi* was not completely new to the sixteenth century, it is not possible sharply to distinguish its immediate influence from the cumulative effects of several centuries of familiarity. Nevertheless, I think one can say that Linacre's translation, as well as several additional factors, resulted in a substantial enhancement in understanding both of the meaning of the text and of its overall importance among Galen's works.

A discussion of the major themes of the text by Giovanni Michele Savonarola, a leading medical teacher of the first half of the fifteenth cen-

---

[7] *Methodus medendi, vel de morbis curandis. Thoma Linacro interprete* (Paris, 1519).

[8] R. J. Durling, "Linacre and Medical Humanism", in Francis Maddison, Margaret Pelling and Charles Webster (eds.), Essays on the Life and Work of Thomas Linacre (Oxford: Clarendon Press, 1977), pp. 103-106; on *Methodus medendi*, see pp. 85, 87-89.

[9] R. J. Durling, "A chronological census of Renaissance editions and translations of Galen", in *J. Warburg and Courtauld Insts.* 24 (1961) 230-305; p. 293.

[10] Ibid., p. 243; cf. also pp. 241-242.

tury, will illustrate my point by way of contrast. Savonarola began his lectures on the practice of medicine with a long introductory tract entitled *De modo processus artificialis medici in medendo.*[11] As we shall see, the basic requirements for a methodical cure are fairly well delineated, but certain general features of the doctrine are missing or understated. First, the term methodus medendi itself is absent, and its place is taken only by a relatively weak equivalent, modus medendi. The latter occurs obliquely in the title of the tract, but there is only one place in the text where it approaches the special meaning of methodus medendi. This follows the discussion of diagnosis, where Savonarola invokes Christ and the Holy Spirit to "open the way to a cautious mode of healing (ad timorosum medendi modum)"[12] and then goes on to discuss many of the central points of *Methodus medendi.*

Also conspicuously absent from Savonarola's discussion are both the phrase and the concept of the curative indication. He simply establishes, first, that a knowledge of the essence and cause of disease is crucial to a rational cure, and then lays down a series of "rules (canones)" regarding the many additional factors that must be taken into account as well. These include, with regard to the disease, its quality, quantity, location, periodicity, and symptoms, and, with regard to the patient, his or her temperament, strength, age, occupation, sex, region, habitude, customs, and repletion, as well as the season and condition of the air.[13] In his later treatise on fevers, Savonarola explicitly referred back to these rules as "curative indications" and there gave quite a good account of the concept.[14] Further research may possibly help to clarify the change—perhaps access to a different translation of *Methodus medendi* may have made the difference, or perhaps in the earlier account he was led astray by the fourth fen of Avicenna, in the Latin version of which these same matters are also discussed without clear reference to curative indications.[15] But his older contemporaries Jacopo da Forli and Ugo Benzi were quite familiar with both the term and the concept,[16] and so it is possible that

---

[11] Giovanni Michele Savonarola, *Practica* (Venice, 1560), fols. 1-8.

[12] Ibid., fol. 5r.

[13] Ibid., fol. 7v.

[14] Giovanni Michele Savonarola, *Practica canonica de Febribus* (Venice, 1552), fol. 17.

[15] E.g., in *Meth. med.*, 2, 4 ἔνδειξις comes out as significatio in Gerard's version, but in 9, 17 it is rendered indicatio in Burgundio's. Cf. X 101-102, and 658, with Galen, *Opera* (Venice, 1490), fols. 387v and 415v, and see also Durling, "Linacre", p. 85. Savonarola seems to distinguish the two versions in the *Practica* when citing "10. therapeuticae, &quarto de ingenio primo ca." (fol. 5r). Avicenna, *Canon*, I, 4, esp. ch. 1: *Libri in re medica omnes* (Venice, 1564), vol. I, pp. 185ff.

[16] Jacopo da Forlì, *In Hippocratis aphorismos, et Galeni super eisdem commentarios, expositio et Quaestiones* (Venice, 1547), fols. 4v-5r, 8v-9v, 116v-118r, 132r-133r; Ugo Benzi, *In septem sectiones Aphorismorum Hippocratis ... expositio* (Pavia, 1518), fols. 8r-9r, 27v-29v;

Savonarola simply was not sufficiently impressed with the idea to bother introducing and explaining it in the earlier work.

Finally, while Savonarola does make several passing references to Galen and to *Methodus medendi*,[17] he gave no hint that the whole modus under discussion was, specifically, that of Galen, much less that it was the special subject of that particular treatise. Indeed, apart from Christ and the Holy Spirit, the only person who is credited with a "modus & ordo rationalis" was Savonarola's teacher, Antonio Cermisone, to whose "mathematical and physical genius" is due the "modus ponendi casum medicinalem in terminis suis."[18] This was a format for organizing the data of a case history, including the description of the symptoms, the account of the essence and cause of the disease, and the listing of the many other factors such as age and temperament that are also relevant to the cure. Savonarola stressed that such an ordering was crucial for every case if the cure was to be based on art rather than chance, though the formula was to be used more particularly when it was necessary to write a formal consilium.

Thus Savonarola was clearly aware of both the substance and the importance of Galen's *Methodus medendi*, but he seems to have had little concern to emphasize either that it was a definite method or especially that it was Galen's method, or to set it forth in Galen's own terms. It would have been most unusual for a comparable figure of the sixteenth century to treat these points with such understatement and indirection. For one thing, the dominant movement within the learned medical profession through much of the sixteenth century was the effort to return directly to the ancient Greek sources as the basis of teaching and practice.[19] Thus it became important not only to draw on Galen's works (as Savonarola himself did) but also to try to get Galen exactly right and to make it quite clear that one was propounding authentic Galenic doctrine. Consequently, as we shall see, the indicationes curativae—both the concept and the term—were widely emphasized, and earlier physicians were criticized for neglect or misunderstanding in this regard.

---

idem, *Expositio super libros Tegni Galeni* (Venice, 1518), fol.89r. However, both show some vacillation between "significatio" and "indicatio". See da Forlì, fol. 2r, and Benzi, *Aphorismorum*, fols. 4v and 29.

[17] Savonarola, *Practica*, fols 5r, 6v, 7r.

[18] Ibid., fols. 7r and 8r.

[19] Durling, "A chronological census", pp. 231-245; idem, "Linacre and Medical Humanism"; J. J. Bylebyl, "The School of Padua: Humanistic Medicine in the Sixteenth Century", in Charles Webster (ed.), Health, Medicine and Mortality in the Sixteenth Century (New York and Cambridge: Cambridge University Press, 1979), pp. 335-370.

Furthermore, another major trend of the sixteenth century helped to ensure that *Methodus medendi* would have an especially exalted place in the hierarchy of Galen's books. This was a virtual obsession, not only among physicians, but intellectuals generally, with "method", in all of its meanings and aspects.[20] The very pervasiveness and complexity of such discussions may to some extent have blurred the meaning of *Methodus medendi*, but this was probably a small price to pay for the heightened interest that resulted.

One major consequence of these changing perspectives was a widespread effort to give greater prominence to *Methodus medendi* within the medical curriculum. As we shall see, this was the uppermost ambition of da Monte, and it was shared in varying degrees by many of his contemporaries. However, they encountered the difficulty that the formal teaching of medicine was still heavily based on commentary on prescribed texts, but that *Methodus medendi* was not commonly included among the texts so authorized.[21] The obvious solution would have been to modify the curriculum to include it, and indeed Linacre himself stipulated *Methodus medendi* as one of the major texts for the new lectureships that he endowed at Oxford and Cambridge.[22] But Linacre was in the unusual position of playing the piper in a country that was, medically speaking, rather underdeveloped. Elsewhere, it might prove difficult or impossible to gain approval for any changes in the two major parts of the medical curriculum, namely the lectures on theory and practice.[23] The Italian medical universities seem to have been especially conservative in this regard, and the significance of this was magnified by the

---

[20] Neal W. Gilbert, Renaissance Concepts of Method (New York: Columbia University Press, 1960); Bates, "Sydenham and method", pp. 324-331.

[21] *Meth. med.* was sometimes used as a teaching text, e.g., at Montpellier in the fourteenth century and at Jena in the sixteenth (Durling, "A chronological census", p. 234, n. 24, and p. 245); and at Bologna in the fifteenth century (C. Malagola, Statuti ... dello Studio Bolognese [Bologna, 1887], pp. 276-277). But the comparative paucity of published commentaries suggests that it was not very much used for this purpose. These apparently include Johann Agricola, *Scholia copiosa in Therapeuticam methodum* (Augsburg, 1543) [on whom see Dilg below] and Francesco Valles, *Commentaria illustria in Cl. Galeni libros subsequentes ... IV. Methodi medendi libri tres* (Cologne, 1594), neither of which I have seen; and Fabio Pace, *Commentarius in sex priores libros Galeni Methodi medendi* (Vicenza, 1598) and *Commentarius in septimum Galeni librum Methodi medendi* (Vicenza, 1608). Pace was president of the College of Physicians at Vicenza, where there was no medical university.

[22] J. M. Fletcher, "Linacre's Lands and Lectureships", in Maddison, Pelling and Webster (eds.), Life and Work of Thomas Linacre, pp. 130, 168, 188.

[23] For examples of both change and conservatism, see Gernot Rath, "Medical education at the south German universities in the fifteenth and sixteenth centuries", in *J. Med. Educ.* 35 (1960) 511-517.

fact that they were generally the largest and most numerous in Europe, and played a major international role in medical education.[24]

Thus apart from private or extracurricular teaching, the approach often had to be that of fitting the subject matter of *Methodus medendi* into the traditional curriculum. With regard to the theory of medicine, this could be done quite readily. The prescribed texts might vary from place to place, but in the Italian schools three were absolutely standard, and they were also in common use elsewhere. These were the first fen of the *Canon* of Avicenna, Galen's *Ars medica*, and the Hippocratic *Aphorisms*, which the professors of theory would expound in a three-year cycle. The first fen of Avicenna is a survey of physiology, and so not directly relevant to *Methodus medendi*, but the other two books offered excellent possibilities. The *Ars medica* is, of course, a survey of all of medicine, and concludes with the basic principles of methodical treatment. Even better, many of the *Aphorisms* take the form of rules for when and under what conditions certain medical procedures should or should not be carried out. In his own commentary on the *Aphorisms*, which heavily influenced most later ones, Galen frequently interpreted such statements in terms of his own doctrine of curative indications, and referred the reader to *Methodus medendi* for a fuller discussion.[25] Thus one could scarcely comment on these two works without saying at least something about the Galenic method of treatment, and some teachers of the sixteenth century availed themselves of the opportunity to say a great deal about it.[26] The commentary on the *Aphorisms* in particular might easily become almost a whole course on the subject of methodical cure.[27]

---

[24] B. Bertolaso, "Richerche d'archivo su alcuni aspetti, dell' insegnamento medico presso l'università di Padova nelle sette- e ottocento", *Acta Medicae Historiae Patavina* V (1958/59) 1-30; Bylebyl, "The School of Padua", pp. 368-369; Pietro Ascanelli, I Fascicoli personali dei lettori artista ... di Bologna (1973), passim.

[25] E.g., XVII B 360-361, 377-378, 422, 426, 429-431.

[26] On the *Aphorisms*, see the following note. For *Ars medica*, see the commentary of da Monte discussed below, and also Martin Acakia, *Galeni Pergameni ars medica.... M. A. interprete & enarratore* (Lyons, 1548), pp. 560-569, 582-597, 626-635; and Salvo Sclano, *Commentaria in tres libros artis medicinalis Galeni* (Venice, 1597), esp. 459-467 and 602-609. Sclano refers (p. 459) to his own commentary on the *Aphorisms* for fuller discussions of curative indications.

[27] For two older commentators who discussed the curative indications but without making them a major theme, see the references to Jacopo da Forlì and Ugo Benzi in note 16 above. Contrast with the commentary of da Monte, discussed below, and that of Capivaccio in his *Opera omnia* (Venice, 1617), pp. 266-395. In his introduction (p. 269), Capivaccio states that it is the view of "Iuniores medici" that Hippocrates "in ipso libro primo de instrumentis medicis loquitur, & de indicationibus, quibus medicus dirigi potest, ut recte instrumentis uti potest". Capivaccio agrees (p. 270) that the subject matter is indeed "de curatione, ac eius indicationibus", and further identifies this with the subject matter of *Methodus medendi*. His commentary contains much on indications—see, e.g., pp. 283-291 and 356-367.

The Italian universities were astonishingly faithful to this mode of teaching medical theory, preserving it intact until the second half of the eighteenth century. For a few decades in the first half of that century, Bologna made the bold experiment of substituting *Methodus medendi* for the first fen of Avicenna, but the latter was eventually restored.[28] In other parts of Europe, however, it became common at an earlier time to relinquish the traditional mode of teaching theory in favor of a straightforward survey of all of medicine, which came to be called the Institutes of Medicine, and was usually based upon the canonical division of the subject into physiology, pathology, semeiology, hygiene and therapeutics. The pattern for these changes was set by two important texts of the mid-sixteenth century, Leonhart Fuchs's *Institutiones medicinae* and Jean Fernel's *Universa medicina.*[29] The two works differ somewhat in scope in that Fernel's text was intended to cover both theory and practice, and therefore deals with both general and special therapeutics, while Fuchs's was meant to be accompanied by a separate course (and text) on the practice of medicine, and so deals only with general therapeutics, in addition to the other four branches of medicine. The two agree, however, in explicitly identifying general therapeutics with the term "methodus medendi". Fernel's account of the latter was based to a considerable degree on the Galenic treatise of that name, while Fuchs's was an explicit precis of it, focussing largely on the concept of the curative indications.[30]

The course on the practice of medicine might also offer some opportunities for a general exposition of the methodus medendi. At some universities the approved texts included the fourth fen of the first book of Avicenna, where he dealt with general therapeutics.[31] At least in the Latin version one can see the methodus medendi only as through a glass darkly, but the commentary provided ample opportunity to present the

---

[28] Ascanelli, I Fascicoli, e.g., pp. 135, 160-161, 206, 216-217, 240.

[29] C. D. O'Malley, "Medical Education During the Renaissance", in C. D. O'Malley (ed.), History of Medical Education (Berkeley and Los Angeles: University of California Press, 1970), p. 101. Leonhart Fuchs, *Institutiones medicinae* (first under that title, Lyons, 1555), Jean Fernel, *Universa medicina* (first under that title, Paris, 1567). Both texts had a long and complex prehistory.

[30] Fuchs, *Institutiones medicinae* (Lyons, 1555), pp. 528-554; Fernel, *Universa medicina* (Paris, 1567), pp. 344-357. See also e.g., Gregory Horst's Institutes in his *Opera medica omnia* (Nuremberg, 1660), pp. 317-323, "De methodo medendi", and Lazarus Riverius, *Institutiones medicae*, Bk. 5, part 1, "De methodo generali medendi" (Lyons, 1672), pp. 381-398.

[31] A number of the leading Italian teachers of the fourteenth and fifteenth centuries commented on Avicenna I, 4, but Bologna is the only university I know of where this text remained in regular use during the sixteenth and seventeenth centuries. See the following note, and Ascanelli, I Fascicoli, passim.

substance of *Methodus medendi* in Galen's own terms.[32] Or, if he chose, the professor of practice might simply begin his course with an overview of the methodus medendi, much as Savonarola did, though in the sixteenth century he would take care to make clear the Galenic basis of his doctrine.[33]

Thus by the second half of the sixteenth century, most European medical students would almost certainly have been made aware that there was a distinctively Galenic method of treatment, and would probably have been exposed at least once to a more or less detailed delineation of its characteristic features. However, the possibility that this would have a deep and lasting influence must be measured against the fact that in the course on practice they would be exposed to an approach to therapeutics that was basically antithetical to the methodus medendi. As noted above, the essential duty of the professor of practice was simply to teach the diagnosis and cure of all the major kinds of disease on a one-by-one basis. For two years, he would lecture on diseases of particular parts of the body, arranged in the head-to-toe order, and, in the third year, on fevers, which were regarded as diseases of the entire body.

The conflicts between *Methodus medendi* and the courses (and textbooks) on practice were at several levels. One of these was organizational, and pertained chiefly to the head-to-toe part of the course. In Galenic terms, this represented an arrangement according to the affected part rather than the nature of the affection, though it was the latter that was of greater moment in *Methodus medendi*.[34] The professor of practice could at least approach the fevers as a large class of diseases to be divided and subdivided in accordance with the method of division that Galen recommended.[35] But, for example, the localized inflammations were scattered throughout the body, and so throughout the whole course, thus making it difficult to discuss them in any sort of methodical way, in terms either of etiology or of therapeutics. This difficulty was clearly perceived by Laurent Joubert, who advocated a complete reorganization of the course on the basis of the kind of affection rather than of the affected part.[36]

On another level, though, the whole course was amethodical precisely because it sought to teach the students specifically how to recognize and cure all of the major diseases, rather than to inculcate a general

---

[32] A. M. Betti, *In quartam fen primi Canonis Avicennae commentarium* (Bologna, 1560). The commentary is replete with references to *Meth. med.* and its characteristic language, notably the "indications", e.g., fols. 7v, 35v, 79r. Betti was a professor at Bologna.

[33] See Altomare, below. The more common practice was simply to plunge into the diseases of the head, with little or no general introduction.

[34] *Meth. med.*, 1, 6-9; 2, 1 = X 48-81.

[35] Ibid., 1, 3; 2, 6 = X 21-28, 115-125.

[36] Laurent Joubert, *Medicinae Practicae priores Libri tres* (Lyons, 1577), pp. 11-12, 17.

therapeutic method. Giovanni Manardi pointed to this difficulty in his *Epistolae medicinales*, one of the fundamental texts of the medical humanist movement. Here he referred to the approach of "common doctors", who discover remedies simply by giving a name to the disease under treatment and then consulting a textbook to find out what should be done for the disease so named. This he contrasted with the approach of "true physicians" who

> "... prosecute their art by method having but scant regard for names [and so] investigate the essences and causes of diseases by division and resolution in order to elicit therefrom therapeutic indications and frame intentions by which they discover means of driving away diseases from human bodies."[37]

The defect to which Manardi called attention is especially apparent in the ninth book of Rhazes's *Ad Almansorem*, which was the primary text on which the head-to-toe part of the course was based.[38] With regard to each disease, Rhazes limited his discussion to just two aspects, namely diagnostic signs and remedies. In other words, the course was patterned on the empiricist approach that was for Galen the antithesis of a methodical treatment, and as we shall see, this point was particularly emphasized by da Monte in his critique of the genre.[39]

Recognition of the deficiencies in Rhazes's approach was by no means new to the sixteenth century, since well before that time the professors of practice had routinely added discussions of the causes of each disease.[40] But inasmuch as they still ended up telling the students how to recognize, explain, and cure every disease, they still obviated the need to learn and apply a general therapeutic method. Much the same objection could be raised against a further elaboration of the genre, whereby some of the older authors on practice would list a series of intentiones which had to be fulfilled in order to achieve a cure. For example, in the late fifteenth century *Practica* of Marco Gatinaria (d. 1496) we read that spasm is often caused by repletion with phlegmatic material, and that its cure is based upon six intentiones: "First, the administration of a proper regimen. Second, the digestion of the material causing the spasm. Third, evacuation. Fourth diversion, Fifth, resolution. Sixth, correction of the symp-

---

[37] Giovanni Manardi, *Epistolae Medicinales* (Basel, 1535), p. 97. The citation and translation are from Wightman, "Quid sit methodus?", p. 371.

[38] The text is included in G. Kraut (ed.), *Opus medicinae saluberrimum* (Hagenau, 1533).

[39] *Meth. med.*, 1, 4; 2, 7 = X 30-32, 126-127. In both the title and the preface of his edition of Rhazes (Basel, 1544), Albanus Torinus claimed that Rhazes had relied on rational "indications" for his cures, but at the beginning of Book 9 of *Ad Almansorem*, he noted that Rhazes had treated each disease "ἐμπειρικῶς" (p. 209).

[40] See, e.g., the commentary of Galeazzo da Santa Sophia, in *Opus medicinae practicae saluberrimum*, ed. Kraut, e.g., pp. 4v-5r.

toms.''[41] This has at least a superficial resemblance to the way in which Galen might summarize curative intentions in *Methodus medendi*, but since Gatinaria simply stipulates all of the intentions for all of the diseases, there is again no clear need for the student to acquire a general method for formulating them on his own.

Thus Leonhart Fuchs may have been exaggerating but he was not off the mark when he dismissed these intentiones in the older texts of practice as a hopelessly watered-down version of the *Methodus medendi*:

> ''For if you consider their curative indications, which they call 'intentions', you will almost never see anything that is properly demonstrated or discovered according to the legitimate method. For they just have something which they imagine is applicable to practically all diseases when they write that first it must be digested (for so they speak), then it must be purged, third it must be strengthened, and finally it must be resolved (primo digerendum ... dein purgandum, tertio roborandum, & ultimo resolvendum). And this indeed is their circle, to which they perpetually return throughout the entire cure. And would that today there were not so many physicians throughout our Germany who think that the stem and stern of the whole art consist in these four things. But how many things that are inept, ridiculous, and far removed from the truth are interspersed through their indications will be easily noticed by anyone who reads their writings judiciously and compares them with Galen's method.''[42]

Fuchs was writing here as the author of his own *Practica*, and he clearly thought that the genre could be brought into conformity with *Methodus medendi* simply by reforming its specific content. However, apart from the difficulties already noted, it seems to me that it was inherently impossible to write or teach in the traditional format without directly violating the Galenic method, inasmuch as the discussion of each disease concludes with a more or less elaborate curatio that is usually based entirely upon the nature and cause of the disease. Galen did, of course, attach great weight to the latter as the first indication of the cure, but he also made it clear that it is an insufficient basis by itself for the discovery of a specific remedy; consideration must also be given to such additional indications as the strength and temperament of the patient, the occurrence of complications in the disease itself, and the state of the air.[43] Indeed, it is precisely the need to adapt therapy to highly individualized sets of circumstances that makes it so important for the individual physician to acquire a general method as the basis of his practice.[44]

---

[41] Marco Gatinaria, *De curis aegritudinum particularium noni Almansoris practica uberrima* (Lyons, 1542), fol. 12. Curative intentions were also provided by Giovanni Arcolani in his commentary on Rhazes, published as *Practica* (Venice, 1560), e.g., pp. 11, 13, 21.

[42] Fuchs, *De curandi ratione libri octo* (Lyons, 1548), preface.

[43] See esp. *Meth. med.* 3, 1-3, 7-9; and 9, 7-17.

[44] Ibid., 3, 3 & 7 = X 181-183, 205-210.

This lack of attention to individualization was singled out by Daniel Solenander as a major defiency in the whole genre of *Practica*. In his many years of practicing medicine, he said, he had sometimes consulted these books, and not without benefit, but he had found far greater utility in the collections of consilia by the great doctors. The problem with the textbooks of practice, he wrote, is that:

"... everything is treated in such a way that it cannot be applied to this or that individual, except with great labor. Yet this has always been judged to be the most difficult thing of all in medicine, namely that those things which are explained in universal terms can be applied to a particular individual. But in the medical consilium that is the primary scope, namely that this person (hic privatus) should be cured, and not always from just one disease, but often from many complicated ones, and sometimes opposed or contrary to one another."[45]

Many authors on practice did, it is true, make more or less dutiful references to the need to adapt therapy to the individual, but I know of only one instance in which the inherent deficiencies of the genre were frankly acknowledged within the genre itself. This is in the introduction to Savonarola's *Practica*, where he gave about as stern and clear a warning as he could that knowledge of the disease is insufficient as the basis of a rational cure[46]—but then proceeded in the traditional manner to explain how to cure each disease on that basis alone!

For the sixteenth century, I have so far found only one author of a traditional *Practica* who even hinted at a possible discrepancy between the genre and a true methodical cure. This was Girolamo Capivaccio, who wrote and lectured at great length on the subjects of method in general, and methodus medendi in particular outside of the framework of his lectures on practice.[47] At the beginning of the latter, he noted briefly that in order to cure disease one must have knowledge of its essence, and that he would deal with the latter at the generic and specific levels. "For the individual essence cannot be taught in the classroom," he said, "but can only be learned by practice at the bedside of the sick."[48] Thus the implication seems to be that the discussions of the diseases that follow should be regarded only as rough approximations of a methodical cure, and not as a complete representation of the method.

It might be argued that in an age when knowledge of *Methodus medendi* itself was widely diffused, Capivaccio's point would have been almost self-evident and therefore did not have to be spelled out in the lectures

---

[45] Solenander, *Consilium medicinalium* (Hanau, 1609), preface.
[46] Savonarola, *Practica*, fol. 5r.
[47] Capivaccio, *Opera*, pp. 205-206, 208-248, 249-258, 870-910.
[48] Ibid., p. 396.

and textbooks of practice. However, one must weigh this possibility against the frequent claims, implicit in titles and explicit in prefaces, that these traditional *Practicae* are the very embodiment or application of the Galenic method of healing. For example, the Parisian Galenist Jacobus Sylvius began the preface of his textbook of practice by pointing out that the curative method consists in universal principles, and that no one would have perfect knowledge of it unless he has been exercised in particulars.[49] Noting that he had just completed a course of lectures on *Methodus medendi* itself, he said that he had decided to publish his textbook in order to provide his students with the necessary exercise "in curing almost all the diseases." However, his book is essentially a paraphrase of the humble little *Practica* by Gatinaria that was discussed above. About all that Sylvius did was to translate Gatinaria's barbarous Latin into a more elegant style, and to replace his references to Avicenna with citations of analogous passages in *Methodus medendi*.[50] It is depressing to think that Sylvius, after having commented his way through the whole of *Methodus medendi*, could actually believe that he had produced a valid application of its principles. I would prefer to suppose that he did it simply for the money (the book apparently sold very well).[51]

A rather more substantive effort was made by Donato Antonio Altomare in his lectures and textbook of practice. He took the same route as had Savonarola, that of prefixing a general method of treatment to his discussion of the individual head-to-toe diseases, but with two major differences: on the one hand, the Galenic basis of his method was openly proclaimed, but on the other hand, he gave no hint of any possible disparity between a true methodical cure and the approach of the traditional *practica*.[52] On the contrary, he began with the assertion that since Galen's time his method had been "untouched up to the present, and brought to light by no one." Altomare, then, proposed to describe this "universal method", so that his treatment of the individual diseases would then be seen as so many applications of it to particulars that Galen had described as the necessary complement to the general method. He discussed at some length the various factors that make up a complete comprehension and cure of a disease on Galenic principles: how to determine the affected part and the nature of the affection through diagnostic signs; how to infer the cause of the disease and to make a prognosis; how

---

[49] Jacobus Sylvius, *Morborum internorum prope omnium brevi methodo comprehensa, ex Galeno praecipue, & Marco Gattinaria* (Paris, 1545), pp. 1-2.

[50] Compare, e.g., Sylvius, p. 54, with Gatinaria, p. 38v.

[51] i.e., it was often reprinted.

[52] Donato Antonio Altomare, *De medendis humani corporis malis: Ars medica* (Naples, 1560), pp. 1-18.

to find a cure for the disease on the basis of the curative indications, including not only the nature of the disease, but also the strength and temperament of the patient, the condition of the air, and so forth; and how to establish priorities in cases involving more than one disease.[53]

Altomare's method consisted in this whole process of diagnosis and treatment, and it would be unfair to judge his claim to have applied it solely on the basis of the curationes that are given for the individual diseases. But at least with regard to the latter, it is difficult to see in what sense they could be regarded as applications of the method he had outlined. Little or nothing is said about the curative indications in relation to the individual diseases. His remedies are drawn heavily from Paul of Aegina, Alexander of Tralles, and the other standard authors who wrote on particular diseases, and they also include not a few elaborate polypharmaceutical preparations.

Moreover, Altomare's occasional remarks about taking account of the nature of the patient only underscore his general disregard of this factor. For example, his treatment for loss of memory included a recipe calling for specific amounts of several dozen possible ingredients. Mention of so many numbers apparently prompted him to recall Galen's statement in *Methodus medendi* that the quantity of remedies is not subject to general rules.[54] Thus, he advised the students, the specific amounts he had just outlined should be regarded only as examples:

> "The quantity of the individual ingredients which we have stated can be increased or diminished in individual affections in accordance with variations in the strength, temperament, nature and age of the patient, as well as of his habits, the region, the time of year, the condition of the heavens, and so forth ... And I advise you always to hold this in your memory."[55]

Perhaps there was a touch of humor in the last remark, but in any event, Altomare did not explain to his students how they are supposed to adjust the amounts of several dozen ingredients in accordance with a dozen or so factors in order to achieve the desired cure of amnesia!

It would be misleading, however, to suggest that *Methodus medendi* never penetrated beyond the titles, prefaces, and introductions of such works. In fact, by the second half of the sixteenth century such teachers of practice as Capivaccio, Massaria, and Rudio routinely discussed the curative indications of each of the diseases in the survey.[56] For some

---

[53] Ibid., esp. pp. 14-18.

[54] *Meth. med.*, 3, 3 = X 182-183.

[55] Altomare, *De medendis*, pp. 22-23; similarly, p. 41, but contrast with pp. 47-48.

[56] Eustachio Rudio, *Ars medica* (Venice, 1608), e.g., Bk. I, fols. 7v-8r, 16v, 142v-144r; Bk. II fols. 7, 22v, 50v, 51r; Girolamo Capivaccio, *Practica medicina*, in *Opera*, e.g., pp. 409-410, 557-558; Massaria, *Practica medica* (Venice, 1617), e.g., pp. 105-106, 125, 142, 357-358; cf. also p. 485.

diseases this might be no more than a perfunctory line or two, but in a significant number of instances, the coverage of just the indications might run to one or even several long folios in the printed editions. This meticulous attention to the curative indications no doubt underscored the importance of this central principle of the Galenic method, and if the discussion had ended at this point these texts would have been reasonably compatible with the latter. But the authors would not have fulfilled their duty as professors of practice if they did not go on to reveal how, specifically, to cure each disease and of course they could do so only by taking their indications chiefly from the disease itself, in violation of the method.

One major medical author who managed to circumvent this difficulty was Jean Fernel, in his *Universa medicina*. He did so simply by taking the traditional survey of individual diseases out of the realm of practice and placing it instead under pathology. The latter section of the book covers two of the canonical five divisions of medicine, namely etiology and semeiology. Fernel first gave general accounts of these two subjects, and then turned to the survey of fevers and head-to-toe diseases, confining his discussion of each to just causes and signs.[57] On the other hand, the division called "Therapeutics" or "methodus medendi" begins with a universal method of treatment, which, while not a straightforward precis of *Methodus medendi*, does incorporate most of its major themes.[58] The subsequent sections on special therapeutics are confined to the instruments of cure, i.e., bloodletting, purgation, and materia medica. Thus at no point did Fernel address the issue of specifically how to cure every disease, and according to his disciple, Plancy, he felt very strongly that this can be learned only at the bedside, under the guidance of an experienced physician.[59] However, in this respect Fernel was bucking a powerful trend, and there are even some late editions of the *Universa medicina* in which the editor thoughtfully provided the curationes for each disease that Fernel had omitted, thus transforming his special pathology into a traditional practica.[60] Indeed, Fernel's whole nosology was plucked out of pathology, and, with the addition of such curationes, was appended to therapeutics.

This example underscores how deeply rooted was the tradition of teaching the practice of medicine primarily through a survey of diseases and remedies, rather than through a general methodus medendi. In fact,

---

[57] Fernel, *Universa medicina*, pp. 176-343.

[58] Ibid., pp. 344-357.

[59] Guillaume Plancy, " 'Life' of Fernel", in Charles Sherrington, The Endeavor of Jean Fernel (Cambridge, 1946), pp. 150-170; pp. 157-158.

[60] Fernel, *Universa medicina* (Geneva, 1679), pp. 321-660.

this sort of course proved to be perhaps the most durable component of the medical curriculum—apart from major changes in nosology it survived into the modern era. The course did not, however, exhaust the possibilities for the teaching of practice because the traditional academic system allowed for a wide range of private teaching, both in the classroom and at the bedside. Depending upon the teacher's point of view, these opportunities could be used to inculcate a method of cure that was more in keeping with *Methodus medendi* than was the public course. Nevertheless, all such efforts would be substantially weakened as long as there continued to be a major public course which was called "the practice of medicine", and which embodied an approach to practice that was basically incompatible with the Galenic method.

It was this central issue that Giovanni Battista da Monte confronted during his brief tenure as first professor of practice at the University of Padua. He came to Padua with excellent credentials as both a practicing physician and a Galenic scholar.[61] He was the general editor of the Giunta edition of the Latin Galen (1541-1542), perhaps the greatest landmark in the whole movement by Renaissance physicians to bring about a rebirth of ancient Greek medicine in their own time. Sources vary as to whether da Monte took up the position at Padua in 1539, 1540, or 1541,[62] but in any case he held the first chair of practice for only a short time, giving it up in 1543 in favor of that of medical theory, in which he continued until his death in 1551.[63] Da Monte's leaving the chair of practice may well have reflected failure to gain acceptance for the changes that he advocated, but in no other sense could he be counted a failure as a teacher. Indeed, he seems to have inspired an admiration among his students that bordered on adulation. He published very little of his own work, but beginning even before his death, and especially afterward, various students brought out a flood of titles based largely on transcripts of his lectures. And since he taught both practice and theory, and gave

---

[61] The fullest biography is Giuseppe Cervetto, Di Giambattista da Monte e della medicina italiana nel secolo XVI (Verona, 1839), which contains many documents and excerpts from contemporary writings pertaining to da Monte.

[62] Da Monte's student Johann Crato, in his edition of da Monte's In nonum librum Rhasis ad R. Almansorem lectiones primi anni publicae professionis in Academia Patavina (Basel, 1562), gave 1541 as the first year of his public teaching, and further specified 3 November 1541 and 5 June 1542 as the beginning and end of his first lectures on Rhazes (pp. 1 & 686). Antonio Riccoboni, De gymnasio patavino (Padua, 1598), p. 22, gives 1540 as the year that he assumed the chair. Giacomo Tomasini, Gymnasium patavinum (Udine, 1654), p. 297, gives 1539. More recently, Bartolo Bertolaso, "Ricerche d'archivio su alcuni aspetti dell'insegnamento medico presso la università di Padova nel cinque- e seicento", Acta medicae historie Patavina 6 (1959/60), p. 24, confirms 1540.

[63] All of the previously cited sources agree on this date, except for Tomasini (p. 292) who gives 1544. Tomasini also states (pp. 292 and 297) that in 1546 da Monte resumed the chair of practice, but none of the other sources confirm this.

many private courses of a more specialized nature, the volume of material is quite large. To my knowledge, this effort to preserve and publish virtually every word that passed his lips was unprecedented for a medical teacher. And what makes this material especially valuable is that it includes a rather large number of what seem to be more or less verbatim transcripts of discourses delivered at the bedsides of patients, both in the Paduan hospital and elsewhere. I shall, of course, have something further to say about these bedside discourses, but first I shall discuss da Monte's public teaching.

Da Monte began by lecturing on the ninth book of Rhazes's *Ad Almansorem*,[64] but instead of being weighed down by this traditional format he infused into it a new approach to teaching practice that gave clear priority to a general methodus medendi. Both in his introductory remarks and at various stages in the commentary he pointed out that Rhazes's method was that of the empiricist sect, i.e., he simply gave signs and cures for each disease, paying no attention to the "indication from the cause" followed by dogmatic physicians.[65] In proceeding to supply the missing rational elements, da Monte did no more than was done by most commentators on Rhazes, although by explicitly raising the methodological issue, he repeatedly impressed upon the students the basic difference between the empirical and the methodical approaches.

But what really sets da Monte's lectures apart is that following this more or less dutiful commentary on each disease according to Rhazes, he then added a second, longer discussion of the same disease in which he sought to build a proper foundation from the ground up.[66] In these sections, he allowed himself to digress freely on general pathological processes such as pain, fluxion, inflammation, sympathy, and contagion.[67] Also quite numerous are methodological digressions—in fact, he continually reminded his auditors that he was trying to teach them not just how to deal with this or that kind of disease, but how to approach any disease by means of a universal method.[68] He criticized the earlier authors on practice for being so preoccupied with enumerating all the particulars about every disease that they neglected to inculcate such a method.[69] There were three major points that da Monte sought to

---

[64] I have tentatively followed the sequence of da Monte's lectures given by Crato in the preface to his edition of da Monte, *In nonum librum Rhasis* (1562). Except where noted, I shall refer to Valentine Lublin's edition of *In nonum librum Rhasis ad Mansorem ... expositio* (Venice, 1554).

[65] *In ... Rhasis* (1554), pp. 4, 6r, 11, 45v, 78r, 94v, 98v.

[66] This intention is explicitly stated in ibid., pp. 6r, 46r, 86r, 104v.

[67] Ibid., e.g., pp. 217v, 219r-227v, 235v-238v, 285v-287r.

[68] Ibid., pp. 94v, 98v-99r, 104v, 106v, 110v, 114v, 165r-169v.

[69] Ibid., pp. 45v-46r, 50v-51r.

convey: first, how to arrive at a knowledge of the essences and causes of diseases by the method of division; second, how to recognize the disease and its causes through the consideration of signs; and third, how to discover the means of treatment through the curative indications.[70]

The method of division was, for da Monte, the medical method par excellence. The failure of his predecessors to use the method and to explain it to the students has led to both confusion and error regarding the species of disease.[71] Thus, to understand a disease such as catarrh, one must first understand the broader class of fluxes, to which it belongs.[72] Catarrh itself is a fairly broad genus which must be properly divided into its constituent species as the basis of diagnosis and treatment. I do not want to give you "confused doctrine" said da Monte, "so I must convey the doctrine through a method so that you will have the sources from which you can take all the distinctions."[73] With regard to catarrhs, they are to be distinguished on the basis of, first, the particular anatomical pathway through which the descent occurs, second, the qualities of the humor flowing down, and third, the affection—of the brain itself or of some remote organ—that is the origin of the humor.[74] Since there are multiple possibilities under each heading there will be a very large number of ultimate species of catarrh, but the provision of this method for dividing them eliminates the need to enumerate them all. And since the lowest divisions are made on the basis of causal factors, this division reveals not only the essence of each species, but also its proximate causes.[75]

Beyond being able to distinguish the various kinds of catarrhs that can occur, one must also be able to recognize which particular kind is present in a given patient by means of appropriate signs. These too must be divided, beginning with those that are common to all catarrhs and extending to those which will permit one to determine the pathway, humor, and source, and so identify the lowest species.[76] However, while signs are very important, da Monte repeatedly cautioned that they do not lead the physician to the cure; rather they lead him to knowledge of the nature and cause of disease, and once that has been accomplished, they are of little further interest.[77]

---

[70] Ibid., pp. 46r, 104v, 211v.
[71] Ibid., pp. 104v-105r.
[72] Ibid., pp. 235v-238v.
[73] Ibid., p. 243v.
[74] Ibid., pp. 243v-246v.
[75] Cf. also ibid., p. 106v.
[76] Ibid., pp. 252r-257r; cf. also 110v, 293v-296v.
[77] Ibid., pp. 110r, 114v, 293v, 302v.

It is here that the curative indications take over. As da Monte stated, everything else is for the sake of these,[78] and he was quite fulsome in discussing the indications, not only for each larger species but for the subdivisions as well.[79] The first time that he came to discuss them, he gave a general explanation of the concept and outlined the sources from which they are taken, and recapitulated these points on several subsequent occasions.[80] He made it clear that while those taken from the disease and its cause are the first and most important, they are not by themselves a sufficient basis on which to treat since regard must also be given to such factors as the temperament and strength of the patient and the condition of the air.[81]

Da Monte scored the earlier writers on practice for their neglect of the indications, though he divided them into two classes in this regard. Worst of all were those who were, in effect, empiricists, since they only described signs and remedies.[82] Physicians who practiced according to these books would simply look up the disease based upon the signs and then prescribe the remedy, whether it was really suitable or not. The second group are in between the empiricists and the true methodical physicians, in that they have tried to follow Galen's method but have done so imperfectly. They are the ones who list the five or so curative intentions and then tell how they are to be fulfilled. Physicians who rely upon these books must also take their lead from the symptoms and then try to fulfill the intentions, again regardless of whether they are exactly right for the particular patient. The only true methodical physicians are those who are not content with signs and intentions, but penetrate to the very source, namely a knowledge of "the nature of the thing" from which alone the true indications can be taken.

Da Monte was quite consistent in discussing the divisions and the causes, the signs, and the indications for each kind of disease, but when it came to cures, his approach varied considerably. In the traditional textbooks of practice, the discussion of each disease routinely concluded with a section on curatio, but da Monte seems to have been concerned to avoid doing what he had criticized in others, namely, the laying down of stereotyped remedies. In some instances, he did not discuss cures at all, but ended with the indications.[83] In a couple of diseases he did follow through and specify means to fulfill the various indications, but since he

---

[78] Ibid., p. 114r.
[79] Ibid., pp. 67r-75v, 114v-121v, 137r-143r, 257v-270v, 302r-336r.
[80] Ibid., pp. 67v-68v; 114v, 302v.
[81] Ibid., pp. 68r, 75v, 114v, 120r, 302v, 336.
[82] Ibid., p. 197.
[83] Ibid., pp. 75v, 121v.

had discussed multiple forms of the disease, and at least several indications for each, these sections grew to enormous length.[84] What he eventually settled on as the most satisfactory way to handle this problem was to limit the discussion to a "curatio particularis", that is, a hypothetical case history in which he would stipulate a patient with a certain set of symptoms, then show how the diagnosis should be made from these, how the indications should be taken, and finally how they should be fulfilled.[85] For example, at the beginning of his discussion of phrenitis, he told the students, "First you will hear all the distinctions of causes...., second the signs, third the indications, fourth the explanation of the cure."[86] After surveying the first three, he stated, "So now that we have taken the indications, and have established the foundation, let us propose a brief cure in Socrates, who is thirty years old."[87] Here as elsewhere the case represents only one of the various forms of the disease, and so could not be taken as a substitute for a general curatio; rather, it exemplifies the process of therapeutic reasoning.

Thus, da Monte managed to transform the commentary on Rhazes into a methodical silk purse by consistently using the diseases in Rhazes's list to exemplify general pathological processes and methodological themes, and by relying chiefly on cases to exemplify how all of this knowledge can be applied to curing disease. However, this was accomplished at a rather heavy price with respect to the traditional duty of discussing every disease, for by the forty-seventh lecture, da Monte had reached only the sixth disease, epilepsy.[88] Rather than abandon his approach for a more economical one, he reaffirmed it with a vengeance, devoting the remaining twenty lectures to just two diseases, catarrh and pleuritis, which were avowedly taken out of the usual order because of their exemplary value.[89]

Ordinarily the course of lectures on Rhazes would extend over two years, but da Monte apparently did not take it up again the next year. Instead, he followed the logic of the position that he had enunciated by commenting instead on a quite different work, namely Galen's *Ars curativa ad Glauconem*.[90] This work is, of course, very closely related to

---

[84] E.g., ibid., pp. 146r-162r.

[85] Ibid., pp. 122r, 143r, 196v, 270v, 337r.

[86] Ibid., p. 104v.

[87] Ibid., p. 122v.

[88] *In ... Rhasis* (1562) divides the text into the individual lectures; p. 465.

[89] *In ... Rhasis* (1554), pp. 234v, 284v.

[90] Giovanni Battista da Monte, *In libros Galeni de arte curandi ad Glauconem Explanationes* (Venice, 1554). On p. 57r, da Monte noted that he was speaking as professor of practice. Book one of *Ad Glauconem* was sometimes used for lectures on fevers, but contrast da Monte's approach with that of Trincavelli, who regarded the opening section on the

Methodus medendi, whose title it often shares.[91] It covers much the same subject matter, though in a shorter format that made it better suited for commenting. At the beginning of these lectures, da Monte warned the students that they should not expect to hear from Galen how to cure each and every disease. His aim was rather to convey a universal method for curing all diseases, and then to apply it to some kinds of fevers and fluxes merely for the sake of exemplifying how the method is to be applied in particular instances.[92] He quoted Galen to the effect that anyone who has acquired the right method and then asks to be told how to cure the individual diseases is like someone who has a statue of Minerva by Phidias and then asks him to carve a thumb.[93] He was equally emphatic, though, in agreeing with Galen that the method alone was not enough; exercise in particulars is crucial to the perfection of its use.[94]

Da Monte devoted the greater part of the course to expounding Galen's method and examples, but he began with a substantial preface of his own. This was necessary because Galen had construed the method of curing rather narrowly as therapeutics per se, but his emphasis on rational indications presupposed a great deal of theoretical insight into the nature and causes of disease. Therefore, in this preface, da Monte gave a comprehensive survey of all of medicine up through semeiotics. He acknowledged that he had taken this all from Galen—"I would be worthy of reprehension if I said anything new"—but he took pride in having set it all forth clearly and distinctly where Galen himself was often diffuse and disjointed.[95] He began with the concept of method in general, and then took up the four methods of ancient philosophy: demonstration, division, resolution, and composition.[96] Of these, the second and third are the most germane to medicine, because the physician must divide the category "disease" down to its lowest species and then resolve the species into its principles and causes, leading to knowledge of its essence.[97] It is this knowledge that will later be shown to provide the first and most important curative indications.

After distinguishing these methods from the similarly-named orders of teaching, da Monte then embarked upon the subject matter of medicine

---

general methodus medendi as a distraction to be gotten over as quickly as possible: *In Galeni libros De differentiis febrium, atque in priorem De arte curandi ad Glauconem explanationes* (Venice, 1575), pp. 85-88.

[91] Da Monte, *In ad Glauconem*, p. 2r, regarded it as a "compendium" of *Meth. med.*

[92] Ibid., pp. 2r-3v.

[93] Ibid., p. 3r; *Pro puero epileptico*, XI 359.

[94] *In ad Glauconem*, pp. 2r-3v.

[95] Ibid., p. 54v; cf. also p. 20.

[96] Ibid., pp. 7v-14r.

[97] Ibid., pp. 9-10, 12v, 13v-14v.

itself. The overall order of his doctrine is that of resolution, beginning
with the concept of health as the end toward which medicine is directed,
but his method of teaching is that of division.[98] Thus the science of
health, or physiology, is divided as usual into elements, temperaments,
humors, spirits, parts, and functions, and of course each of these
headings has at least one further level of subdivisions. Then in turn he
went on to divide hygiene, etiology, and semeiology along appropriate
lines. In the preface there is no comparable treatment of the fifth division
of medicine, therapeutics, because that is of course the subject of Galen's
Ad Glauconem and of da Monte's commentary on it. The preface and commentary thus form a logical whole, beginning with the general question
of method and ending with the methodus medendi itself.[99]

Among the themes that da Monte sounded in the preface was one that
he took up from Galen and which would recur throughout his own
teaching, namely that the central problem for the physician is that of
establishing the relationship between the universal and the particular, or
between the general methodus medendi and the treatment of an
individual patient. For example, at the end of his survey of physiology,
he noted that in going on to discuss hygiene and therapy he would be
leaving the purely contemplative part of medicine and entering that
which is oriented toward action.[100] However, one can only act on particular individuals, and if one is to do so rationally, one must have
knowledge of their particular natures. The problem is that one cannot
arrive at such knowledge through any of the four established methods—
demonstration, division, resolution, or composition—because these are
applicable only at some level of generality at or above that of the lowest
species.

If we cannot have knowledge of the individual by any method, asked
da Monte, "Then by what art?" His answer was:

---

[98] Ibid., pp. 115v-116v, 26r, 48v.

[99] However, John Caius published a paraphrase of just the preface under the title *De
medendi methodo libri duo, ex. Cl. Galeni Pergameni & Jo. Baptistae Montani ... sententia* (Basel,
1544). This is a misnomer, because the preface does not include a discussion of methodus
medendi, as distinct from "method" in its broader senses. Subsequently, Johann Crato
published a more authentic version of the preface, but he helped to perpetuate the confusion by calling it *Methodus therapeutica* and by reinforcing its separation from the commentary on *Ad Glauconem* (in *Opuscula varia ac praeclara* [Basel, 1558]). Recent efforts to analyze
da Monte's views on method without reference to his views on methodus medendi have
been less than satisfactory even to their authors. See Wightman, "Quid sit methodus",
esp. p. 373, and Wear, "Galen in the Renaissance", esp. p. 243. Bates, "Sydenham and
method", pp. 328-330, has stressed the need to keep in mind the specific meaning of
methodus medendi when evaluating the contributions of Renaissance physicians to the
more general debates on methodology.

[100] *In ad Glauconem*, pp. 26v-27v.

"The individual is known through accidents and through sensation, because sensation has particular objects, and so it is necessary to have signs and particular appearances which offer themselves to the senses, because knowledge of the nature of the body cannot be had otherwise. These [signs] are the functions and operations of each individual man, and from these we know the nature of each person. We consider the natural and the animal functions, and whatever else is apparent to the senses, and from these particulars we make universal judgments. Thus we have begun to show as under a cloud how universals are applied to particulars. The art of the physician turns on this relationship and is applied through signs."[101]

Da Monte is not, of course, here advocating a radical clinical empiricism. The universals to which he refers are the explanatory principles of Galenic medicine, in which he has implicit faith. These must be firmly fixed in the physician's mind, which is why it is so important for them to be taught in a clear and orderly manner.[102] The relationship between the signs and the universals is also one that is preestablished, based upon an understanding of how the universals and the signs are related to one another as causes and effects.[103] For this reason, in teaching it is necessary to discuss etiology before semeiology, whereas in practice the sequence is reversed; one must begin by carefully studying the signs and symptoms of this particular patient in order to discover which ones of the possible universals are present in his nature, and hence relevant to the cure.[104]

We have seen, though, that da Monte had a certain wariness about signs lest they be thought of as the direct source from which the cure is taken. This may be why, in the preface to *Ad Glauconem*, he went directly from his account of the differences and causes of disease to a summary account of the curative indications, after which he took up the signs, rather than following the order causes, signs, and indications that he had used in the lectures on Rhazes.[105] By closely linking the indications with the differences and causes of diseases, da Monte might have risked giving the impression that they are to be taken only from the latter, but he tried to make it clear, both here and at greater length in the commentary itself, that this is not the case.[106] Indeed, sometimes those taken from such things as the temperament or age of the patient, or the condition of the air, can completely negate those taken from the disease, and physicians might even kill their patients by neglecting their individual differences.[107]

---

101 Ibid., pp. 26v-27r.
102 Ibid., p. 427r.
103 Ibid., pp. 64v-65r.
104 Ibid., p. 92.
105 Ibid., p. 57.
106 Ibid., pp. 58v-64v.
107 Ibid., p. 124v.

As he put it, "Nowadays many errors are committed because modern physicians try to fit everyone with the same pair of shoes."[108]

Given the influence of da Monte as an individual and of the University of Padua as an institution, his example might have paved the way for a lasting and more widespread reform of the course on medical practice but this was not to be. In 1543, da Monte transferred to the chair of medical theory, changing places with his near-namesake, Pamphilo Monti.[109] Possibly the change was not completely voluntary on da Monte's part. He noted in the lectures on *Ad Glauconem* that he was being criticized by many for delving into matters more appropriate to the professor of theory,[110] and one wonders if he may not have also met the opposite criticism of neglecting to cover the usual subject matter of the course on practice. In 1540, Pamphilo Monti had published a thoroughly traditional text on head-to-toe diseases (called, however, *Methodus medendi*) and so could probably have been counted on to lecture accordingly.[111]

For his part, da Monte began his lectures as professor of theory by denouncing the custom of splitting the medical doctrine into these two parts.[112] Medicine itself can, of course, be divided into theory and practice, or into speculation and action, but the action is nothing other than the exercise of the art of curing, and the speculation should itself be wholly oriented toward the same end.[113] In other words, the speculative part of medicine is, simply, the habit of mind, or the universal principles, that will permit one to practice the art according to a definite method. The supposition that the speculative part can itself be divided into theory and practice, to be taught by separate individuals, has led to the deplorable situation of having professors of practice who do nothing but hand out "recipes and secrets", and professors of theory who "occupy themselves with empty questions and neglect the true methodus medendi."[114] The implication seems to be that da Monte, as professor of theory, would provide the students with all of the general knowledge that they need to practice medicine; the separate course of lectures on practice is an irrelevancy.

In this respect, da Monte's purposes were actually served rather well by the traditional curriculum of medical theory. He began by lecturing

---

[108] Ibid., p. 124r.

[109] See note 63 above.

[110] *In ad Glauconem*, p. 57r.

[111] Panfilo Monti, *Methodus medendi* (Augsburg, 1540). In the preface, Monti describes the methodus medendi as simply a matter of being able to recognize the disease, and knowing the appropriate remedy. Another edition was published at Venice in 1545.

[112] Da Monte, *In artem parvam Galeni explanationes* (Lyons, 1566), pp. 1-32.

[113] Ibid., pp. 18-20, 27-32.

[114] Ibid., p. 3.

on Galen's *Ars medica* which is, as noted, a survey of the whole of medicine. The famous opening lines permitted da Monte to discuss the general question of "method" to his heart's content and then go on to survey physiology, pathology, and semeiology, and finish up with the methodus medendi.[115]

The following year, da Monte lectured on the Hippocratic *Aphorisms*, a work that he interpreted in accordance with its essentially clinical character. In fact, he indicated in his lectures that he was now receiving the reverse of the earlier criticism, namely that he was delving far too deeply into practical matters than was appropriate for the professor of theory.[116] Yet the course as a whole was vintage da Monte in embracing all of medicine, both theory and practice. He accepted Galen's contention that Hippocrates was a dogmatic physician who professed, implicitly if not explicitly, most of the principles of Galen's own system. Thus as a preface to the lectures, he took the students through a schematic survey of "Hippocratic" medicine, beginning with elements, temperaments, humors, and so forth.[117]

The first aphorism, beginning "life is short, the art is long", provided the occasion for the inevitable lengthy methodological discussion. Here the dominant themes are that the crucial problem for the physician is that of applying universal theories to particular cases, and that once the universals have been acquired, prolonged practice and exercise are the indispensable means of learning to apply them.[118] It is in this sense that the art is long in relation to one man's life: not, as Galen thought, because "the discovery of the art (artis inventionem)" took many generations, but because "the art even as it has now been discovered (artem iam inventam)" cannot be perfectly mastered in the course of an entire lifetime.[119] What makes the art of the physician so peculiarly difficult relative to that of, say, the blacksmith, is that the latter can count on the immutability of the iron on which he works, whereas the physician must allow for the constant change of the human body in response to all manner of circumstances.[120]

Nevertheless, all is not hopeless. There is the promise of increasing skill through practice, and there is also the methodus medendi: "If the physician wishes to act distinctly with regard to the human body, he must

---

[115] Ibid., passim.
[116] Da Monte, *In primam & secundam partem Aphorismorum Hippocratis Lectiones* (Venice, 1555), p. 141v.
[117] Ibid., pp. 1-16.
[118] Ibid., pp. 25r-32r.
[119] Ibid., pp. 32v-34v.
[120] Ibid., p. 28r.

take distinct indications.''[121] Ostensibly, the *Aphorisms* might seem to be in conflict with the latter because Hippocrates does not begin by laying down a method nor does he seem to base his precepts on rational indications.[122] But da Monte is confident that Hippocrates had the method in his mind if not in his book, so that he did indeed draw his precepts "from the method itself", rather than from simple experience.[123] This then prepared the way for da Monte to follow Galen's lead in interpreting the rest of the *Aphorisms* on the basis of the doctrine of curative indications.[124] In fact, the commentary is almost as much an exposition of *Methodus medendi* as of the *Aphorisms*.

Thus in his lectures on both the *Ars medica* and the *Aphorisms*, da Monte managed to cover essentially the same range of topics (though in differing proportions) as he had in the preface and commentary on *Ad Glauconem*. Only in the third year, when he came to the first fen of the *Canon* of Avicenna, did he have to confine himself chiefly to physiology.[125] I shall not discuss the remainder of his public teaching, except to note that in 1550 he retired, but returned a year later to give another course of lectures, in the midst of which he died. These last commentaries were on the third book of the Hippocratic *Epidemics*, a choice that was avowedly based upon the opportunity for detailed analysis of its case histories.[126] In choosing to focus on cases in this last course, da Monte did in his public lectures what he had been doing in his private teaching throughout his tenure at Padua—and not just on written case histories, but on living patients.[127] Unfortunately, I have as yet found no place in da Monte's methodological discussions where he comments explicitly on this method of teaching. This was perhaps because he would not have regarded it as either "method" or "teaching (doctrina)" in the strict senses of those

---

[121] Ibid., pp. 34r-35r.

[122] Ibid., p. 39r.

[123] Ibid., pp. 39r-43r.

[124] Ibid., pp. 42-46, and passim to end.

[125] Da Monte, *In primam fen libri primi Canonis Avicennae explanatio* (Venice, 1554).

[126] Da Monte, *In tertium primi Epidemiorum sectionem explanationes* (Venice, 1554), pp. 1v-2r.

[127] To my knowledge, the most detailed discussion of da Monte's bedside teaching is that in Comparetti, da Monte, pp. 42-72. For a recent summary, see L. Münster, "Die Anfänge eines klinischen Unterrichts an der Universität Padua im 16. Jahrhundert", *Med. Mon. schr.* 23 (1969) 173. I have discussed it in "The School of Padua", pp. 346-352 and in Lloyd G. Stevenson (ed.), A Celebration of Medical History (Baltimore: The Johns Hopkins University Press, 1982), pp. 204-208. I hope to publish a fuller analysis, with selected texts and translations. The transcripts of da Monte's consultations and bedside discourses are interspersed in various editions of his written consilia. These editions are many, and their relationships complex. That of Johann Crato, *Consultationes medicae Ioannis Baptistae Montani* (Basel, 1572) appears to be the most comprehensive, and all of my references will be to it.

terms, because for him both of these were, by definition, concerned with universal principles.[128] Even the formal analysis of an individual case would be a matter of applying a universal method or doctrine to a particular instance, or, in other words, a form of "exercise" or "practice".[129] And da Monte did say a great deal about the latter as the crucial counterpart of the acquisition of a universal method. Individuals do not always translate their general precepts into concrete actions, but as we have seen, he did follow the logic of his position in trying to reorient the public lectures on practice toward the inculcation of a general methodus medendi, and an equal emphasis on bedside teaching would have been the logical way of completing the program.[130] Thus a near contemporary of his was probably quite right in saying that da Monte's reason for taking his students to the Paduan Hospital was, simply, "to carry out what Galen prescribed and declared to be very necessary, namely that what he had clearly explained from the lectern should be applied to particular cases, thereby developing the skills of his students."[131]

The transcripts show that da Monte not only gave analyses of the diseases of charity patients in the hospital, but also engaged extensively in formal consultations with two or more physicians in cases of well-to-do patients. It was sometimes explicitly acknowledged that the latter also served a didactic function, as for example, when da Monte began by addressing his fellow consultants, "Excellent doctors, we are about to consult for the sake of this young nobleman, and we will also say much that will benefit the students, and so we will profit both of them."[132] Da Monte certainly did not invent the bedside consultation, nor was he the first to use it for didactic purposes. In one of his hospital discourses, he noted that he had himself attended such consultations as a medical student, but he was quite dissatisfied with the proceedings: the doctors generally failed to conduct a proper examination of the patient, and also neglected to give due consideration to the temperament of the patient, the disease, and the disposition of the air, i.e., the three main sources of curative indications according to the Galenic method.[133] Whether, as is commonly said, he was the first to conduct clinical lectures in the hospital

---

[128] On method not being applicable to individuals, see In ad Glauconem, p. 26r. See also In ... Rhasis (1554), p. 261r., where he distinguishes doctrina from historia.

[129] See In ad Glauconem, p. 59r: "Haec omnia post paucos dies exercebimus, & examinabimus circa aegrotos."

[130] Da Monte was fond of quoting Galen, Meth. med., 9, 6 = X 628-629 that a universal method and exercise in particular examples are the two legs of any art. E.g., da Monte, In Aph. lect., p. 25v.

[131] Girolamo Donzellini, in the preface to his edition of da Monte, Consilia (1559).

[132] Consultationes (1572), col. 489.

[133] Col. 938; Meth. med., 9, 14 = X 645-649.

must, I think, be considered an open question.[134] The sixteenth-century sources do not state that he was, though this was later inferred from the absence of earlier evidence of the practice. But we know so little at all about practical precepting before da Monte that it would be unwise to reach any definite conclusions on the basis of the evidence presently available. There is no doubt, however, that he did cultivate bedside teaching so assiduously as to leave behind a substantial record of his activities, and it is not unreasonable to suppose that this example helped prepare the way for the decree of 1578 which officially sanctioned formal clinical teaching at Padua on a daily basis.[135]

I have already suggested that the pursuit of bedside teaching was the logical counterpart to da Monte's emphasis on inculcating a general therapeutic method in his public lectures, and there is also a great deal from the lectures that is reflected in the specific content of the consultations and clinical discourses. One of these is a strong emphasis on careful observation of signs and symptoms as the crucial first step in each case. Of course, we must not expect da Monte to behave like a clinician of the nineteenth-century Paris school in this regard; he was a convinced Galenist for whom observation served only as the point of entry into the Galenic theoretical system on which the diagnosis and cure would be based. Nevertheless, to be of value for this purpose, the observations must be carefully collected through a discrete process that is anterior to and independent of theoretical deductions. Thus even before asking the patients any questions, one should first make a systematic survey of those things that are apparent of themselves; in da Monte's words, one should "make a catalogue" or "construct a simple history."[136]

A second striking feature of da Monte's consultations and clinical lectures is his pervasive use of the method of division that is also so prominent in his classroom lectures. In fact, from this perspective one can see why it is often difficult, in reading his general methodological discussions, to determine whether he is speaking about the method of teaching medicine or about the method of practicing it. For in his approach to practice, one must have the whole Galenic system fixed in one's mind in an orderly arrangement of divisions and subdivisions. In dealing with a particular case, one in effect runs through the system and makes a whole series of yes-or-no or either-or decisions based upon the signs and symptoms that are present. Thus the first stage in the observation of the patient is the consideration of the disturbed functions (func-

---

[134] I have discussed this issue in "The School of Padua", pp. 347-348, and in Stevenson (ed.), A Celebration, pp. 204-208.

[135] "The School of Padua", pp. 349-350 and A Celebration, p. 207.

[136] *Consultationes* (1572), col. 938; also cols. 76, 756, 901, 956.

tiones laesae), "since a disease is nothing other than a preternatural disposition that clearly disturbs the functions."[137] To make this survey one must divide the functions into the animal, the vital, and the natural, and in turn into the subdivisions of these, and then consider the functions of the patient with regard to each.[138] For example, with regard to the animal functions, does the patient reason coherently? Does he recognize old friends when they appear? Are there any sensory or motor distur-bances, either generally or in some part of the body? Again, with regard to the vital functions, what is the state of the bodily heat? What are the characteristics of the pulse? And with regard to the natural functions, what is the state of the digestive organs, both functionally and as felt by palpation?[139] What are the characteristics of the excreta?

After surveying these and other functional disturbances as well as other signs and symptoms, the next stage is to interpret the data to determine the nature and cause of the underlying bodily affection. The approach used is generally that of *De locis affectis*, in which one reasons from the disturbed function to the affected part, then in turn to the nature of the affection, and finally to its causes, both proximate and remote.[140] For example, da Monte summarized the results of one such inquiry: "So from the pulse we determine that the affection is in the heart; from the increased heat, that it is a fever; and because of the inequality of the pulse, that it is a humoral fever."[141] The next step is to determine which one, or combination, of the four humors is involved:

"The proper signs must be taken from the disturbed functions: a pulse that is vehement, great, rapid, frequent, and unequal indicates that this is a fever resulting from a hot putrefying humor. Because the humor is hot, it must be either blood or bile. In addition, the fever is interrupted by periods of manifest cold, lasting for about an hour. But a putrid fever that begins with chills cannot arise from blood which putrefies within the veins. There-fore the cause must necessarily be yellow bile."[142]

And once all the causes have been traced, then the final step in this phase is to reverse the process to show that all of the symptoms can indeed be explained by the affection and its cause, either as the direct result of the latter, or as the result of sympathetic involvement of some other organ.[143]

A third major theme from da Monte's classroom lectures that is also quite evident in the bedside discourses is that of the methodus medendi

---

[137] Col. 901.
[138] Ibid., and also, e.g., cols. 62, 629, 895-896, 940, 956.
[139] Palpation: E.g., cols. 629, 916, 943, 954, 964, 981.
[140] E.g., cols. 62, 76, 78, 629, 756, 896.
[141] Col. 901.
[142] Col. 902.
[143] Ibid.

itself, i.e., the process of reasoning from the theoretical understanding of the disease and the patient to an overall therapeutic strategy and then to a specific therapeutic regimen. Explicit reference is made to curative "indications" in a number of the cases ad the concept is implicit in most of them.[144] In one instance he made it a point to show how the same method of division that reveals the disease also yields the indications:

> "We have therefore a putrid fever depending upon a humor, whence there arises the general indication that it must be evacuated. But we do not yet know which humor we ought to evacuate. We must therefore make this determination for if we have distinct divisions, we will also have distinct indications for the cure."[145]

After determining that the humor in question is a mixture of bile and phlegm, he then faced another division, namely is it putrefying in the veins or out of them? "And from this will arise indications, for we will act one way if the putrefaction is in the veins, and another way if it is out." Thus he continued to divide until he arrived at a definite indication of "quid agendum".

Here as generally, first importance is attached to the nature of the disease and its causes; indeed, the most frequently recurring refrain in the discourses is that the overall intention is to cure the disease and that one cannot do this without knowledge of its nature and causes.[146] However, the diseases that da Monte tends to discover are the complicated ones, involving more than one affection, that are so prominent in *Methodus medendi*.[147] These are the kind for which no general rules can be followed, so that careful consideration must be given to whether they are independent or causally related, and if the latter, which is primary and which secondary. Again, with regard to therapy, one must decide which to attack first, and, if they are contrary in their indications, how the conflict is to be resolved.

While the nature and causes of the disease usually claim the center of da Monte's attention, he also made generous reference to most of the other curative indications of the Galenic method. Thus many (though not all) of the cases include a separate section devoted to reconstructing the natural temperaments of the whole patient and, often, of his principal organs.[148] Account is als frequently taken of the patient's age, occupa-

---

[144] E.g., cols. 756, 925, 960, 964-965, 968.
[145] Cols. 958-959.
[146] E.g., cols. 76, 901, 912, 930, 975, 981, 984.
[147] E.g., cols. 79-81, 908, 914, 916, 926-927, 930-932, 937, 968.
[148] E.g., cols. 77-79, 756, 908-910, 914-915, 916, 925, 938-940, 951-952, 954-955, 975, 987-988, 995, 999.

tion, habits with regard to the six non-naturals, as well as of the present strength of his faculties and of the condition of the surrounding air.[149] These data figure variously in the diagnostic and etiological analyses, as predisposing and precipitating causes, as well as being factors which must be taken into account, along with the disease and its proximate causes, in the choice of therapy. There are, indeed, a number of instances in which da Monte first shows that a certain treatment would be indicated by the disease but then rejects it on the grounds of the patient's age or strength or some other such circumstance.[150]

Finally, with regard to the specific treatments that da Monte prescribes, I shall note only that they are usually rather elaborate, but that almost nothing is done without a clear explanation of its rationale relative to the curative indications and to the other remedies. That is exactly as we should expect, because these cases were supposed to be models of methodical treatment. They may also give us some idea of how da Monte himself practiced medicine under less public circumstances, but they probably do not tell us how the average physician of the period arrived at his prescriptions.

Nevertheless, on the basis of Linacre's translation and its many editions, of da Monte's bedside discourses and public lectures, and of the countless other more or less faithful explanations of the principles of *Methodus medendi*, I think we can say that the latter was alive and well in the Renaissance at least as the highest ideal of what therapeutics should be. It was not, however, the only basis on which the practice of medicine was taught, probably because of the inherent difficulty of the true methodus medendi. This situation would not have surprised Galen himself, who was ever ready to assert that his approach was not that of the vast majority of physicians.[151] The medical teachers of the Renaissance were not in a position to adopt quite so elitist an attitude, because although the inspiration of their teaching was Galenic, it was carried out within a framework that was already highly bureaucratic. Those who received a university medical degree formed, it is true, a social elite among all practitioners, but there was no guarantee that those who had the wherewithal to attend university would all be willing or able to attain the highest level of methodical practice. Da Monte acknowledged this fact at the beginning of his last course of public lectures where he (characteristically) divided medical students into two groups: those who

---

[149] E.g., cols. 76, 78, 92, 756, 908, 916, 920, 932, 938-939, 976, 982, 984, 988-989, 995.

[150] E.g. cols. 98, 913, 914-915, 928, 943, 959, 968, 985, 999.

[151] *Meth. med.*, 1, 1 = X 4-5. Indeed, as noted at the outset, Galen himself did not always observe the method fully.

have a natural talent for speculative thought and who, provided they choose a good teacher, go on to become great physicians; and those who lack this talent and who, if they do not receive special attention, either drop out of medicine or end up practicing some form of empiricism.[152]

Da Monte said that he hoped to be able to benefit both groups by his commentary on the Hippocratic Epidemics, but I suspect that the second group, at least, probably derived more profit from the traditional course on practice, which was something of a compromise between empiricism and the *Methodus medendi*. The persistence of this course prevented the latter from ever becoming the sole basis of medical practice, though it could not prevent individual teachers and students from trying to live up to the higher standard that Galen had set.

---

[152] Da Monte, *In tertium primi Epidemiorum*, p. 1v.

PETER DILG

JOHANN AGRICOLA AMMONIUS' KOMMENTAR ZU GALENS *METHODUS MEDENDI*

Im Jahre 1534 erschien bei Philipp Ulhard zu Augsburg ein über 600 Seiten starker (unpaginierter) Oktavband mit dem Titel 'Scholia copiosa in therapeuticam methodum, id est, absolutissimam Claudii Galeni Pergameni curandi artem. Qui liber hoc nomine magni habetur, quod consummationem totius medicinae complectatur, sive indicationes curativas, sive theorematum enarrationes respicias'. Als Autor zeichnete der Professor der Medizin und der griechischen Sprache an der Ingolstädter Universität: Johann Agricola, genannt (H)Ammonius (ca. 1490-1570),[1] der damit sein erstes wissenschaftliches Werk vorlegte[2] und zugleich die Reihe seiner Galen-Kommentare eröffnete.[3] Was dieses Buch vor allem bedeutsam macht, ist indes die Tatsache, daß es sich dabei um den ersten Kommentar zu Galens *Methodus medendi* aus der frühen Neuzeit — vielleicht sogar überhaupt — handelt.

In dem Brief, den Agricola stolz seinen Scholien vorangestellt hat, wird dieser Anspruch denn auch durch keinen Geringeren als Erasmus von Rotterdam bestätigt: "... tua virtus multo erit celebratior, quod primus [!] strenuam operam navaris in hac therapeutica Galeni methodo elaboranda" (A 2ʳ).[4] Nicht zuletzt stützt Agricola selbst diese Behaup-

---

[1] Zu Leben und Werk Agricolas vgl. meinen Artikel in: Die Deutsche Literatur. Biographisches und Bibliographisches Lexikon. Reihe II: Die Deutsche Literatur zwischen 1450 und 1620. Hrsg. von Hans-Gert Roloff. Bd. I. Bern (im Druck). — Dort auch über den (auf griech. [h]ammos [= Sand] zurückgehenden) Beinamen (H)Ammonius.

[2] Ein Jahr zuvor hatte Agricola zwar schon einen Pesttraktat herausgebracht, der jedoch — in deutscher Sprache abgefaßt und ganz der Tradition solch populärer Regimina verpflichtet — gleichsam außerhalb seiner sonstigen, humanistisch-philologisch geprägten Veröffentlichungen steht: 'Ain grüntlicher fleissiger außzug/ auß allen bewerten Kriechischen und Lateinischen lerern × ... Von ursachen/ zaichen/ fürsehung/ und haylung der grewlichen pestilentz ...' (Augsburg [1533]).

[3] In den folgenden Jahren publizierte Agricola u.a. noch Kommentare zu Galens *De locis affectis* (Nürnberg 1537), *De inaequali intemperie* (Basel 1539) und *Ars medica* (Basel 1541); davon wird letzterer kurz erwähnt bei William P. D. Wightman: Quid sit Methodus? "Method" in Sixteenth Century Medical Teaching and "Discovery". Journal of the History of Medicine and Allied Sciences 19 (1864), 360-376, hier S. 376. — Eine zusammenfassende Studie über Agricola als Kommentator Galens befindet sich in Vorbereitung.

[4] Anlaß für dieses Schreiben vom Mai 1533 waren einige "quaestiones" inhaltlicher und sprachlicher Art gewesen, die Agricola an Erasmus mit der Bitte um Klärung gesandt und die dieser — da in großer Zeitnot und "plus quam obrutus negotiis" — eilig (und deshalb auch nur zum Teil) beantwortet hatte.

tung, wenn er in seinem Widmungsschreiben an den herzoglichen Kanzler Leonhard v. Eck u.a. davon spricht, daß "... intacta prioribus saeclis fuit hec methodus curativa ob immensos, qui devorandi erant, labores", weshalb ihm "τῷ πρωτοπείρῳ" jeder vernünftige "philiatros" etwaige Irrtümer sicherlich nachsehen werde. Im übrigen ist er davon überzeugt, daß die Philologen "expositionem nostram super difficillimas voculationes atque orationes inaestimando labore ex immenso Graecorum et Latinorum codicum acervo allatam conflatamque" (A 8ᵛ) billigen werden, zumal er sich auf die dabei geleistete Unterstützung durch Erasmus und Albanus Torinus berufen kann. Als bemerkenswert an diesem weitschweifigen Schreiben, das im wesentlichen ein einziges, zitatenreiches Lob Galens enthält, erscheint lediglich noch Agricolas Äußerung, wonach er bewußt darauf verzichtet hat, dem Beispiel seiner Zeitgenossen folgend "Avicennam interim ... flagellare", da die Lektüre von Galens *Methodus* gerade auch denjenigen nützlich sei, "qui Arabicis medicis sunt affecti" (A 5ʳ).[5] — Betont als Gegengewicht zum Arabismus betrachtet indes der Augsburger Stadtarzt Gereon Schoenopoeus (Sailer) die ihm zur Beurteilung vorgelegten Scholien, wenn er in dem — anschließend abgedruckten — Brief an seinen Lehrer Ambrosius Jung d.Ä. den verderblichen und namentlich durch die "Arabes" verschuldeten Verfall der Heilkunst in den voraufgegangenen Jahrhunderten beklagt[6] bzw. sein eigenes Zeitalter preist, das "veterem illam purissimam medicinam, non quidem novam, sed postliminio reflorescentem" (B ʳ/ᵛ) wiedererstehen lasse: ein Erfolg, den man Männern wie Agricola zu verdanken habe, durch dessen Kommentar ein für jeden wahren Arzt unverzichtbares Werk Galens erschlossen worden sei, das "universae tractationis medicae quasi ἐπιγραφὴν quandam complectitur". So verdienten

---

[5] Eine solch diplomatisch-zurückhaltende Einstellung gegenüber den geschmähten "Arabes" (vgl. Anm. 6) ist bei einem humanistisch gebildeten Mediziner in der Tat ungewöhnlich und steht vollends im Gegensatz zu der erbitterten Art und Weise, in der etwa Leonhart Fuchs — Agricolas Amtsvorgänger an der Ingolstädter Hochschule — den Arabismus bekämpfte. Vgl. hierzu Gerhard Baader: Medizinisches Reformdenken und Arabismus im Deutschland des 16.Jahrhunderts. *Sudhoffs Archiv* 63 (1979), 261-296, hier S. 276-282.

[6] Als ein typisches Zeugnis für die damals übliche Beurteilung der mittelalterlich-arabischen Medizin seitens der Humanisten sei diese Briefstelle hier in vollem Wortlaut wiedergegeben: "Subit enim superiorum saeculorum miserari casum et calamitatem, per quae studiosis artis medicae vix pauci olim atque iidem depravatissimi libri obtingere poterant, qui aliquando ipsissimam rei medendi πανολεθρίαν fuerant invecturi, nisi nostrum saeculum longe foelicius fuisset successurum. Hoc enim ipso nostro aevo scaturire et fluere coeperunt fontes eruditionis limpidissimi. E quibus depravatissimis libris mendose versis, quae Arabes emendicarunt, confuderunt cum barbaris et frivolis suis symmyctis. Quibus omnibus huiusmodi dispositionem accomodarunt (quantum ad tradendi artificium attinebat), ut sursum ac deorsum omnia versantes, infima suprema, magna et minima quasi in unum chaos mihi coegisse semper sunt visi. Qua confusanea doctrina bonam orbis partem in sua castra pertraxerunt ..." (Bᵛ).

diese Scholien größtes Lob, da es mit ihrer Hilfe möglich sein werde, "paulatim ad artis fastigium ascendere ..., quod quidem per Arabicos scriptores impediretur potius quam promoveretur" (B 2r).

Nach einer kurzen "Vita Galeni" aus der Feder des Johannes Manardus folgt die Vorrede an den Leser, in der Agricola die formale Anlage seiner Scholien erläutert bzw. einige Hinweise für die Benutzung des Buches gibt, das er vor allem "in studiosorum immensam ... utilitatem" verfaßt hat. Dabei war es ihm — wie er zunächst ausführt — hauptsächlich darum zu tun, seinen Kommentar nicht ausufern zu lassen, weshalb er sich im Falle des ersten und des zweiten Buches mit Absicht zurückgehalten habe: teils weil die dort behandelten Gegenstände einer näheren Auslegung nicht zu bedürfen schienen; teils weil Galen selbst "in convellendis iis, quae impudenter asseruerat Thessalus" bereits "nimis multum aquae ... insumpsit". Auch sonst seien manche "difficilia loca" — soweit schon von Galen erklärt — unberücksichtigt geblieben bzw. könnten über den das Buch beschließenden "Index scholiorum" aufgefunden werden: "Nam quorsum attineret perpetua tautologia rem eandem tum in scholiis, tum in verborum Galeni contextu nunquam non repetere?". — Ferner macht Agricola den Leser darauf aufmerksam, daß er die 14 Bücher "iuxta antiqui translatoris institutum" (B 4v) in Kapitel eingeteilt und den einzelnen Nummern der besseren Übersicht wegen jeweils die Anfangsworte hinzugefügt habe; eine Maßnahme, die künftig alle Übersetzer und Drucker praktizieren sollten "propter ingentem confusionem discutiendam et discendi gratam facilitatem promovendam". Dabei verweist er einerseits auf eine fehlerhafte, durch Beatus Rhenanus[7] bezeugte Einteilung in der 'Historia mundi [bzw. naturalis]' des Plinius, andererseits auf das Vorbild eines Hugo[8] "opinor theologus, qui vetus et novum instrumentum salutis nostrae πρῷραν καὶ πρύμνην in capita dissecuit". Dies ist um so bemerkenswerter, als er im folgenden durchaus Kritik an der mittelalterlichen Form der Kommentierung übt: Denn während er davon absah, "per continuationes omnia verba Galeni retexere", und sich vielmehr darauf beschränkte, lediglich "argumen-

---

[7] Vgl. Beatus Rhenanus: In C. Plinium. Basel 1526, S. 101, wo an der zitierten Stelle (Lib. X, Cap. XXXIX) verschiedene Lesarten einer bestimmten Textzeile diskutiert werden mit dem Ergebnis: "Estque haec clausula haud dubie praeparatio ad caput sequens. Quam non intellexisse videtur, qui Plinium primus in capita secuit. Ego sane malim ab ea quadragesimi capitis initium facere. Nam cohaerent, quae sequuntur ..."

[8] Es handelt sich dabei um den Augustiner Hugo von St. Victor (gest. 1141), der in seinem 'Didascalicon' (Lib. IV, Cap. II: De ordine et numero librorum) die Hl. Schrift zwar nicht in Kapitel eingeteilt, jedoch eine Übersicht über die Reihenfolge der einzelnen Bücher des Alten und des Neuen Testaments gegeben hat. Vgl. die Ausgabe von C. H. Buttimer. Washington 1939.

tum et scopum capitis cuiusvis" anzuführen, pflegten die Glossatoren, "qui paulo supra nostram aetatem vixerunt", alles "per ecphrasin" zu wiederholen, wodurch sie dem Leser die Lektüre verleideten oder ihn sogar gänzlich davon abhielten. — Unter Berufung auf Galens eigene Angaben empfiehlt Agricola des weiteren allen, die sich "huic nobili therapeuticae methodo" (B 5ʳ) zuwenden wollen, als Voraussetzung für eine gewinnbringende Lektüre die Kenntnis bestimmter Bücher,[9] geht sodann kurz auf die Entstehungsgeschichte jenes Werkes ein und nennt endlich noch Plinius, hauptsächlich aber Dioskurides — da mit Galen in den meisten Fällen übereinstimmend — als diejenigen Autoren, deren er sich "in simplicium medicaminum viriculis enarrandis" (B 6ᵛ) bedient hat.

Bevor Agricola nun mit der eigentlichen Kommentierung beginnt, charakterisiert er zunächst in einer "Perioche"[10] zusammenfassend den Inhalt der 14 Bücher, um anschließend in einer Art Vorkapitel die zentralen Begriffe "methodus"[11] und "therapeutica"[12] sowie die "sectae medicorum ... methodicorum,[13] empiricorum et dogmaticorum" zu erörtern. Die folgenden, nach der erwähnten Einteilung geordneten Scholien behandeln die verschiedensten Stichwörter und enthalten mehr oder

---

[9] Im einzelnen sind dies folgende Werke Galens: *De elementis, De temperamentis, De inaequali intemperie, De naturalibus facultatibus, De animae affectibus* (*De propriorum animi cuiusque affectuum dignotione et curatione*), *De particularum usu* (*De usu partium*), *De morborum differentiis, De symptomatum differentiis*.

[10] Eine weit ausführlichere Inhaltsübersicht (allerdings nur zu Buch 1-7) veröffentlichte im selben Jahr Antoine de Mery: Perioche septem librorum primorum methodi Galeni, cum quibusdam tum ab eodem, tum aliis authoribus traductis (ut vocant) receptionibus. Paris 1534. — Noch umfangreicher, da den Inhalt jedes einzelnen Kapitels zusammenfassend, ist das entsprechende Werk des Johannes Crato: In Cl. Galeni divinos libros methodi therapeutices perioche methodica, in qua perspicua brevitate obscura explicata esse et, quae reprehensionem habuerunt, confirmata videbit lector. Accessit his demonstratio, quo modo ex generali methodo exercitatio sive singulorum morborum curatio petenda sit. Basel 1563.

[11] "Methodus Graecis viam brevem et μεταφορικῶς disciplinam significat. Unde Galeni sententia methodo aliquid inquirere aut invenire ex adverso opponitur ei, quod est fortuito temereque reperire. Est autem id cum via quadam et ordine, ita ut in disquisitione aliquid primum sit, aliquid secundum et tertium, atque ita de reliquis omnibus deinceps, quoad demum ad ipsum, quod ab initio est propositum, sit perventum. Porro finem methodi illius scribit esse invenire cuiusque morbi remedia. Principium vero cognitionem morbi, qualis videlicet is natura sit. Atqui alio nobis authore ad hanc rem perdiscendam opus non erit quam Galeno. Quod si etiamnum haeres in methodo intelligenda reputabis tecum, quod ... prodidit in hunc modum ..." (B 8ᵛ).

[12] "Therapeutica Graecis θεραπεία idem est, quod Latinis remedium vel medela. Et θεραπεύσιμος i[dem] sanabilis. θεραπεύω curo, medeor, concilio, in precio habeo. θεραπευτικός curativus, sanativus" (Cʳ).

[13] Dazu merkt Agricola u.a. an: "Galenus autem librum hunc nobilem admodum non ab illis, sed a vera rationali methodo therapeuticam methodum appellavit, recte sane, illi vero perperam hoc nomen affectarunt, cum fuerint ab omni methodo alieni. Quippe solus ille medicamentis recte uti potest, qui certa methodo curat" (Cᵛ).

minder ausführliche Anmerkungen zu Personen, zu Pflanzen- und Krankheitsbezeichnungen, zu Herkunft, Zubereitung, Wirkung und Anwendung einzelner Arzneistoffe u.a.m., wobei die Erläuterungen teils formal-sprachlicher, teils inhaltlich-sachlicher Natur sind. Neben zahlreichen Querverweisen auf einschlägige Belegstellen bei Galen selbst wird ansonsten das übliche humanistische Literatur- und Bildungsgut ausgebreitet, d.h. eine Fülle alter, neuerer und zeitgenössischer Autoren zur Interpretation herangezogen, unter denen sich gelegentlich auch ein Name aus dem Mittelalter — z.B. "Marbodeus Gallus", also Marbod von Rennes — findet. Darüber hinaus verwendet Agricola in einigen Fällen auch schon graphische bzw. tabellarische Mittel, um etwa geometrische Termini zu veranschaulichen oder die Klassifizierung ähnlicher Erkrankungen übersichtlicher darzustellen.

Den Abschluß des Bandes bildet eine (wie der gesamte übrige Text in Wortwahl und Syntax schwierige) "Peroratio", in der sich Agricola nochmals an die — vorwiegend studentischen — Leser wendet. Sich seiner vollbrachten Leistung als "scholiographus" durchaus bewußt, bekennt er gleichwohl, daß ihm manches unklar geblieben sei "propter expectationem reliquorum tomorum operum Galeni. Quos quom adsecuti fuerimus ..., neque in hoc labore neque alibi unquam defuturus sum studiosorum commodo iuvando" (n 2^r). Zu diesem Zweck wolle er auch in Kürze ein "compendiosum syntagma" in Druck geben, "in quo omnia me ita depinxisse opinor, ut ante oculos veluti in tabella exposuerim, quae diffusius in his XIIII artis curativae libris sunt scripta. Quo instructi trium aut quatuor horarum spacio totam hanc therapeuticam methodum oculis lustrare poteritis". Ferner sei den Studenten künftig ein weiteres Werk zugedacht, das er deshalb "Tituli memorabiles"[14] genannt habe, "quod, quicquid in Galeni monumentis curandis morbis inserviat, in ordinem redigere in hoc libro conati simus, ne quid in posterum habeant Galenomastyges, quo tam insignem medicinae artificem dicant opificio medico utilitatis minimum conciliare" (n 2^v). Gilt ihm doch der Per-

---

[14] Dieses hier angekündigte Buch ließ sich unter den Schriften Agricolas ebensowenig nachweisen wie das zuvor genannte und offenbar schon abgeschlossene "syntagma". Eine solch einprägsame, in Form von Tabellen mit Klammerbifurkationen gestaltete Synopse — allerdings von Galens *De morborum symptomatumque differentiis et causis* — brachte hingegen wenige Jahre später Leonhart Fuchs (1537) sowie Iacobus Sylvius bzw. Jacques Dubois (1539) heraus. Vgl. Eberhard Stübler: Leonhart Fuchs. Leben und Werk. München 1928 (Münchener Beiträge zur Geschichte und Literatur der Naturwissenschaften und Medizin, Heft 13/14), S. 16 (180) und S. 115 (279); Gerhard Baader: Jacques Dubois as a practitioner. In: The medical renaissance of the sixteenth century. Ed. by A. Wear, R. K. French and I. M. Lonie. Cambridge 1985. S. 146-154, hier S. 147f.; ferner Karl Josef Holtgen: Synoptische Tabellen in der medizinischen Literatur und die Logik [Rudolf!] Agricolas und Ramus'. *Sudhoffs Archiv* 49 (1965), 371-390, hier S. 372f.

gamener unstreitig als der größte Arzt und demzufolge jeder als ungelehrt, dem "ille non sapit"! Dagegen verdienten alle diejenigen Anerkennung, durch deren Mühe und Fleiß die erhaltenen Werke Galens "hodie renascuntur", wobei die lateinische Welt namentlich Linacre, Copus und Guinterius[15] zu Dank verpflichtet sei. Was schließlich ihn selbst betreffe, meint Agricola, so werde er sich im Falle eines Irrtums nicht schämen, diesen einzugestehen "praecipue in eo ministerio, quod utilitatis causa posteris traditur ..." (n 3r).

In der Tat sollten seine Scholien nicht von allen so beifällig aufgenommen werden wie beispielsweise von Gereon Sailer. Denn fünf Jahre später sah sich Agricola veranlaßt, in einer elf Seiten umfassenden Verteidigungsschrift "Ad scholiomastiga quendam magni nominis virum ..."[16] zu Angriffen Stellung zu nehmen, die er — wiewohl darin nicht genannt — gekränkt auf sich bezogen hatte. Obschon in Agricolas Replik dieser Kritiker ebenfalls anonym bleibt, äußerte bereits Konrad Gesner die Vermutung, es könne sich dabei um Ianus Cornarius handeln.[17] Tatsächlich hatte sich dieser im Widmungsbrief zu seinem 1537 erschienenen Galen-Kommentar[18] ebenso rigoros wie selbstgefällig von gewissen Onomastica, Pandekten, Thesauri, Scholien und Episteln sowie anderem derartigen Flickwerk distanziert, wobei er auch den Vorwurf des Plagiats nicht scheute und namentlich die Scholien und Episteln als müßige Possen bezeichnete.[19]

---

[15] Bezüglich deren Übersetzungen — wovon Agricola hauptsächlich die zuerst 1519 in Paris erschienene *Methodus medendi*- Übertragung des Thomas Linacre seinem Kommentar zugrunde gelegt hat — vgl. Richard J. Durling: A chronological census of Renaissance editions and translations of Galen. *Journal of the Warburg and Courtauld Institutes* 24 (1961), 230-305, hier S. 296 u. 297.

[16] Neben weiteren kleineren Arbeiten abgedruckt in: Liber aureus Claudii Galeni ... de inaequali intemperie ... Cui ... familiares adiecit commentarios Ioannes Agricola Ammonius ... Basel 1539.

[17] Vgl. Konrad Gesner: Bibliotheca universalis. Zürich 1545 (Neudruck Osnabrück, 1966), S. 382.

[18] Ianus Cornarius: Commentariorum medicorum in decem libros Galeni de compositione medicamentorum secundum locos conscriptorum libri decem... [2.Teil zu: Opus medicum practicum, varium, vere aureum et postremae lectionis. Claudii Galeni ... de compositione pharmacorum localium sive secundum locos libri decem, recens fideliter et pure conversi a Iano Cornario medico physico]. Basel 1537. — Der an Landgraf Philipp von Hessen gerichtete Widmungsbrief ist mit 1535 datiert, wurde also ein Jahr nach dem Erscheinen von Agricolas Scholien verfaßt.

[19] Als Beispiel für einen damaligen Gelehrtenstreit sei diese Kritik hier in vollem Wortlaut wiedergegeben: "Caeterum quod studiosorum iudiciis informandis adiiciendum putavimus, hoc est, ne putent nobis in his commentariis quicquam commune esse cum quorundam huius seculi onomasticis medicis, pandectis medicis, thesauris medicis, scholiis etiam atque epistolis medicis aliisque eiusmodi centonibus speciosis titulis inscriptis. His enim permittimus, ut undecumque et alba et nigra, numeroque modoque sine omni, tum lecta, tum audita, intellectaque et non intellecta, omnia in unum chaos coacervent ac confundant, iamque nihili homines, sui tamen quam similimos ad astra

Obwohl diese Invektive keineswegs persönlich, vielmehr ganz allgemein gehalten war, fühlte sich Agricola doch unmittelbar angesprochen[20] und zu einer Erwiderung aufgerufen.[21] Unter Hinweis auf die ihm zuteil gewordene Anerkennung stellt er darin zunächst fest, er habe sich immer gewünscht, daß der eine oder andere Gelehrte Kommentare "pro libris Galeni obscurioribus intelligendis" (S.2) veröffentlichte. Nachdem nun allmählich die meisten Werke Galens sowohl lateinisch als auch griechisch erschienen seien, sich jedoch niemand — ausgenommen Manardus[22] — dieser Aufgabe unterziehen wollte, habe er begonnen, sich selbst mit solchen Kommentaren zu befassen, "quibus excirem etiam alios in harenam, ut idem opus adorirentur et hic vires ingenii intenderent". Indes sei ihm hierbei nur ein einziger gefolgt — eben sein Widersacher: "ex cavea incubantem leonem excivi". Gegenüber dessen Kritik rechtfertigt sich Agricola anschließend einmal damit, in der "Peroratio" deutlich erklärt zu haben, "quaedam nobis in scholiis manere suspensa et non explicata, donec reliquos operum Galeni tomos adepti ea, in quibus defecimus, simus resarcturi" (S.3); im übrigen beanspruche auch er das Recht, sein Werk in einer zweiten, verbesserten Auflage herauszubringen. Den Vorwurf des Plagiats hingegen weist Agricola entschieden von sich: Habe er doch lediglich an einigen Stellen "e translationibus duorum librorum abs te versorum" (S.4) zitiert, es dabei allerdings für überflüssig erachtet, jeweils den Namen des Übersetzers

---

laudibus vehant et mox non paulo praestantiores mordicus proscindant et, quod in aliis reprehendunt, in sese longe gravius admittant. Concedimus etiam, ut scripta nostra hinc inde expilent, ex integris orationum ac praefationum nostrarum periodis sibi praeliminares epistolas concinnent et, si adeo placet, totum filum retextum sibi pro novo syrmate induant, interim mei nusquam mentionem facientes; neque enim sic legi laboro; modo sciant studiosi verae et syncerae veteris medicinae, talia onomastica nihil aliud quam inanes bullas et nomenclaturas maxima parte falsas esse, tales pandectas per antiphrasin accipiendas esse, scholia et epistolas vere ociosas nugas esse, et quales podagricum molestum videlicet ocium decent, thesauros carbones aut potius carbonum esse favillas ...''. Cornarius (wie Anm. 18), S. 373.

[20] "Inter eos autem, quibus is labor displicet, insurgit adversus scholia translator quidem atque idem commentator et vir medicus multa eruditione conspicuus, Graiae Romanaeque linguae cognitione nulli cedens, qui scholia tum a me, tum ab aliis in Galenum scripta ita contemptim perstringit, ut opinetur illis nusquam apud studiosos locum relinquendum esse. Quanquam vero hoc suppresso meo nomine agit, attamen ita manifeste illum suum fastidiosum contemptum in me torsisse indicavit se, ut nemo lector non possit deprehendere, cui illud doctissimus medicus" (S. 1).

[21] Darin geht es Agricola indes weniger um die in der Überschrift angekündigte "Enumeratio causarum, propter quas Ioannes Agricola Ammonius scholia in 14 libros therapeuticae methodi scripserit" als vielmehr darum, die Vorwürfe des Cornarius im einzelnen zu entkräften bzw. die Mängel seines Kommentars zu erklären und zu entschuldigen — so, wie es der Kolumnentitel treffend charakterisiert: "Excusat[io] script[oris] scholi[orum] in Gale[ni] meden[di] method[um]".

[22] Agricola nimmt hierbei Bezug auf des Johannes Manardus: Galeni ars medicinalis ... versa divinisque commentariolis ... illustrata. Rom 1525.

anzuführen. Bezüglich der Originalität der einleitenden Briefe schließlich, "quas ... tu fictas aut ex tua vel alterius phrasi concinnatas dicis", könne er sowohl Zeugen als auch die betreffenden Autographen vorweisen. Was indes das Widmungsschreiben an Leonhard von Eck angehe, müsse er freilich zugeben, im Zitieren aus Galens Werken unmäßig gewesen zu sein, wenn auch nicht ohne Grund: "nempe ut redderem candidum lectorem magis attentum et avidiorem ad relegenda monumenta Galeniana" (S.5). Im übrigen handle es sich um ein Verschulden des Druckers, der die am Rand vermerkten Zitatstellen einfach weggelassen habe und — da in Eile[23] — nicht zu bewegen gewesen sei, "ut renovaret primum quaternionem vel meis expensis et adnotationes citationum marginibus apponeret" (S.6); so konnte der Eindruck entstehen, als wollte er sich Galens Worte selbst zuschreiben — weshalb Agricola im folgenden nun alle "loci" im einzelnen nachträgt. Ferner nimmt er auch seine Gewährsmänner: Hermolaus Barbarus, Nicolaus Leonicenus, Johannes Manardus, Virgilius Marcellus, Georgius Agricola und Euricius Cordus vor der geübten Kritik, nur "meras nugas" verbreitet zu haben, in Schutz, um anschließend seinerseits zum — allerdings maßvollen — Angriff auf Cornarius überzugehen. Sich dessen bewußt, den an Galen Interessierten durch seinen Kommentar "gustum quendam rationalis medicinae" (S.8) vermittelt zu haben, hält Agricola dem "rigidus censor" vor, daß dieser nur Hippokrates unter den Ärzten gelten lasse, sich gleichwohl aber auf dieselben Autoren stütze wie er. Im Grunde liegt ihm jedoch nicht an einer Auseinandersetzung; vielmehr erinnert er Cornarius in versöhnlichem Ton daran, daß auch Cicero geringere Redner geduldig angehört und selbst "noster Galenus" unbedeutendere Ärzte nicht verschmäht habe. Endlich sei er nicht der einzige, dem die zur Schau gestellte "immodestia" mißfalle: "incides brevi in multos, qui leoni utcunque ferocienti barbam vellere audebunt" (S.10). Zum Beweis gibt Agricola abschließend den Brief eines Kollegen[24] wieder, worin dieser einerseits seine Hochachtung für Cornarius nicht verhehlt, andererseits aber ebenfalls dessen "ambitio" und "temeritas" tadelt; dies um

---

[23] Der hier als "festinabundus typographus" bezeichnete Philipp Ulhard hatte in seinem — mit "VII.Idus Martii 1534" datierten — Schlußwort zu die 'Scholia' die vielen (über sechs Seiten umfassenden!) Errata in der Tat damit entschuldigt, daß das Buch noch zur Frankfurter Messe fertiggestellt werden mußte. — Agricola hat im übrigen aus diesen schlechten Erfahrungen mit seinem Augsburger Drucker die Konsequenz gezogen und seine Werke fortan bei anderen Verlegern erscheinen lassen.

[24] Da Agricola aus einem Privatbrief zitiert, muß die Frage letztlich offen bleiben, wer der ungenannte Verfasser (Leonhart Fuchs?) ist, über den nur mitgeteilt wird, daß er "eruditione multiiuga et lucubrationibus elegantibus in publicum editis conspicuus est" und "in praeclara quapiam Germaniae academia Galenianam atque Hippocraticam medicinam interpretatur inter rei medicae sitientissimos auditores". Vgl. Stübler (wie Anm. 14), S. 103f. (267f.).

so mehr, als auch des Cornarius Kommentar "insignes errores" enthalte
und man überhaupt das "perversum iudicium" jener Menschen nicht
billigen könne, die nur das Vollkommene gelten ließen, "quasi vero hu-
manum non sit, interdum aberrare ..." (S.11).

*   *

Offensichtlich ist es zu einer zweiten Auflage der 'Scholia copiosa' nicht
gekommen; vielmehr gerieten sie wohl ebenso bald in Vergessenheit wie
Agricolas übriges Werk. Doch bleibt dem Ingolstädter Professor immerhin das Verdienst, damit nicht nur den ersten, sondern — wie es scheint
— auf Jahrzehnte hinaus auch einzigen Kommentar zu Galens *Methodus
medendi* veröffentlicht zu haben.[25]

---

[25] Jedenfalls ließ sich bisher ein eigenständiger Kommentar zu diesem Werk erst wieder gegen Ende des Jahrhunderts nachweisen, der — wiewohl äußerst umfangreich (über
1500 Folio-Spalten!) — allerdings nur Buch 1-7 berücksichtigt und in zwei Teilen veröffentlicht wurde von Fabius Pacius: Commentarius ... in Galeni libros methodi medendi.
Pars prima triplici donata indice ... [zu den ersten sechs Büchern]. Vicenza 1597; Commentarius in septimum Galeni librum methodi medendi quaestionibus physicis et medicis refertus ... Vicenza 1608.

LIST OF ABBREVIATIONS

AAW	Abhandlungen der Akademie der Wissenschaften
ABA	Abhandlungen der Berliner Akademie (der Wissenschaften)
BL	British Library
BN	Bibliothèque Nationale
CIG	Corpus Inscriptionum Graecarum
CMG	Corpus Medicorum Graecorum
HSS	Handschriften
L.	Littré (Hippokrates-Editor)
LSJ	Liddell-Scott-Jones (editors of the Greek-English Lexicon)
MS	Meyerhof-Schacht (editors of Galen's treatise on medical names)
MS(S)	Manuscript(s)
NAW	Nachrichten der Akademie der Wissenschaften
n.d.	no date
N.S.	New Series
o.c.	opus citatum
Sextus M	Sextus Empiricus "Adversus Mathematicos"
Sextus PH	Sextus Empiricus "Pyrrhoneioi Hypotheseis"
Suppl. Or.	Supplementum Orientale (des CMG)

INDEX OF NAMES
(ANCIENT AND MODERN)

STUDIES IN ANCIENT MEDICINE

The *Studies in Ancient Medicine* deals with the medical traditions of ancient civilizations. The Graeco-Roman tradition forms the focus of the new series, but later medical practice (Byzantine and Islamic) will be considered, as will medicine in the Egyptian, Armenian and other related traditions.

The series consists of monographs and multi-author volumes on the theory and practice of public and private medicine in Antiquity, Late Antiquity and the Early Middle Ages drawing on written sources, and also on other historical and archaeological evidence. The series will also contain translations of ancient texts with philological and medical commentaries, annotated bibliographies of published works relevant to particular subfields and lexica of medical terms in the various ancient traditions.

1. F. KUDLIEN and RICHARD DURLING (eds.). *Galen's Method of Healing.* Proceedings of the 2nd International Galen Symposium. 1991. ISBN 90 04 09272 2
2. HIPPOCRATES. *Pseudepigraphic Writings.* Letters — Embassy — Speech from the Altar — Decree. Edited and translated by WESLEY D. SMITH. 1990. ISBN 90 04 09290 0

In preparation:

JODY RUBIN PINAULT. *Hippocratic Lives and Legends.*

ROBERT I. CURTIS. *Garum and Salsamenta.* Production and Commerce in Materia Medica.